AF764029

Essentials of Radiology Physics

Essentials of Radiology Physics

by

Charles A. Kelsey, Ph.D., F.A.C.R.

Chief of Biomedical Physics
Professor of Radiology
The University of New Mexico
Medical Center
Albuquerque, New Mexico

WARREN H. GREEN, INC.
St. Louis, Missouri, U.S.A.

Published by

WARREN H. GREEN, INC.
8356 Olive Boulevard
St. Louis, Missouri 63132, U.S.A.

All right reserved

©1985 by WARREN H. GREEN, INC.

ISBN No. 87527-354-8

Printed in the United States of America

PREFACE

This book is the outgrowth of lectures over the past nineteen years to Radiology Residents and Technologists. The same topics were covered in both series of lectures, but the emphasis and depth of coverage were adjusted for the two classes. The purpose of this book is to provide an entry level textbook which assumes no recent physics courses. It starts from first principles so that everyone in the class will have the same background and a uniform terminology. Those students who feel somewhat weak in mathematics are advised to thoroughly review the elementary concepts presented in the first chapter. Some physics concepts have been simplified for better understanding. This book is not designed as a do-it-yourself textbook. It was designed for study with a competent instructor.

The initial motivation of many physics students in radiology is passing the National Board or Registry Examination. The primary purpose of this text is to develop an understanding of the physics principles of radiology so that they can be used to produce quality radiographic examinations. The text contains all the essential material needed to pass the National Board and Registry Examinations. The vast majority of students using these physics lectures notes have readily passed their examinations.

SI units are used throughout the textbook. "Old-fashioned" units such as the Roentgen, rad, rem and mCi, however, are a fact of life in today's Radiology Departments, and will continue in use for some time into the future. Consequently, both the "old" and SI units are presented in most example problems.

The problems are an integral part of the text. Students should carefully work through the example problems and also the problems at the end of each chapter. A calculator with the square root, logarithm and exponential functions is essential.

I would like to acknowledge the good-humored assistance of Debbie Suttie who suffered through the many typing revisions. I want to thank the students and residents, particularly Drs. A.M.

Landry and R.R. Spencer, who caught innumerable errors and omissions. Any which remain are my responsibility. I welcome any suggestions and comments on how this text could be improved. Finally I'd like to acknowledge the support of both my family and my Chairman, Dr. Robert Moseley, who have encouraged me and suffered through the pangs of authorship with me.

CONTENTS

page

Preface v

Chapter

1 BASIC PHYSICS AND MATHEMATICS 3
Questions 29

2 ATOMIC AND MOLECULAR STRUCTURE 34
Questions 43

3 ELECTRICITY AND MAGNETISM 46
Questions 59

4 ALTERNATING CURRENT AND ELECTRICAL CIRCUITS 64
Questions 74

5 X-RAY GENERATORS 77
Questions 85

6 X-RAY TUBES 89
Questions 106

7 X-RAY PRODUCTION 110
Questions 118

8 X-RAY INTERACTIONS 122
Questions 137

9 STATISTICS 144
Questions 154

10 CONTRAST AND IMAGE FORMATION 157
Questions 179

11 X-RAY FILM 184
Questions. 194

12 INTENSIFYING SCREENS 199
Questions. 208

13 SCATTER AND SCATTER REDUCTION. 211
Questions. 224

14 RADIATION DETECTORS 227
Questions. 239

15 FLUOROSCOPIC IMAGING 243
Qeustions. 262

16 DIGITAL IMAGING. 266
Questions. 279

17 COMPUTERIZED TOMOGRAPHY 282
Qeustions. 300

18 SPECIAL RADIOGRAPHIC TECHNIQUES 303
Questions. 314

19 NUCLEAR DECAY 317
Questions. 335

20 NUCLEAR MEDICINE IMAGING 340
Questions. 353

21 DIAGNOSTIC ULTRASOUND IMAGING. 358
Questions. 381

22 MAGNETIC RESONANCE IMAGING. 390
Questions. 409

23 RISK FACTORS IN DIAGNOSTIC RADIOLOGY. 413
Questions. 421

24 RADIATION PROTECTION 424
Questions. 434

ANSWERS 439

ABBREVIATIONS 448

INDEX 455

Essentials of Radiology Physics

CHAPTER 1

BASIC PHYSICS AND MATHEMATICS

Physics is the study of the physical world around us. It makes use of fundamental laws to describe the interactions in mathematical terms. Physics deals in measured values of the physical world. Every measured value has both a quantity (how much) and a unit (what kind). There are two kinds of units, *fundamental* and *derived.*

FUNDAMENTAL UNITS

The fundamental units are *length, mass* and *time.* Length measures the space an object occupies. Length is measured in meters. The meter is defined as 1650763.73 times the length of one of the emission waves from the Krypton atom. Mass measures how much matter an object contains. Mass is measured in kilograms. The kilogram is defined in terms of a platinum-iridium cylinder kept in a vault in Sevres, France. Time measures how long an event occurs. Time is measured in seconds. The unit of time is defined as 9192631770 vibrations of a Cesium atom.

DERIVED UNITS

Derived units are such quantities as area, volume, density, specific gravity, velocity or temperature which are made up of combinations of the fundamental units. There are two systems of units in general use in the United States, the English and the Metric or the SI (Systeme International) Systems. Table 1.1 compares the SI and English Systems for some of the most commonly used quantities.

TABLE 1.1
FUNDAMENTAL AND DERIVED UNITS IN SI AND ENGLISH SYSTEMS

Fundamental Units	*SI*		*English*		*Conversion*
length	meter	m	foot	ft	1 m = 3.281 ft
mass	kilogram	kg	slug	–	1 kg = .0685 slug
time	second	s	second	s	–
Derived Units					
Area	square meters	m^2	square feet	ft^2	1 m^2 = 10.76 ft^2
Volume	cubic meters	m^3	cubic feet	ft^3	1 m^3 = 35.3 ft^3
Force	newton	N	pound	lb	1 N = .2247 lb
Energy	joule	j	foot pound	ftlb	1 J = .7375 ftlb
Energy	joule	j	electron volt	ev	1 ev = 1.6 x 10^{-19} j
Power	watt (j/s)	W	horsepower	hp	1 hp = 746 W
Exposure	Coulomb per kilogram	C/kg	Roentgen	R	1 R = 2.58 x 10^{-4} C/kg
Dose	gray	Gy	rad	rad	1 Gy = 100 rad
Dose Equivalent	sievert	Sv	rem	rem	1 Sv = 100 rem
Activity	becquerel	Bq	curie	Ci	1 Ci = 3.7 x 10^{10} dps
Frequency	Hertz	Hz	cycles/second	cps	1 Hz = 1 cps

REVIEW OF BASIC MATHEMATICS

Fractions

Fractions to be added or subtracted must have a common denominator (bottom number).

$$\frac{1}{3} + \frac{1}{4} = \frac{4}{12} + \frac{3}{12} = \frac{7}{12}$$

Example 1.1:

What is $\frac{2}{3} + \frac{1}{5}$?

$$\frac{2}{3} + \frac{1}{5} = \frac{10}{15} + \frac{3}{15} = \frac{13}{15}$$

Multiplication of Fractions

To multiply fractions the numerators (top numbers) are multiplied as are the denominators (bottom numbers).

$$\frac{2}{3} \times \frac{1}{4} = \frac{2}{12} = \frac{1}{6}$$

Example 1.2:

What is $\frac{2}{3}$ of $\frac{4}{5}$?

$$\frac{2}{3} \times \frac{4}{5} = \frac{8}{15}$$

Division of Fractions

To divide fractions invert the second (or bottom) term and multiply.

$$\frac{2}{5} \div \frac{3}{7} = \frac{2}{5} \times \frac{7}{3} = \frac{14}{15}$$

Example 1.3:

$$\text{What is } \frac{7}{8} \div \frac{1}{3}?$$

$$\frac{7}{8} \div \frac{1}{3} = \frac{7}{8} \text{ x } \frac{3}{1} = \frac{21}{8}$$

$$= 2\ 5/8$$

Scientific Notation

Very large or very small numbers are more easily written in scientific notation. A curie is 37000000000 disintegrations per second. This is written in scientific notation as 3.7×10^{10} disintegrations per second (dps). To convert a number greater than one into scientific notation:

a) place a decimal point to the right of the first numeral and
b) count the number of places between the new decimal point and the previous location of the decimal point. That number is the exponent of 10 in scientific notation.

$$7530000 = 7.53 \times 10^6$$

For numbers less than one, put a decimal point to the right of the first numeral and then count the number of places between the previous decimal point location and the new decimal point location. This value is the negative exponent of 10 in the scientific notation.

$$.0000693 = 6.93 \times 10^{-5}$$

To add or subtract numbers in scientific notation, the exponents of 10 must be the same.

Multiplication of Numbers in Scientific Notation

To multiply numbers in scientific notation, we multiply the numbers in front of the 10's and add the exponents of 10.

$$(7.53 \times 10^{6}) \times (6.93 \times 10^{-5})$$

$$= 52.2 \times 10^{1}$$

$$= 5.22 \times 10^{2}$$

$$= 522$$

Example 1.4:

What is $(4.7 \times 10^{2}) \times (8.4 \times 10^{3})$?

$$(4.7 \times 10^{2}) \times (8.4 \times 10^{3}) = 39.48 \times 10^{5}$$

$$= 3.948 \times 10^{6}$$

$$= 3{,}948{,}000$$

To divide numbers in scientific notation, divide the numbers in front of the factors of 10 and subtract the exponents.

$$(64 \times 10^{8}) \div (4 \times 10^{3}) = 16 \times 10^{5}$$

$$= 1.6 \times 10^{6}$$

$$= 1{,}600{,}000$$

Example 1.5:

What is $(48 \times 10^{5}) \div (3 \times 10^{3})$?

$$(48 \times 10^{5}) \div (3 \times 10^{3}) = \frac{48}{3} \times 10^{2}$$

$$= 16 \times 10^{2}$$

$$= 1.6 \times 10^{3}$$

$$= 1{,}600$$

In scientific notation, we have given prefixes to the various powers of ten. Table 1.2 gives some of the commonly used prefixes together with their abbreviations.

TABLE 1.2
PREFIXES AND ABBREVIATIONS OF POWERS OF TEN

Value	*Prefix*	*Abbreviation*
10^{-12}	pico-	p
10^{-9}	nano-	n
10^{-6}	micro-	μ
10^{-3}	milli-	m
10^{-2}	centi-	c
10^{3}	kilo-	k
10^{6}	mega-	M

Example 1.6:
How many volts can be obtained from a 150 kilovolt generator?

$$150 \text{ Kilovolt} = 150 \text{ KV}$$
$$= 150 \times 10^3 \text{ v}$$
$$= 150{,}000 \text{ v}$$

Percentages

Before working with percentages, first convert the percentage to conventional fractions by dividing the percentage number by 100.

$$45\% = \frac{45}{100} = .45$$

Example 1.7:

What is 15% of 80?

$$80 \times .15 = 12$$

Geometry

In radiology, the most important application of geometry is in the use of similar triangles. Similar triangles have identical shape but different sizes. Similar triangles have the same angles and the ratio of their sides are equal.

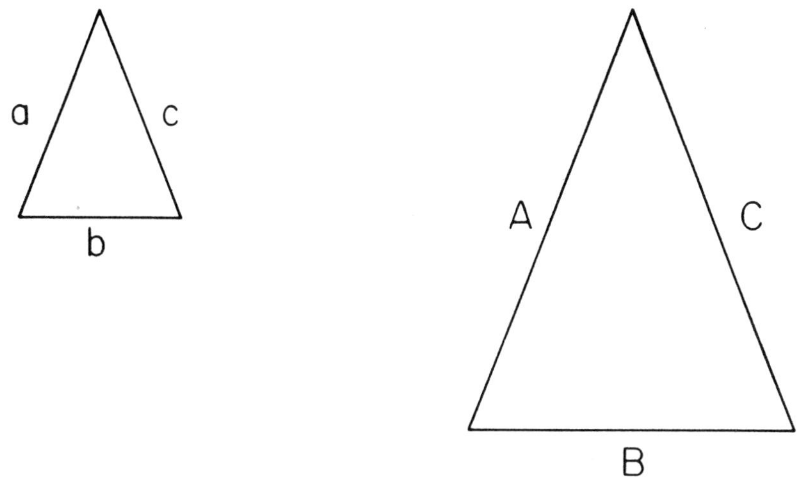

Figure 1.1. Similar triangles.

$$\frac{a}{A} = \frac{b}{B} = \frac{c}{C} \qquad 1.1$$

Example 1.8:

If the large triangle has sides A, B and C equal to 6, 8 and 10 respectively and side a of the small triangle is 4, what is the length of sides b and c?

Side b

$$\frac{4}{6} = \frac{b}{8}$$

$$b = 8 \times \frac{4}{6}$$

$$= 5.3$$

Side c

$$\frac{4}{6} = \frac{c}{10}$$

$$c = 10 \times \frac{4}{6}$$

$$= 6.7$$

In radiology, similar triangles are often used to calculate the object size if we know the image size. Figure 1.2 illustrates application of similar triangles to determine the object size.

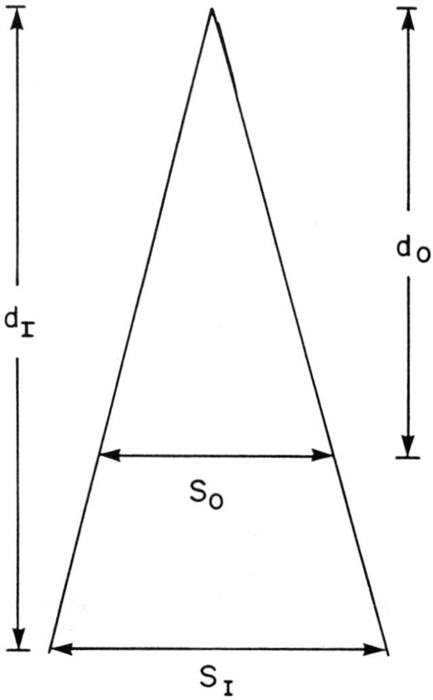

Source

object size = S_o
Source object distance = SOD
image size = S_I
Source image distance = SID

Object

$$\frac{d_o}{d_I} = \frac{SOD}{SID} \qquad 1.2$$

And $$\frac{S_o}{S_I} = \frac{SOD}{SID}$$

or

Image

$$\frac{d_o}{SOD} = \frac{d_I}{SID}$$

Figure 1.2. Similar triangles made up of the Object and Image.

Example 1.9:
What is the image size of a 10 cm (4") wide object if the source image distance (SID) is 100 cm (40") and the distance from the source to the object is 80 cm (32")?

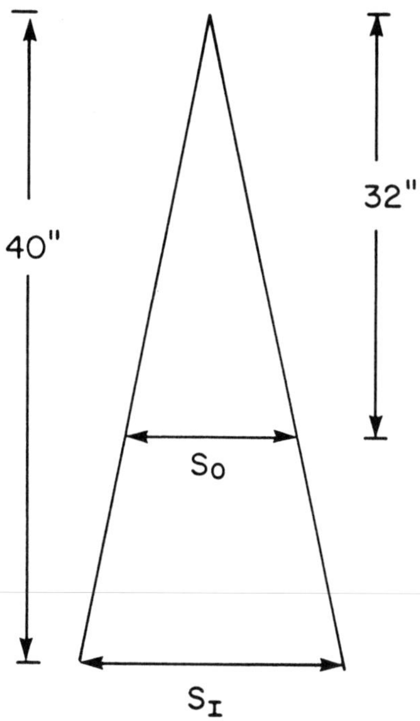

$$\frac{S_I}{100} = \frac{10}{80}$$

$$S_I = 10 \times \frac{100}{80}$$

$$= 12.3 \text{ cm}$$

Figure 1.3. Geometry for Example 1.9.

It is much more likely that we know (or can estimate) the distance from the object to the image plane. This adds another step to the calculations. It always is helpful to make a sketch of the problem geometry.

Example 1.10:
What is the size of an object whose image is 3" long if the object is 4" from the image and the SID is 48"?

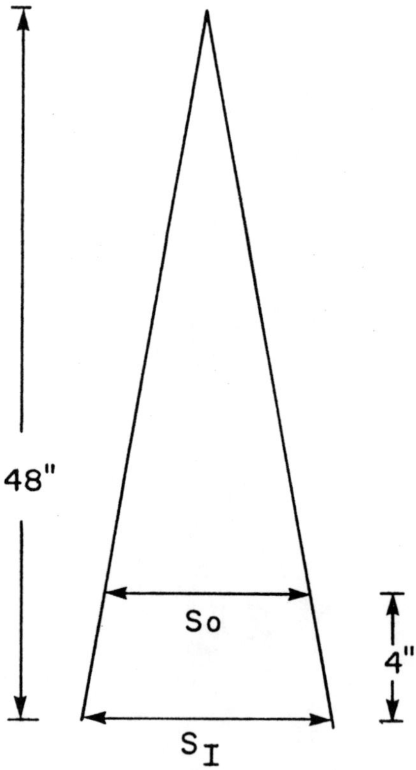

$$SOD = 48 - 4 = 44''$$

$$\frac{So}{S_I} = \frac{SOD}{SID}$$

$$So = 3 \times \frac{44}{48} = 2.75''$$

Figure 1.4. Geometry for Example 1.10.

Magnification

The ratio of image size to object size is called the **magnification.** Large magnifications require short source–object distances and large SID's.

$$m = \frac{S_I}{S_o} \equiv \frac{SID}{SOD} \qquad 1.4$$

Newton's Laws of Motion

Sir Isaac Newton in 1686 published three general laws of motion. They are:

I. *Newton's Law of Inertia.* A body at rest will remain at rest and a body in motion will remain in motion unless acted on by an external force.

II. *Newton's Law of Force.* The force on a body is given by its mass times its acceleration.

$$F = ma$$

III. *Newton's Law of Equal Reactions.* For every action there is an equal and opposite reaction.

Objects in Motion

The description of objects in motion is given in terms of velocity and acceleration. Acceleration is a change in velocity. The velocity, v, of an object describes the distance, d, it has traveled in a certain amount of time, t.

$$d = v \times t \qquad 1.5$$

Example 1.11:
If a ball moves 40 meters in two seconds what is the velocity?

$$d = v \times t$$

$$10\ m = (v\ m/s) \times (2s)$$

$$v = \frac{40m}{2s} = 20m/s$$

Both the quantity and the units must be correct to obtain the correct answer. Often the solution to a problem can be obtained by knowing the units of the answer.

Velocity

The fundamental equation of velocity for a body whose initial velocity is v_o and whose acceleration is a is given by:

$$v = v_o + at \qquad 1.6$$

Accelerations are measured in units of m/s^2 or ft/s^2.

Example 1.12:
A ball starts out with an initial velocity of 2m/s. After 4 seconds of acceleration the velocity is 12m/s. What was the acceleration?

The units of acceleration are m/s^2

$$v = v_o + at$$

$$12m/s = 2m/s + at\ m/s$$

$$10m/s = a\ m/s^2 \times 4s$$

$$a = \frac{10}{4}\ m/s^2$$

$$a = \frac{5}{2}\ m/s^2$$

$$a = 2.5\ m/s^2$$

This means that the velocity changes by 2.5 m/s during every second of the acceleration.

An object which has **constant velocity** has an **acceleration** of **zero.**

Mass and Weight

Newton's second law relates a body's mass to the body's weight. A body's mass is a property of the body. A body's **weight** is the **force** on a body due to gravitational attraction.

TABLE 1.3
UNITS OF MASS AND FORCE

	Mass	*Force*	*Acceleration Due to Gravity*
English	Slug	Pound	32 f/s^2
SI	Kilogram	newton	9.8 m/s^2

Table 1.3 gives the units of mass and force in the English and SI Systems.

The English unit of mass is used only in physics and engineering courses and in scientific trivia games.

The SI unit of force, the newton, is equal to one kg m/s^2.

Force Due to Gravity

From Newton's Second Law:

$$F = ma \quad 1.7$$

We can write:

$$Wt = mg \quad 1.8$$

where Wt is the weight, F, the force of gravity and g is the acceleration due to gravity.

In space, a body is weightless because g = O but the body still has mass.

Example 1.13:
What is the weight of an 80 kg person on the surface of the moon if the acceleration of gravity on the moon is 1.6 m/s^2?

On Earth	On Moon
Mass = 80 kg	M = 80 kg
Wt = mg	Wt = mg
Wt = 80 kg x 9.8 m/s^2	Wt = 80 kg x 1.6 m/s^2
Wt = 784 N	Wt = 128 N

On the moon, a person weighs only 1/6 their earth weight.

Work and Energy

The term **work** has a very specific physics definition. Work is the action of a force through a distance.

$$W = F \times d \qquad 1.9$$

Work is measured in units of **foot-pounds** in the English System and **Newton-meters** in SI Units. One Newton-meter equals on joule.

Example: How much work is done by a 6 lb. force acting through 3 ft?

$$W = F \times d$$

$$W = 6 \text{ lb} \times 3 \text{ ft}$$

$$W = 18 \text{ ft-lb}$$

Example 1.14:
How much work is done lifting a 2 kg object 3 meters in the air?

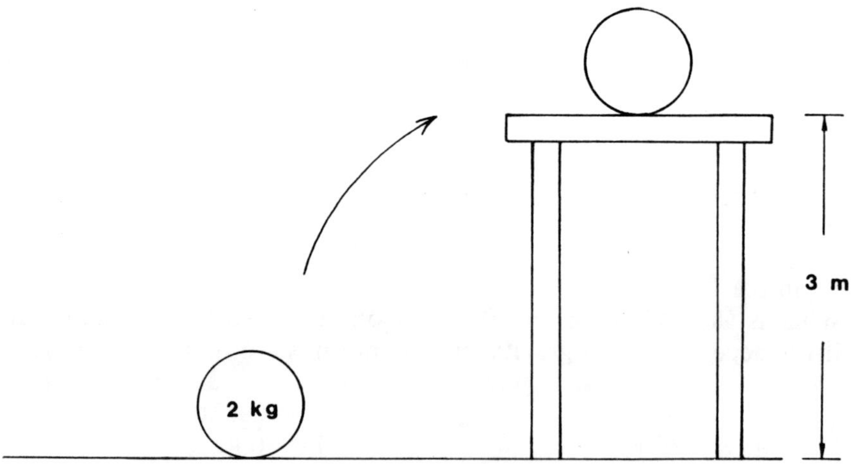

Figure 1.5. Work required to lift a 2 kg object 3m.

First, we must calculate the force required to lift the object: For lifting problems, the force required is the weight of the object

$$F = mg$$

$$F = m \times 9.8\ m/s^2$$

or

$$F = 2kg \times 9.8 = 19.6\ kg\ m/s^2$$

$$F = 19.6\ N$$

The force required to lift the object is 19.6 newtons. This force will act through a distance of 3 m.

$$\begin{aligned} Work &= F \times d \\ &= 19.6\ N \times 3m \\ &= 58.8\ Nm \text{ (newton-meters)} \\ &= 58.8\ j \quad \text{(joule)} \end{aligned}$$

Energy

Energy is defined as the **ability to do work.** In radiology, we are concerned with both **electrical** and **mechanical** energy. There are two types of mechanical energy, **potential** and **kinetic** energy. Potential energy is the stored ability to do work. Kinetic energy is the energy of motion. The Conservation of Energy Law says that energy can be converted from one form to another but it can neither be created nor destroyed.

If a bowling ball is carried up to a 10th floor window, it gains a potential energy equal to the force (mg) exerted times the height of the window (h). This is just the work done in getting the ball up to the window. If the ball is dropped out the window, its kinetic energy ($\frac{1}{2}mv^2$) at the bottom of the fall will be equal to its original potential energy.

Kinetic Energy = Potential Energy

$$\tfrac{1}{2}mv^2 = mgh \qquad 1.10$$

Example 1.15:
A 7 kg bowling ball is carried up to a 10th floor window whose height is 36m. If the ball is dropped out the window what is the velocity of the ball as it hits the ground?

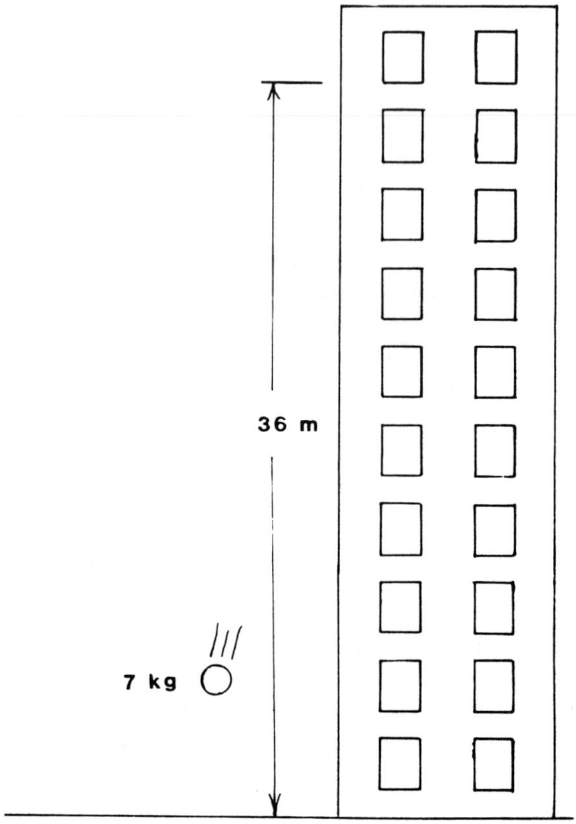

Figure 1.6. The kinetic energy of ball as it reaches the ground is equal to the potential energy at the top.

$$\text{Potential Energy} = \text{Kinetic Energy}$$

$$mgh = \tfrac{1}{2}\, mv^2$$

$$7 \times 9.8 \times 36 = \tfrac{1}{2} \times 7 \times V^2$$

$$V^2 = 705.6\ m^2/s^2$$

$$V = \sqrt{705.6}$$

$$V = 26.6\ m/s$$

Notice that this result says that **any** body dropped out of a 36m high window will strike the ground with the same velocity. In the absence of air resistance this is true. Galileo is reported to have dropped two different sized balls off the Leaning Tower of Piza to prove this law in 1590.

Momentum

Momentum (p) is the product of the mass times the velocity.

$$p = mv \qquad 1.11$$

Momentum is conserved in collisions; that is the momentum before a collision is equal to the momentum after a collision.

$$mv)_{before} = mv)_{after} \qquad 1.12$$

Momentum is measured in units of kg m/s.

Heat

Heat is energy of molecular motion. Heat transfer can occur through three processes:

1. Conduction
2. Convection
3. Radiation

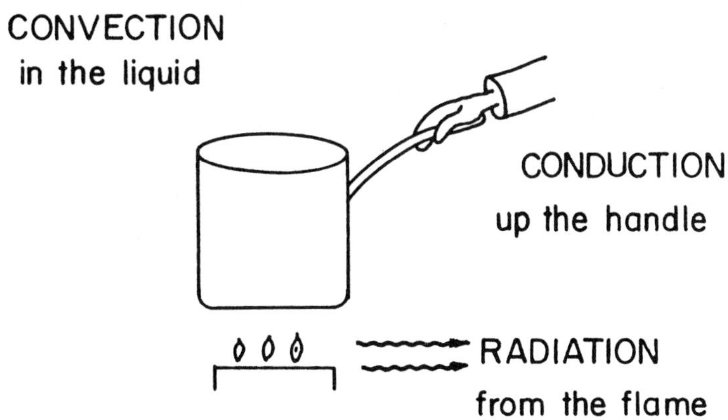

Figure 1.7. Example of the three heat transfer processes.

Conduction is the transfer of heat through a solid material. The metal pot handle transfers heat to your hand through the process of conduction. **Convection** is transfer of heat through motion of the material. Convection transfers heat throughout a pot of water through motion of the water. **Radiation** is emission of energy from a body. Radiation energy can be transferred through a vacuum and depends on the temperature of the body. Radiation is the principle means of heat transfer from x–ray anode to the tube housing.

Temperature

Temperature is used to describe whether a body is hot or cold. Temperature can be measured using thermometers which measure the expansion or contraction of a liquid column. Mercury or colored alcohol are commonly used. The most common temperature scales are the **Celsius** and the **Fahrenheit** scales.

In order to define a temperature scale a high point, a low point, and the number of degrees between high and low points

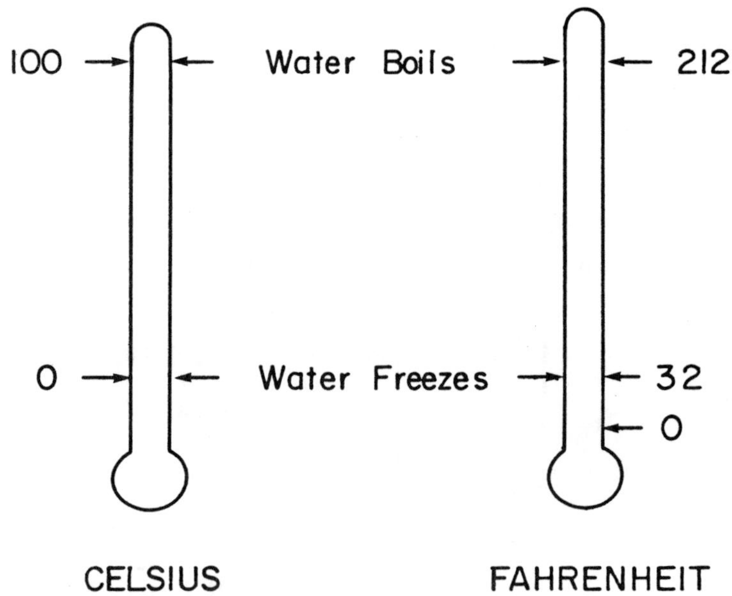

Figure 1.8. Comparison of Celsius and Fahrenheit scales.

must be specified. The Celsius scale is defined as 100° between the low point 0° (freezing point of water) and the high point 100° (boiling point of water).

When Gabriel Fahrenheit developed his thermometer in 1700, he chose 0° as the coldest temperature attainable by man (a mixture of salt, water and ice) and for the 100° point he chose the body temperature of a healthy horse. These convert into a boiling point of water of 212° Fahrenheit and a freezing point of water of 32° Fahrenheit.

Conversion of Temperatures

The easiest way to convert temperatures is to remember that there are 180° between the freezing and boiling points of water on the Fahrenheit scale and 100°C on the Celsius scale. A Celsius degree is almost twice as large as a Fahrenheit degree.

To convert Celsius to Fahrenheit, we multiply by the ratio of the degree sizes and then add 32° to make up for the change in the low point on the scale.

$$°F = \frac{180}{100} \times °C + 32 \qquad 1.13$$

Example 1.16:

Convert 37°C to Fahrenheit

$$37°C \times \frac{180}{100} = 66.6$$

0°C = 32°F so we must add 32°F

$$66.7 + 32 = \mathbf{98.6°F}$$

To convert from Fahrenheit to Celsius we first must remove the extra 32° and then multiply by the ratio of the degrees.

$$°C = (°F - 32) \times \frac{100}{180} \qquad 1.14$$

Example 1.17:

Convert 180°F to Celsius

32° F = 0°C

so we must first subtract 32°

$$180° - 32°F = 148°$$

$$148 \times \frac{100}{180} = 82.2°C$$

If there is ever any question about whether to multiply first and then subtract 32°, or vice versa, just convert 0°C to 32°F or vice versa as a test.

Example 1.18:

$$0°C \times \frac{180F}{100C} = 0°F + 32° = 32°F$$

$$32°F - 32 = 0° \times \frac{100C}{180F} = 0° C$$

Electromagnetic Radiation

All forms of electromagnetic radiation travel with the speed of light, 3×10^8 m/s. The energy of electromagnetic radiation is related to its frequency f by

$$E = hf \qquad 1.15$$

where he is Planck's constant ($h = 6.6 \times 10^{34}$ j-sec). Note that higher frequency waves have higher energy.

Electromagnetic radiation is transmitted by electromagnetic waves. Figure 1.9 presents the electromagnetic spectrum from long wavelength low energy radio waves to high energy short wavelength gamma rays.

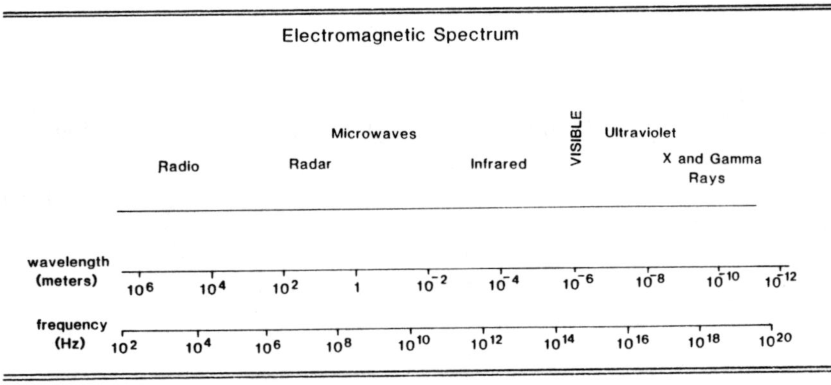

Figure 1.9. The electromagnetic spectrum.

Only x–rays and gamma rays have enough energy to separate one or more electrons from the atom to produce an ion pair. X–rays and gamma rays are classified as **ionizing radiation.** The wave length (λ) is the distance between corresponding parts of succeeding waves. It is the distance from one peak to the next peak or from one valley to the next valley.

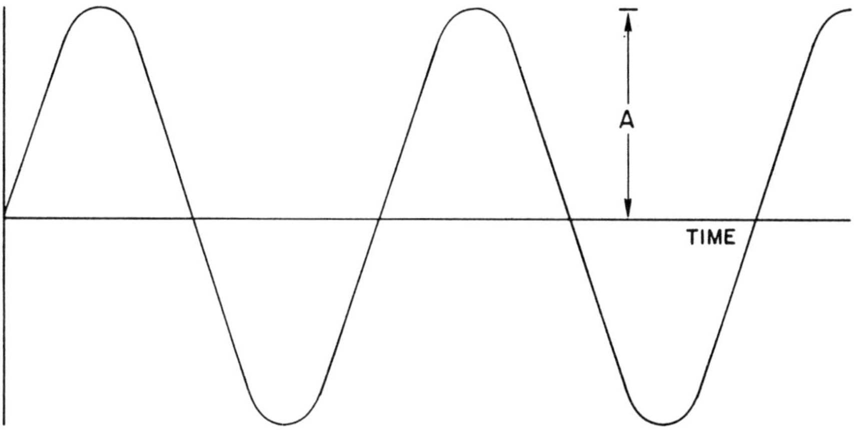

Figure 1.10. An electromagnetic wave.

The **frequency** f is the number of complete cycles passing a given point per second. Frequency is measured in Hertz or cycles per second (1 Hz = 1 cps). The **period** T of the wave is given by:

$$T = {}^{1}/_{f} \qquad 1.16$$

The **amplitude** A is the magnitude of the wave from 0 to the maximum (either positive or negative). The velocity v of the wave is related to the wave length and frequency by:

$$V = f\lambda \qquad 1.17$$

The relationship between the energy carried in the wave the frequency or wave length which is given by equation 1.8. For **electromagnetic radiation**

$$c = f\lambda \qquad 1.18$$

where c = velocity of light 3×10^8 m/sec). All electromagnetic radiation travels with the speed of light. Combining Equations 1.15 and 1.18 we find

$$E = hf = hc/\lambda \qquad 1.19$$

If the energy is measured in keV and the wave length is measured in Angstroms ($1\text{Å} = 10^{-10}$m), then

$$E\ (\text{KeV}) = \frac{12.4}{\lambda(\text{Å})} \qquad 1.20$$

or

$$\lambda(\text{Å}) = \frac{12.4}{E(\text{keV})}$$

Intensity

Intensity is defined as the energy passing through a unit area. It is measured in joules per meter^2. The intensity of an x–ray beam is obtained by multiplying the number of photons passing through a given area by the energy of each x–ray photon.

Radiation Units

When a patient has an x–ray examination, it's important to know how much radiation is used. The photon **fluence** measures the number photons per square centimeter. A more convenient measure of radiation is a measure of the ionization produced in air (the **exposure**). The Roentgen was defined as the amount of radiation which would produce 2.58×10^{-4} coulombs per kilogram of dry air. Although the Roentgen is not officially recognized as the scientific unit, it is still in widespread use today. The SI unit of exposure is the coulomb per kilogram (C/kg). 1 R = 260 μ C/kg

Radiation Dose

A unit more closely linked to biological effects is a measure of energy deposited in a medium – the **dose.** The unit of dose measures the radiation energy deposited in the patient's body. A **gray** is defined as a deposition of one joule of energy per kilogram. The older unit of dose is the **rad.** One rad equals 100 erg/gm (1 erg = 10^{-7}j) (1 Gy = 100 rad). If a radiation beam deposits

1 j of energy in a 1 kgm block of tissue the dose is 1 gray. If the same beam deposits 2 j energy in a 2 kgm tissue block, the dose is still 1 gray (2 j/2 kgm).

Other Radiations

Alpha particles and beta particles are products of natural radioactive decay. Alpha particles are very highly ionizing with very short ranges in tissue. Protons and neutrons can be obtained from particle accelerators. These other radiations have different properties than x and gamma rays. They are not electromagnetic radiation and they deposit their energy over a much shorter range.

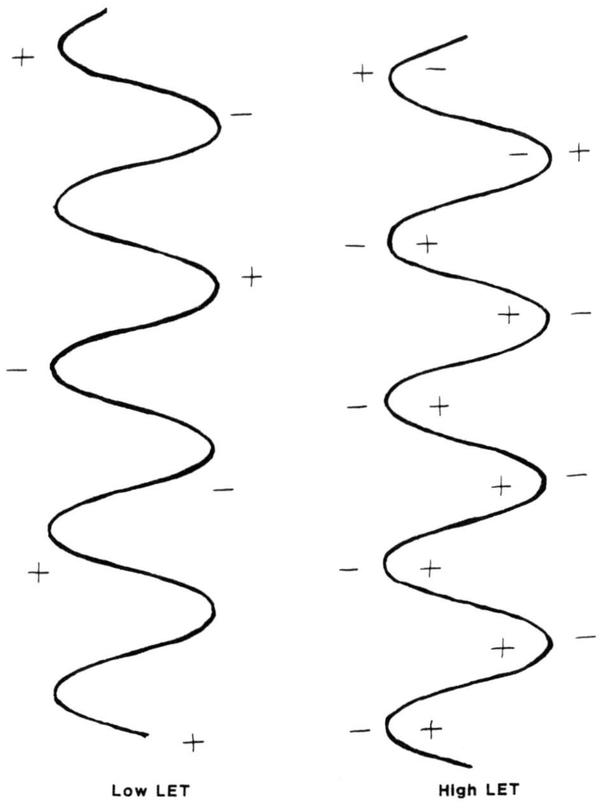

Figure 1.11. Different Linear Energy Transfer particles.

Linear Energy Transfer

One method of describing the amount of ionization or energy deposition along a particle track is in terms of Linear Energy Transfer (LET). LET is measured in KeV per micron. The biological effect of a particle depends on its LET. Higher LET particles have larger biological effects.

Example 1.19:
If an alpha particle deposits 4 MeV over a track length of 20 microns, the LET is:

$$\text{LET} = \frac{4000}{20\mu}\ \text{KeV} = 200\ \text{KeV}/\mu$$

Quality Factor

Radiation beams of neutrons, alpha particles, pions or other exotic forms of radiation have biological effects different than x-rays. We have to "adjust" the dose with a quality factor to obtain the dose equivalent. The dose equivalent is designed to relate the biological effects of different types of radiation. It is measured in sieverts or rems.

$$1\ \text{sievert} = \text{QF} \times \text{Gray} \qquad 1.21$$

$$1\ \text{rem} = \text{QF} \times \text{rad} \qquad 1.22$$

The quality factor is designed to account for the different biological effectiveness of different types of radiations. Table 1.4 presents quality factors for representative particles of different LET values.

TABLE 1.4
LET VALUES

Radiation	*LET KeV/μ*	*Quality Factor*
X and Gamma Rays Beta Particles	1	1
Neutrons 〉 10 keV	50	10
Protons	100	10
Alpha Particles	200	20

For medical x-rays QF = 1 and the units have been adjusted so we can assume:

$$1\text{R} = 1 \text{ rad} = 1 \text{ rem} \tag{1.23}$$

and

$$1 \text{ Gy} = 1 \text{ Sv} \tag{1.24}$$

Inverse Square Law

If a point source of radiation as shown in Figure 1.12 is located at point P, then the same amount of energy passes through the place A B C D as through the plane E F G H. That is, the same number of photons and total energy passing through the two planes are equal. However, the energy in the number of photons

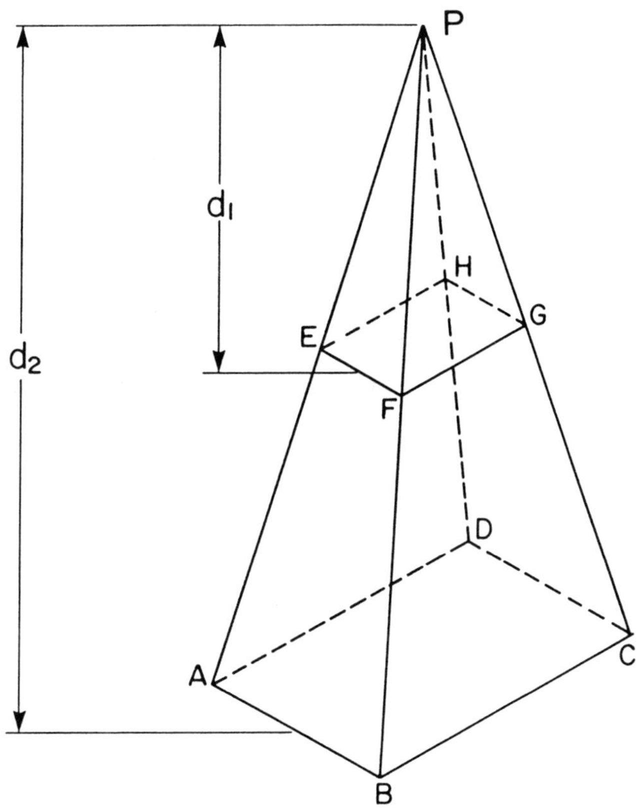

Figure 1.12. Inverse Square Law Geometry.

passing through E F G H are spread over a larger area. Thus, the intensity (energy per unit area) is less at a greater distance from the source. The relationship between the intensity at A B C D and the intensity of E F G H is given by the equation:

$$I_{E\,F\,G\,H} = I_{A\,B\,C\,D} \qquad 1.25$$

and

$$E_2(d_2)^2 = E_1(d_1)^2 \qquad 1.26$$

Example 1.20:
Calculate the exposure rate two meters from a source whose exposure rate is 100 mR per hour at one meter.

$$E\,(2m) = 100\,(½)^2 = 25 \text{ mR/hr}$$

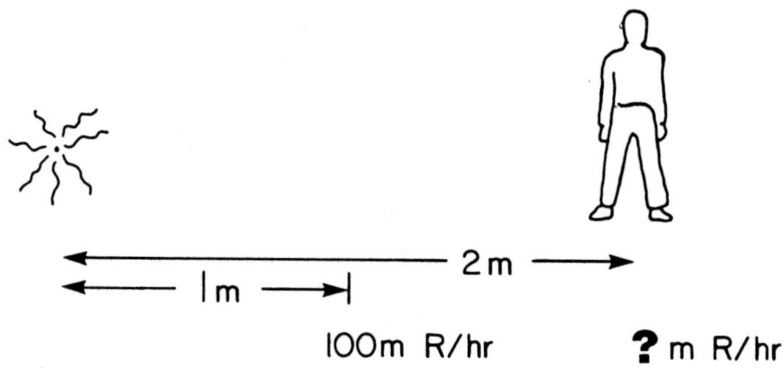

Figure 1.13. Inverse Square reduction in exposure.

CHAPTER 1 QUESTIONS

1. How far does an object moving with a velocity of 12 m/s travel in 4 seconds?

2. An object is initially moving with a velocity of 4 m/s. What is the acceleration if its final velocity is 25 m/s after 7 seconds?

3. A ball travels 24 m in 4 seconds. What is its velocity?

4. An acceleration of 2 m/s^2 acts on an object for 6 seconds. If the final velocity is 21 m/s what was its initial velocity?

5. If a body is at rest how long does an acceleration of 3 m/s^2 have to act in order to have the body's final velocity equal 12 m/s?

6. A force of 6 N acts on a 3 kg body. What is the acceleration?

7. A force of 8 N acts on a 2 kg body. What is its acceleration?

8. A force of 12 N produces an acceleration of 3 m/s^2 on a body. What is the mass of the body?

9. What force will produce a 12 m/s^2 acceleration of a 2 kg body?

10. What is the gravitational force (weight) on a 3 kg body?

11. What is the mass in slugs of a 64 lb (weight) body?

12. What is the gravitational force (weight) on a 4 kg body?

13. What is the mass (in slugs) of a body which experiences a gravitational force of 128 lb? (weighs 128 lb)

14. Write the expression for work in terms of force F and distance d.

15. A force of 18 lb moves a body through a distance of 3 ft. How much work was done?

16. A man lifts a 24 lb weight 2 ft in the air. How much work does he do?

17. What is the gravitational force (weight) on a 6 kg body?

18. How much work in joules is done lifting a 6 kg body through a distance of 3 m? (Hint 1 j = 1 Nm)

19. Write the expression for gravitational potential energy in terms of mass, height and the acceleration of gravity.

20. A 7 kg ball is lifted 3 m in the air. What is its potential energy?

21. Write the expression for kinetic energy in terms of mass and velocity.

22. A 3 kg object is moving with a velocity of 4 m/s. What is its kinetic energy?

23. A 4 kg object is moving with a velocity of 3 m/s. What is its kinetic energy?

24. A 3 kg object has a kinetic energy of 24 j. What is its velocity?

25. A 4 kg object has a kinetic energy of 72 j. What is its velocity?

26. A 5 kg object has a kinetic energy of 10 j. What is its velocity.

27. A 2 kg object has a kinetic energy of 12 j. What is its velocity?

28. A 4 kg object is carried to the top of a 12 m tower. What is its potential energy?

29. If the ball is dropped from the 12 m tower what is its velocity just as it strikes the ground?

30. What form of heat transfer involves the motion of a fluid?

31. What form of heat transfer brings heat from the sun?

32. What form of heat transfer brings heat from one end of a metal rod to the other end?

33. What is the momentum of a 3 kg ball moving with a velocity of 4 m/s?

Add or Subtract these fractions:

34. 1/2 + 1/3
35. 5/6 - 1/5
36. 1/3 + 5/9
37. 7/8 - 1/4
38. 2/7 + 1/3

Multiply or Divide these fractions:

39. 1/2 x 2/5
40. 3/5 ÷ 1/4
41. 5/7 x 2/3
42. 1/2 ÷ 1/4
43. 2/3 x 3/4

Write in Scientific or Conventional Notation

44. 6×10^5
45. 4000000
46. .00205
47. 17500
48. 314000000
49. 6.67×10^{-2}
50. 3.00×10^7
51. .0103
52. 22×10^4
53. 7.32×10^{-3}

54. What is 12% of 125?

55. What is 70% of 250?

56. What is 30% of 620?

57. What is 45% of 220?

58. What is 1% of 250?

59. What is the object size that produces an image 3.5" long if the object is 6" from the film and the SID is 42"?

60. What image size is produced by an object 2" long if the source object distance is 64" and the SID is 72"?

61. Give an example of Newton's First Law of Motion from everyday life.

62. What is the weight of a person on the planet Krypton ($g = 12\ m/s^2$) if the person weighs 60 kg on earth?

63. With what force does a 70 kg individual push back on an airplane seat during takeoff if the plane's acceleration is $3\ m/s^2$?

64. What is the potential energy of a 16 lb. ball after it has been lifted to the top of a 50 ft. tower?

65. What is the potential energy of a 30 kg bowling ball which has been raised to the top of a 125 m building?

66. How many minutes could this energy light a 40 watt light bulb?

67. What is the momentum of an 8 kg ball moving with a velocity of 7 m/s?

68. How fast is a 3 kg ball moving if its momentum is 33 kg m/s?

69. What form of heat transfer is used to cool a room with electric fan?

70. What form of heat transfer brings the sun's energy to the earth?

71. Convert 50°F to °C.

72. Convert 50° C to ° F.

73. What is the amplitude of this wave?

74. What is the frequency of this wave?

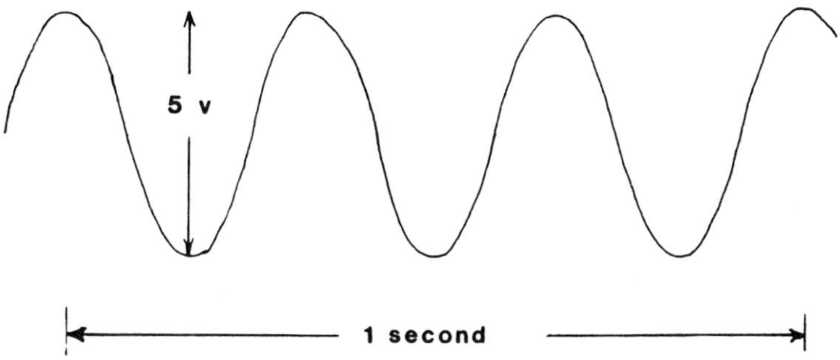

75. What is the period of this wave?

76. What is the exposure 6 m from a source if the exposure 3 m from the source is 400 m R/hr?

77. What is the exposure of 2 m from a source which is 100 m R/hr at a distance of 3 m?

78. Which of the following is NOT one of Newton's Laws of Motion?
   A. A body at rest will remain at rest and a body in motion will remain in motion unless acted on by an external force.
   B. $F = ma$
   C. $E = mc^2$
   D. For every action there is a reaction.

79. Which radiation is not electromagnetic radiation?
   A. Ultrasound
   B. Radio
   C. X-rays
   D. Light

80. Heat can be transferred by:

1. collection.	A. 1, 2, 4
2. convection.	B. 1, 2, 3
3. conduction.	C. 1, 3, 4
4. radiation.	D. 2, 3, 4

81. What is the mass of a body if a 14 N force produces a 1 m/s^2 acceleration? The acceleration due to gravity is 9.8 m/s^2 or 32 ft/s^2.

CHAPTER 2

ATOMIC AND MOLECULAR STRUCTURE

The Bohr model of the atom describes the neutral atom as a dense positive nucleus surrounded by negative electrons moving in definite orbits or shells.

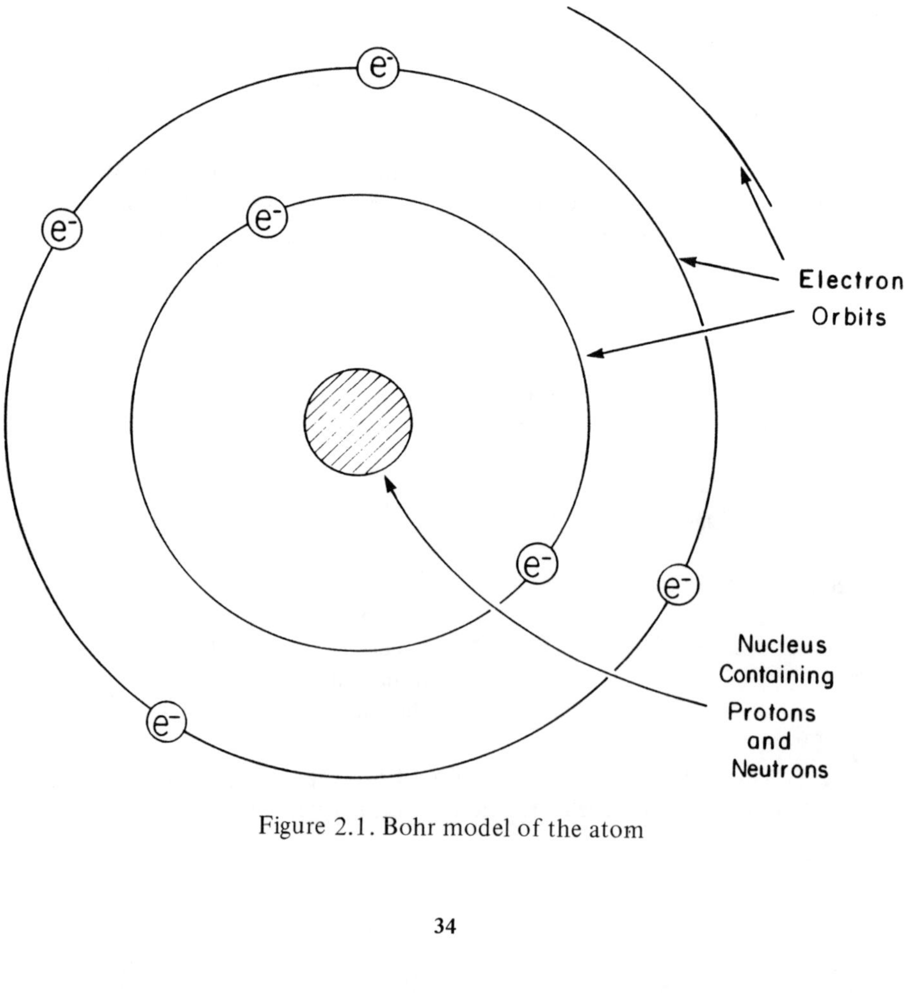

Figure 2.1. Bohr model of the atom

An electron can be in one orbit or another but it can't be in between.

The nucleus is made up of **nucleons**. Nucleons are either **protons** having a positive charge or **neutrons** which have zero charge. Atoms are neutral, the number of orbital electrons surrounding the nucleus is equal to the number of protons within the nucleus. The atomic number, Z, of an atom is equal to the number of protons in the nucleus. Because the weight of nucleons and nuclei are very small numbers when experssed in kilograms, it is convenient to use a scale based on atomic mass units. The atomic weight, A, is measured in AMU. The atomic mass unit is based on the mass of the most common nucleus of carbon (carbon–12). One AMU is 1/12 the mass of the carbon–12 nucleus.

$$1\text{AMU} = 1.6606 \times 10^{-27} \text{ kgm}$$

Table 2.1 presents the masses of the electron, proton, neutron, deuteron and alpha particle in AMU and in kilograms.

TABLE 2.1
CHARACTERISTICS OF SOME NUCLEAR PARTICLES

Particle	*Charge*	*AMU*	*Mass kgm*
electron	-1	5.48×10^{-4}	9.1×10^{-31}
proton	+1	1.00728	1.6726×10^{-27}
neutron	0	1.00867	1.6749×10^{-27}
deuteron	+1	2.01355	3.3444×10^{-27}
alpha	+2	4.001507	6.6463×10^{-27}

The proton is the nucleus of a hydrogen atom, the deuteron is a combination of one proton and one neutron and the alpha particle is the nucleus of a helium atom, it contains two protons and two neutrons.

Periodic Table

Elements have similar chemical characteristics when arranged in order of increasing Z. Figure 2.2 presents the first rows of the Periodic Table. Elements H, Li, Na and K in the left most column of the Periodic Table are very reactive.

A new row is started whenever one of the orbital shells is filled. Atoms with filled orbital shells occupy the right hand

Hydrogen H							Helium He
Lithium Li	Beryllium Be	Boron B	Carbon C	Nitrogen N	Oxygen O	Fluorine F	Neon Ne
Sodium Na	Magnesium Mg	Aluminum Al	Silicon Si	Phosphorus P	Sulfur S	Chlorine Cl	Argon A

Figure 2.2 First three rows of the Periodic Table

column of the Periodic Table. They are chemically inert gases and are called the noble gases.

Isotopes

Isotopes are nuclei with the same number of protons and a different number of neutrons, i.e., same Z different A. Isotopes have very similar chemical properties. Table 2.2 shows four different isotopes of carbon together with the atomic weight A in AMU, the number of protons Z and the number of neutrons, N.

TABLE 2.2
ISOTOPES OF CARBON

		$^{11}_{6}C$	$^{12}_{6}C$	$^{13}_{6}C$	$^{14}_{6}C$
	A --	11	12	13	14
	Z --	6	6	6	6
number of neutrons	N --	5	6	7	8

The word **isotope** comes from the Greek words "iso" meaning "the same" and "tope" meaning "place." Isotopes occupy the same location on the Periodic Table. The convention is to write the atomic number Z to the lower left and the atomic weight A to the upper left of the chemical symbol.

Atoms with the same atomic weight A but different atomic number Z are called **isobars** (the same weight).

$$^{12}_{5}B \quad ^{12}_{6}C \quad ^{12}_{7}N$$

are examples of isobars. Atoms with the same number of neutrons (A − Z) are called **isotones.**

$$^{11}_{5}B \quad ^{12}_{6}C \quad ^{13}_{7}C$$

are examples of isotones.

Types of Forces

There are three types of forces in nature, **gravitational, electrostatic and nuclear.** Gravitational forces are attractive. Electrostatic forces are attractive between unlike charges and repulsive between like charges. There are only positive charges in the nucleus so electrostatic forces would cause the nucleus to fly apart were it not for the even stronger attractive nuclear force. The nuclear force operates only at extremely short ranges (10^{-15} m).

Atomic Orbital Structure

As the number of protons increases, the orbital structure of the electrons becomes more complex. The number of electrons which an orbit can hold depends on how close it is to the nucleus and other complex factors. Figure 2.3 is a schematic representation of the first three atoms in the Periodic Table.

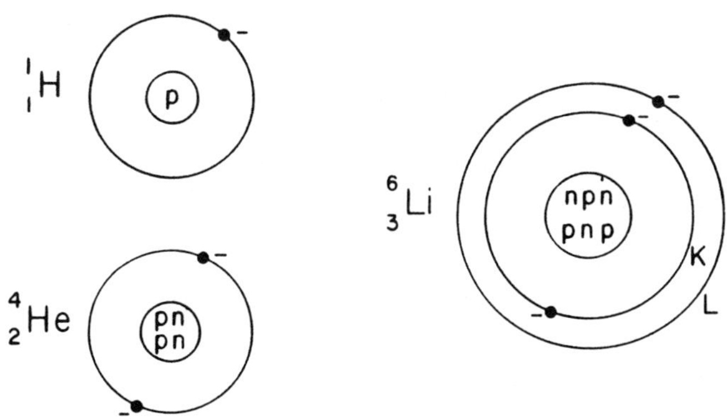

Figure 2.3. Orbits of the first three elements.

The K shell which is closest to the nucleus, can hold only two electrons. The next shell, the L shell, can hold eight electrons, and the next, the M shell, can hold 18 electrons. When a particular shell is completely filled, it forms an extraordinarily stable element. Filling of the K, L and M shells results in the noble gases helium, neon and argon with atomic numbers of 2, 8 and 18 respectively.

Energies

The ordinary unit of energy, a joule (1 joule = 1 newton meter), is much larger than the energies of atomic transitions and so a more convenient unit, the electron volt is used. The electron volt is defined as the energy which a particle with one electron charge gains in moving through a potential of one volt. If an electron moves through a potential difference of 100,000 volts (100 kVp), it will gain an energy of 100 keV. Notice that **kVp** measures the peak applied potential and KeV measures the energy of the particle. One electron volt is equal to 1.6×10^{-19} joules. A joule is an "every day sized unit of energy." One watt is one joule per second. Thus a 40 watt light bulb expends energy at the rate of 40 joules per second or $25 \times 10^{+17}$ KeV per second.

Binding Energies

Electrons in orbits closer to the nucleus are more strongly attracted to the nucleus. The energy required to remove an electron from its orbit is called the binding energy of that electron. Different electron orbits have different binding energies. Orbits further from the nucleus have smaller binding energies.

Nuclei with higher Z (more protons), have higher binding energies. As an example, hydrogen has a K shell binding energy of 13.2 electron volts. Tungsten with a Z of 78 has a K shell binding energy of 69,500 eV. Binding energies are an example of potential energy. Potential energy can be positive or negative but binding energies are always negative. A negative potential energy indicates that energy must be supplied to release the electron in the orbit. The outer shell binding energy of all atoms is a few ev.

Energy Mass Equivalence

Einstein's Equation

$$E = mc^2$$

relates the mass and energy through the velocity of light, c. All electromagnetic radiation travels at the velocity of light, 3×10^8 m/sec.

Example 2.1:
What is the energy equivalent of one electron mass?

$$E = mc^2$$

$$m = 9.1 \times 10^{-31} \text{ kgm}$$

$$c = 3 \times 10^8 \text{ m/sec}$$

$$E = (9 \times 10^{-31} \text{ kgm})(3 \times 10^8 \text{ m/sec})^2$$

$$= 8.19 \times 10^{-14} \text{ joule}$$

$$1 \text{ MeV} = 1.6 \times 10^{-13} \text{ j}$$

$$E = 0.511 \text{ MeV}$$

The mass of one electron is equivalent to 0.511 MeV.

We can also calculate the binding energy of a nucleus. This is equal to the difference in mass, expressed as energy between the nucleus and its constituent nucleons. This mass difference is also called the **mass defect**.

As an example we can calculate the binding energy of the deuteron.

Mass of Proton	1.00728
+	
Mass of Neutron	1.00867
	2.01595 AMU
Mass of Deuteron	−2.01355 AMU
Mass Defect	.00239 AMU

$$.00239 \text{ AMU} \times 931 \text{ MeV/AMU} = 2.23 \text{ MeV}$$

This is the energy holding the deuteron together. It is also the energy required to separate the deuteron into a proton and a neutron.

Energy Level Diagrams

In order to relate the binding energies of the various electron orbits, it is useful to present them in the form of a schematic energy level diagram. The energy levels of tungsten are shown in Figure 2.4. Here, the binding energies are shown as negative energies to indicate the electron is bound to the nucleus and that energy must be supplied in order to remove the orbital electron. For example, to remove a K shell electron we must supply 69,500 electron volts. Such removal would leave a vacancy in the K shell. This vacancy could be filled by an L shell electron dropping into the empty orbital space. Because the L shell electron has a smaller negative binding energy, the energy difference between the K and L shell binding energies will be radiated as a 58.2 KeV (69.5 – 11.3) $K\alpha$ characteristic x-ray. If the vacancy is filled by an M shell electron, a 66.7 KeV $K\beta$ characteristic x-ray will result.

A vacancy in the K shell is most likely to be filled from the L shell. Such a jump of orbital electrons from the L to the K shell will leave a vacancy in the L shell which will then be filled by an electron from one of the outer most orbits. Thus, there can be a whole series of characteristic x-ray emitted following the removal of a single K shell electron. The x-rays from this process are called **characteristic x-rays** because they are characteristic of the atoms.

Auger Electron Emission

Ejection of an Auger Electron is an alternate to characteristic x-ray production. Instead of emitting a characteristic x-ray all the difference in orbital binding energies is given to one of the orbital electrons. This **Auger** electron carries off the energy that would have gone to a characteristic x-ray less the binding energy of the electron.

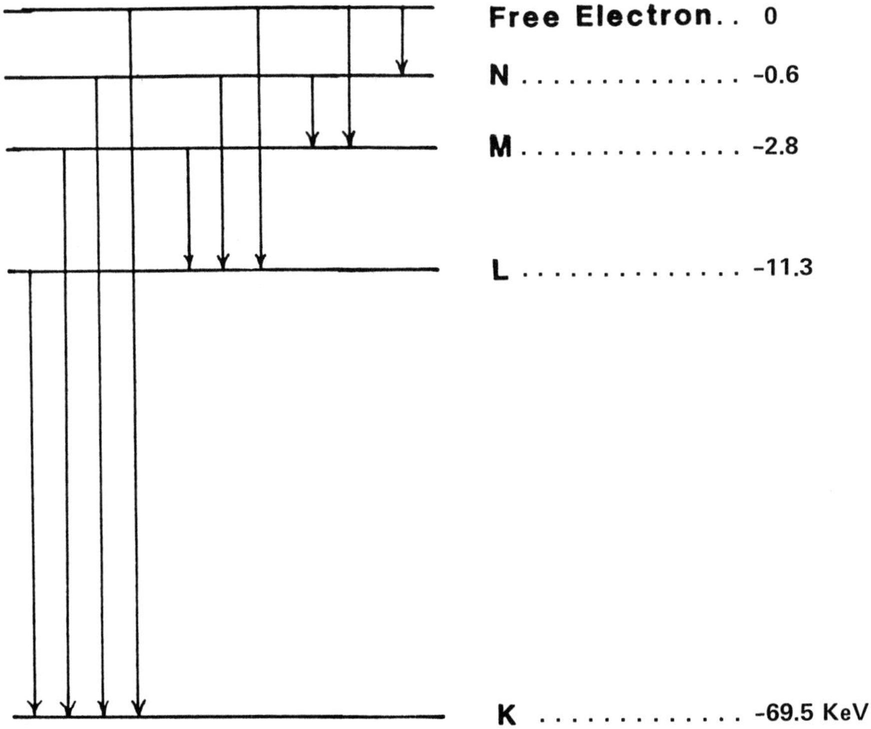

Energy Levels of Tungsten

Binding Energies
of Orbital Electrons

K	69.5	KeV
L	11.3	KeV
M	2.8	KeV
N	0.6	KeV

Figure 2.4. Transitions to produce characteristic x-rays.

Example 2.2:
What is the energy of an M shell Auger electron from a L–K transition in an atom whose binding energies are:

$$K = 55 \text{ KeV}$$

$$L = 8 \text{ KeV}$$

$$M = 0.75 \text{ KeV}$$

Energy available from L–K transition

$$E = 55 - 8$$

$$= 47 \text{ KeV}$$

Energy required to remove M shell electron

$$E = 0.75 \text{ KeV}$$

Energy available to Auger electron

$$E = 47 - .75$$

$$= 46.25 \text{ KeV}$$

Structure of Matter

Matter is anything which has inertia and occupies space. Most matter in nature is a mixture of different **substances.** A substance has a definite composition and can be made up of either **compounds** or **elements.** Elements are the most basic building blocks of nature which cannot be broken down by ordinary chemical means. Compounds are combinations of elements which can be broken down into their constituent parts by chemical reactions. Compounds are a form of two or more elements in definite proportions. A molecule of salt is made up of one atom of sodium (Na) and one atom of chlorine (Cl). The compound is called sodium chloride.

The elements in compounds are held together either by **ionic bonding** or by **covalent bonding.** In ionic bonding, the outer or valence electrons are donated by one element and accepted by another element of the compound. In convalent bonding, the valence electrons are shared by the elements in the compounds.

CHAPTER 2 QUESTIONS

1-3, Match

1. Isotope	A. Same A Different Z
2. Isobar	B. Same Z Different A
3. Isotone	C. Same (A+Z)
	D. Same (A-Z)

4. One AMU is equal to ________.
   A. Mass of Hydrogen Atom
   B. One kgm
   C. 1/12 mass of Carbon Atom
   D. 1/16 mass of Oxygen Atom

5-7, Match

5. Gravitational	A. Act only at short ranges.
6. Electrostatic	B. Are always attractive.
7. Nuclear Forces	C. Force the isotopes apart.
	D. Are attractive for unlike charges and repulsive for like charges.

8-11, A for True or B for False

8. Nuclei with higher Z have higher binding energies.

9. One AMU is equivalent to 931 MeV.

10. Nuclei with a mass defect are radioactive and unstable.

11. Removal of an orbital electron can produce characteristic x-rays or Auger electrons.

12. The total number of nucleons in an atom is equal to ___________.
    A. the number of electrons.
    B. the number of protons.
    C. the number of neutrons.
    D. the sum of the number of neutrons and protons.

13. An atom has orbital binding energies of 60, 35 and 15 KeV. The possible transitions are ______________.
    A. 15, 35, 60
    B. 20, 25, 45
    C. 15, 20, 35, 45, 60
    D. 15, 20, 25, 35, 45, 60

14–17, Match

14.	+2 charge, 4 AMU mass	A. electron
15.	0 charge, 1 AMU mass	B. neutron
16.	+1 charge, 1 AMU mass	C. proton
17.	-1 charge, 5 x 10^{-4} AMU mass	D. alpha particle

18–20, Match the pairs

18.	Isotopes	A. $^{99}_{43}Tc$ - $^{99m}_{43}Tc$
19.	Isobars	B. $^{12}_{6}C$ - $^{13}_{6}C$
20.	Isotones	C. $^{12}_{6}C$ - $^{13}_{7}N$
		D. $^{13}_{6}C$ - $^{13}_{7}N$

21. The L shell binding energy is __________ KeV if a 32.1 KeV M shell Auger electron is emitted from an L-K transition in an atom with a K shell binding energy of 40 KeV and an M shell binding energy of 0.9 KeV.

A. 7
B. 31.2
C. 33
D. 40.9

22. How many nucleons are in a molecule of carbon monoxide (CO) made up of $^{12}_{6}C$ and $^{16}_{8}O$?

A. 14
B. 28
C. 36
D. 42

23. How many protons in carbon monoxide?

A. 14
B. 28
C. 36
D. 42

24. How many neutrons in a water molecule H_2O?

A. 10
B. 8
C. 6
D. 4

25. The M Shell can hold ________ electrons.

A. 8
B. 12
C. 18
D. 24

26. Emission of an Auger electron is an alternative to

A. an isomeric transition.
B. a characteristic x-ray emission.
C. absorption of a photon.
D. emission of an alpha particle.

CHAPTER 3

ELECTRICITY AND MAGNETISM

Static Electricity

Static electricity deals with stationary electrical charges. Static electricity can be demonstrated by running a plastic comb through a cat's fur. The comb will become charged and it is possible to attract small pieces of paper to the comb. As soon as the tiny pieces of paper touch the comb, they fly away. The comb picks up electrons from the cat's fur and becomes negatively charged. The charges on the comb exert a force on the paper through an electric field. When the paper pieces touch the comb, they pick up some of the electrons from the comb and become charged. The fact that they fly away from the comb illustrates the first law of electrostatics.

Like charges repel; unlike charges attract

Figure 3.1 illustrates two charges separated by a distance r. The force between the charges is:

$$F = \frac{Q_1 Q_2}{r^2}$$

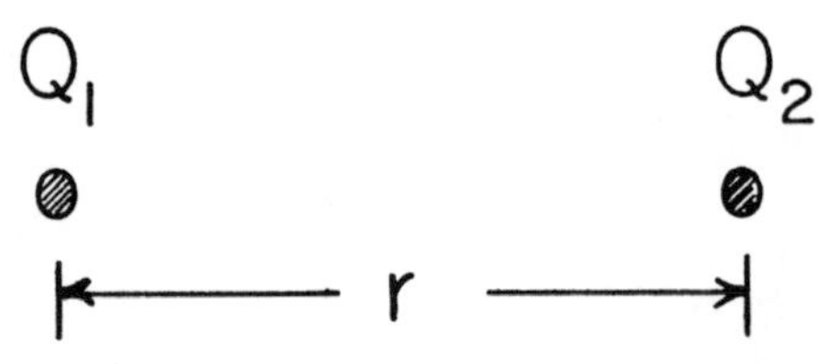

Figure 3.1. Two charges Q_1 and Q_2 separated by a distance r.

Electrostatic Charging

There are three ways to charge objects:

a. friction
b. contact
c. induction

The experiment with the comb and the pieces of paper demonstrated charging by friction and contact. When the comb passed through the cat's fur, friction removed some of the electrons from the fur and they stayed on the comb. The cat has a slightly positive charge and the comb is negatively charged. When the tiny pieces of paper contact the comb, they can pick up some of the charges from the comb and also become negatively charged.

Charging by induction makes use of the fact that different materials have different conductivities. Charging by induction is illustrated in Figure 3.2

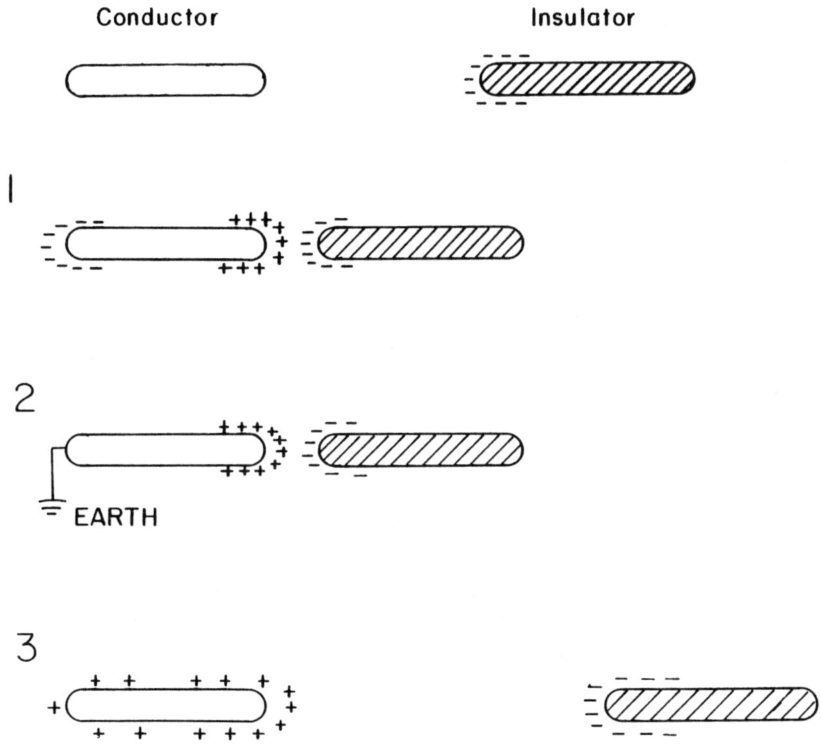

Figure 3.2. Steps in charging by induction.

A charged insulator is brought near to but not touching an uncharged conductor. The charges on the insulator attract opposite charges in the metal to the end closest to the insulator. The like charges in the conductor are repelled to the far end.

If the conductor is connected to ground or earth potential, all the like charges will be drained off. The opposite charges will be held in place by the attraction of the insulator charges. After disconnecting the earth connection, the conductor will remain charged even after the insulator is removed.

All metals are **conductors** which allow electrical charges (electrons) to move freely within them. **Insulators** hold the charge tightly where it is located and do not allow charges to move. Glass, wood, leather and most plastics are good insulators. Semiconductors are materials which are neither good insulators nor conductors.

MAGNETISM

Magnets have both a north and south pole and set up a magnetic field in their vicinity. Figure 3.3 illustrates some of the magnetic field lines near a pair of magnets.

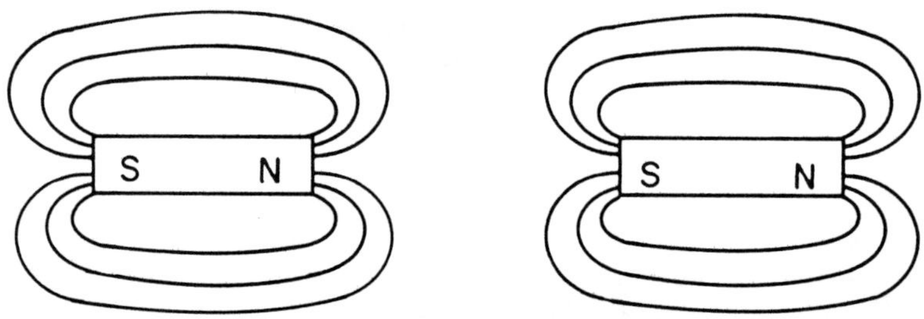

Figure 3.3. Field lines near a pair of permanent magnets

The first law of magnetism states that opposite poles attract, and like poles repel. there are three kinds of magnetic materials:

a. ferromagnetic material
b. paramagnetic material
c. nonmagnetic material

Ferromagnetic are strongly magnetic materials and can be magnetized to produce powerful magnets. Paramagnetic materials are weakly magnetic. Nonmagmetic materials such as wood, paper, plastic and glass experience no forces when placed in a magnetic field. Ferromagnetic materials have groups of atoms called **domains** which can be lined up within the material by placing the ferromagnetic material in an external magnetic field. These domains act like tiny magnets inside the material. A nonmagnetized bar of iron has its domains pointing in all directions. Placing a bar of iron in a magnetic field will line up some of the domains in the direction of the magnetic field. Heating or gently tapping the bar **while in the magnetic field** will align more of the domains and produce a stronger permanent magnet. Figure 3.4 illustrates how the magnetic domains are aligned to produce a permanent magnet.

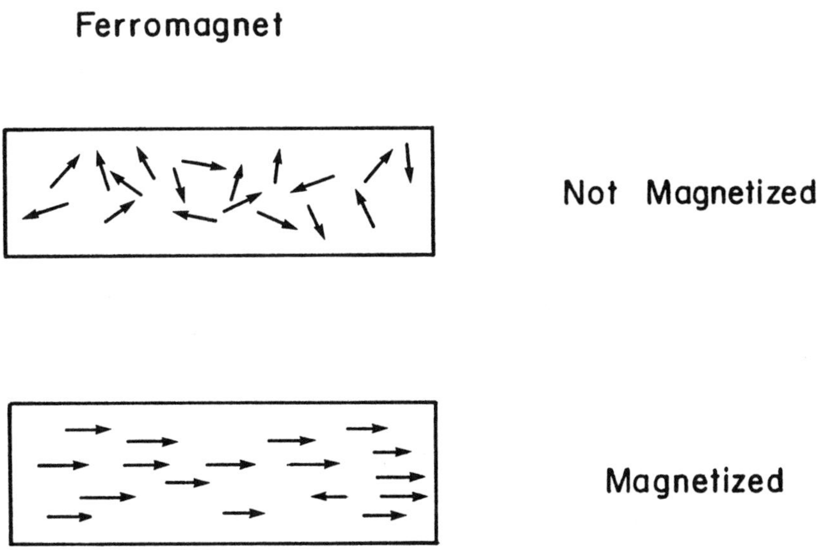

Figure 3.4. Magnetic domains can be aligned in a ferro magnet to produce a permanent magnet.

Simple Electrical Circuits

Figure 3.5 illustrates the simplest form of electric circuit which contains a voltage source, a load (lightbulb) and conductors connecting the source to the load. There are two types of sources available, 1) a battery which makes use of chemical energy to produce an electrical potential and 2) a generator which makes use of mechanical energy to produce an electrical potential. In Figure 3.5, the lightbulb presents a resistance to the flow of electric current and heats up when the current flows through the thin filament of the lightbulb.

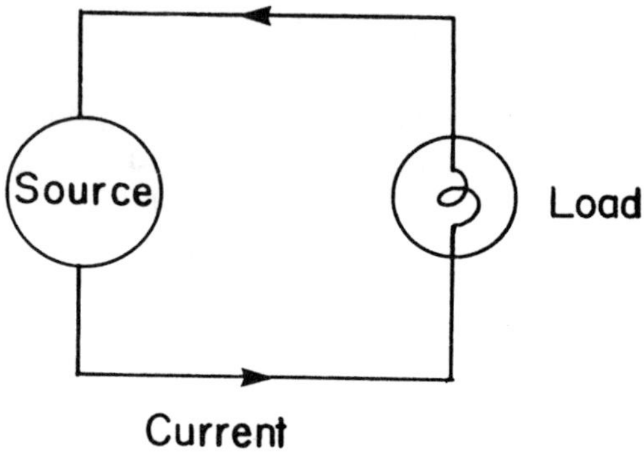

Figure 3.5. Simple electrical circuit containing source and load.

Direction of Current Flow

When Benjamin Franklin was working with batteries, he guessed that the current flow was from the anode (the positive terminal) to the cathode (the negative terminal) of the battery. He guessed wrong. We now know that in most conductors current flow is caused by electrons which move from the negative terminal to the positive terminal. By convention, all electrical circuits are drawn as if positive charges were moving in the wires from the positive to negative terminals.

There must be a continuous path for current to flow from the positive terminal of the source to the negative terminal to have a **complete circuit**. If there isn't a complete circuit or continuous path, the circuit is an **open circuit**.

Electrical current flow is analogous to water flow. Larger pumps, bigger batteries or bigger generators produce a greater pressure and a higher potential. Larger pipes with less resistance allow more flow, just as larger wires allow more current flow. Narrow pipes or valves in a water line restrict the flow as resistors restrict the current flow in electrical circuits.

Voltage

A volt is a measure of electrical potential or pressure and an ampere is a measure of electrical current flow. Ohm's Law:

$$V = I R \qquad 3.1$$

relates the voltage, the current, and the resistance in the circuit. The voltage is measured in volts – the current in amperes and the resistance in ohms.

Example 3.1:
If the 6v battery in Figure 3.4 is connected to a lightbulb with a resistance of 3 ohms, how much current flows in the circuit?

$$V = I R$$

$$6 = I \times 3$$

$$I = 6/3$$

$$I = 2 \text{ amperes}$$

Series and Parallel Circuits

Resistors can be connected together either in series or in parallel. Figure 3.6 illustrates resistors connected in series.

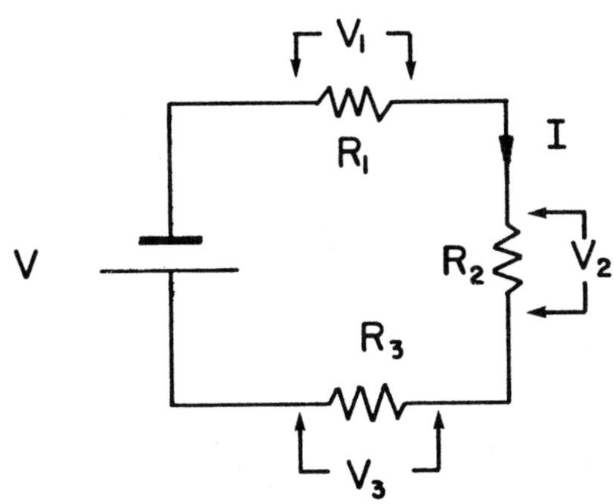

Figure 3.6. Simple series circuit showing the location of the voltage drops across the resistors.

Notice that the same current flows through all the resistors. Resistors in series can be added together to form an "equivalent resistance," R_{eq}.

$$R_{eq} = R_1 + R_2 + R_3 \qquad 3.2$$

The equivalent resistance could be substituted for all the other resistors with no resulting change in current or voltage.

Example 3.2:
If R_1 = 3 ohms, R_2 = 4 ohms, and R_3 = 5 ohms in Figure 3.6, what is the equivalent resistance, current flow and voltage drop across each resistor if the voltage source is a 24 volt battery?

$$\text{Equivalent Resistance} = 3 + 4 + 5 = 12$$

$$V = I\,R$$

$$24 = I \times 12\Omega$$

$$I = \frac{24}{12} = 2 \text{ amperes}$$

Voltage Drop Across R_1

$$V = I\,R$$

$$= 2 \times 3 = 6V$$

Voltage Drop Across R_2

$$V = I\,R$$

$$I = 2 \text{ amperes}$$

$$R = 4\,\Omega$$

$$V = 2 \times 4 = 8V$$

Voltage Drop Across R_3

$$V = I\,R$$

$$I = 2 \text{ amperes}$$

$$R = 5\,\Omega$$

$$V = 2 \times 5 = 10V$$

$$\text{Check } V_1 + V_2 + V_3 = 24V$$

$$6 + 8 + 10 = 24V$$

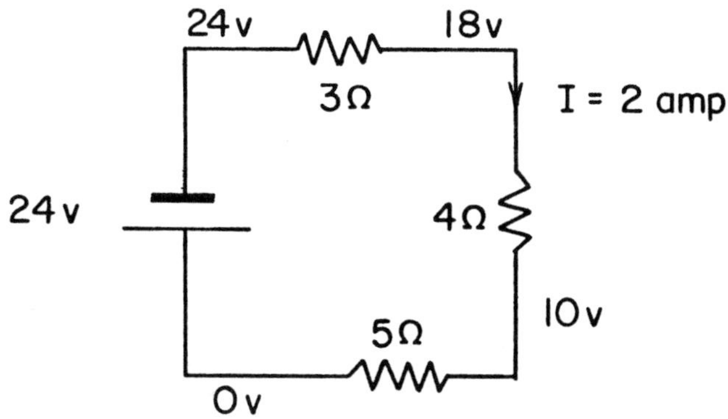

Figure 3.7. Series circuit showing current and voltage at various points around the circuit.

The voltage drop across the entire circuit is the sum of the voltage drops across the individual resistors .

Figure 3.7 illustrates the voltage at each point in the circuit and the voltage drop across each resistor. Between the battery and the 3 Ω resistor the voltage is 24v. The 2 amp current produces a 6v drop across the 3 Ω resistor. Thus the voltage between the 3 Ω and the 4 Ω resistor is

$$24 - 6 = 18 \text{ v}$$

The voltage between the 4 and 5 Ω resistors is 10v because there is an 8v drop across the 4 Ω resistor.

Parallel Circuits

Figure 3.8 illustrates resistors connected in parallel. The voltage across each resistor is the same. This means that the current through each resistor is different and is given by Ohm's law. The total current flowing through the circuit is given by the sum of the currents through each of the resistors.

The equivalent resistance R_{eq} of resistors in parallel is given by

$$\frac{1}{R_{eq}} = \frac{1}{R_1} + \frac{1}{R_2} + \frac{1}{R_3} \qquad 3.3$$

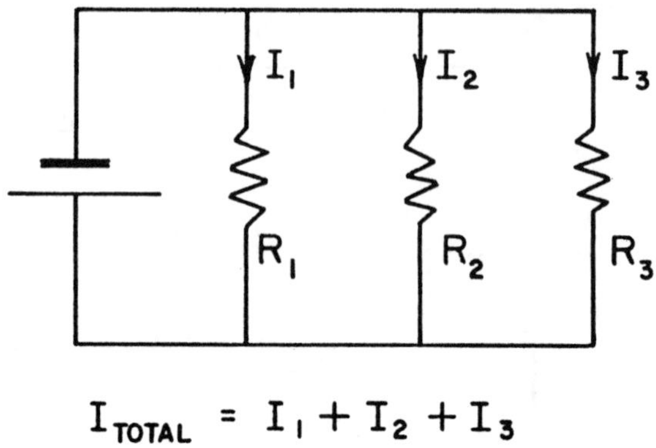

Figure 3.8. Electrical circuit with resistors in parallel.

Example 3.3:
What is the total current flowing through the parallel circuit of Figure 3.8 if R_1 equals 3 ohms, R_2 equals 4 ohms, and R_3 equals 5 ohms and the voltage source is a 24v battery?

1) Calculate the current through R_1

$$V = I R$$
$$24 = I \times 3$$
$$I = 8 \text{ amp}$$

2) Calculate the current through R_2

$$V = I R$$
$$24 = I \times 4$$
$$I = 6 \text{ amps}$$

3) Calculate the current through R_3

$$V = I R$$
$$24 = I \times 5$$
$$I = 4.8 \text{ amps}$$

Total Current = 8 + 6 + 4.8 = **18.8 amperes**

An alternate way to calculate the total current in a parallel circuit is to first calculate the equivalent resistance and then calculate the current using Ohm's Law.

1) Calculate the equivalent resistance R_{eq}

$$\frac{1}{R_{eq}} = \frac{1}{R_1} + \frac{1}{R_2} + \frac{1}{R_3}$$

$$\frac{1}{R_{eq}} = \frac{1}{3} + \frac{1}{4} + \frac{1}{5}$$

$$\frac{1}{R_{eq}} = \frac{20}{60} + \frac{15}{60} + \frac{12}{60}$$

$$\frac{1}{R_{eq}} = \frac{47}{60}$$

$$R_{eq} = \frac{60}{47}$$

$$R_{eq} = 1.276$$

What is the total current through the circuit?

$$V = I\,R$$

$$I = {}^{V}/_{R}$$

$$I = {}^{24}/_{1.276}$$

$$I = 18.8 \text{ amps}$$

The answer is the same in either case.

Some Christmas lights are connected in series and some in parallel. The entire string goes out if one of the series connected lights burns out. If a light burns out in a parallel string all the rest continue burning.

Measurement of Current Values

Ammeters are used to measure the current through a circuit and volt meters are used to measure voltages across a resistance.

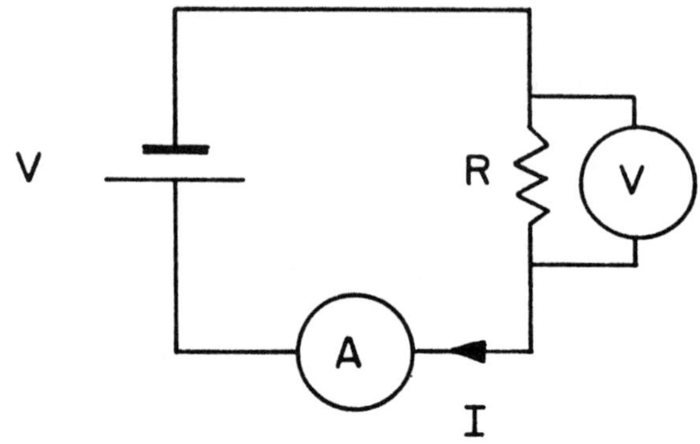

Figure 3.9. Simple circuit with ammeter A to measure current and voltmeter V to measure the voltage drop across R.

Figure 3.9 illustrates the application of both an ammeter (A) and a volt meter (V) in a circuit. Notice that the ammeter is always placed **in** the circuit and the volt meter is always placed **across** the resistor or load. All the current in the circuit flows through the ammeter and none (or practically none) flows through the volt meter.

Capacitor

The simplest form of a capacitor (sometimes called a condensor) is two conducting plates separated by a thin insulating layer as shown in Figure 3.10. If a charge is placed on one of the plates, an equal amount of opposite charge will be attracted to the other plate. If the capacitor is disconnected from the charging circuit, the charge will still remain on the plates, held by mutual attraction. Thus a capacitor can be used to store charge.

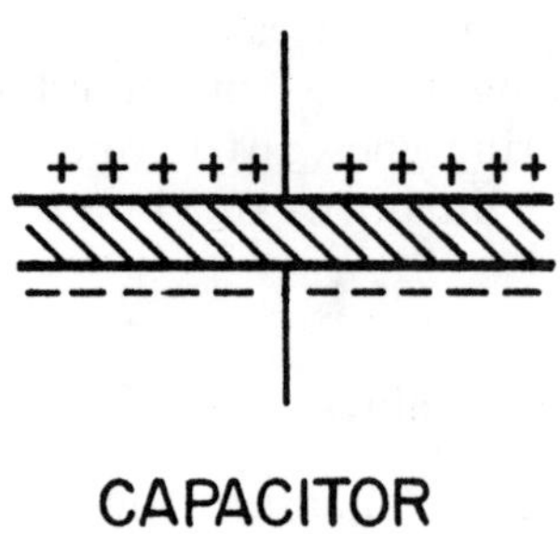

Figure 3.10. Schematic illustration of a capacitor.

Capacitors can be connected in series or in parallel. Capacitors in parallel all have the same voltage across them.

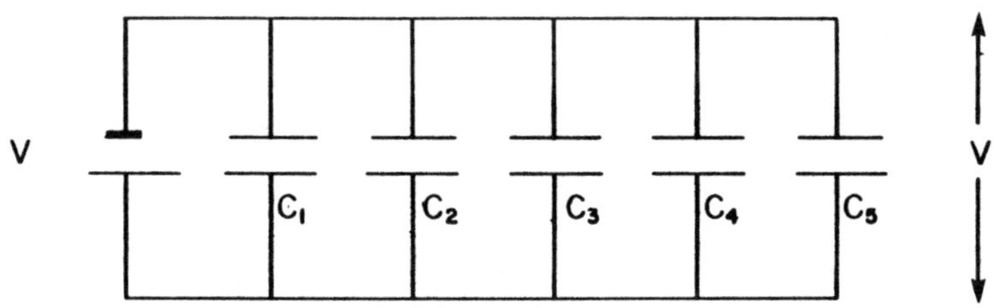

Figure 3.11. Capacitors in parallel. The voltage across each capacitor is the same.

The voltage across a group of capacitors connected in series is the sum of the individual voltages on the capacitors.

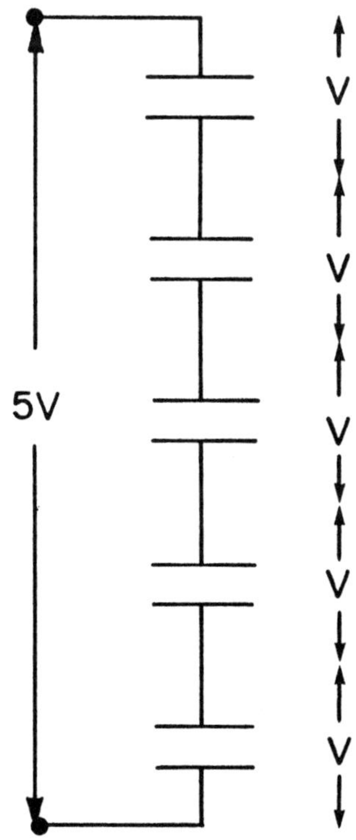

Figure 3.12. Capacitors connected in series. The voltage across the series is the sum of the individual voltages.

Power

Power is a measure of the rate of energy use or doing work. It is measured in watts (1 watt equals 1 joule per second). Volts x amperes also equals watts. Figure 3.13 illustrates a 120v source applied across a 40 watt load.

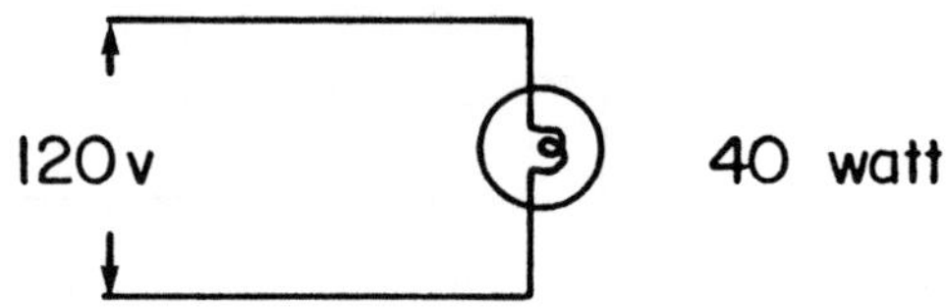

Figure 3.13. A 120v source applied across a 40 watt load.

Example 3.4:
What current flows through a 40 watt lightbulb which is in a 120 volt circuit?

$$\text{Power} = VI$$

$$40 = 120\,I$$

$$I = \frac{40}{120} = \frac{1}{3}\text{ amps}$$

CHAPTER 3 QUESTIONS

1. The force between two like charges
   A. is attractive and varies as $1/r$.
   B. is attractive and varies as $1/r^2$.
   C. is repulsive and varies as $1/r$.
   D. is repulsive and varies as $1/r^2$.

2. Which is NOT a way to charge objects?
   A. Friction
   B. Conduction
   C. Induction

3. A conductor
   A. is usually made of glass, plastic or wood.
   B. is usually a metal.
   C. allows electrons to move only in the dark.
   D. allows electrons to move only in the light.

4. Insulators
   A. hold charges so they cannot move easily.
   B. hold charges so they can move easily only in the dark.
   C. hold charges loosely so they can move easily.
   D. hold charges so they can move only in the light.

5. When charging by induction
   A. the object being charged must be an insulator.
   B. the two objects must be brought close enough to touch.
   C. the conductor will have a charge opposite that which was nearby.
   D. None of the above.

6. Magnetic domains

A. are found only in ferromagnets.
B. are responsible for paramagnetic materials.
C. are usually found in materials such as plastic, wood or glass.
D. are present only in magnetized material.

7. Heating a magnet while in an external magnetic field

A. will randomize the domains.
B. will reduce its paramagnetism.
C. will make it stronger.
D. will change its resonance frequency.

8. If the resistance in a circuit is increased with constant voltage

A. the resistance will decrease.
B. the voltage will increase.
C. the current will increase.
D. the current will decrease.

9. Ohm's Law is

A. $V = I/R$
B. $I = VR$
C. $I = V/R$
D. $R = VI$

10–15, A for series, B for parallel

10. The voltage across resistors in ________ is the same.

11. The current through resistors in ________ is the same.

12. The equivalent resistor for a group of resistors in ________ is the sum of the resistors.

13. If a string of Christmas tree lights continues to burn when one light burns out, the string is connected in ________.

14. The voltage across capacitors in __________ is the sum of the individual voltages.

15. When capacitors are connected in __________ the voltage across them is the same.

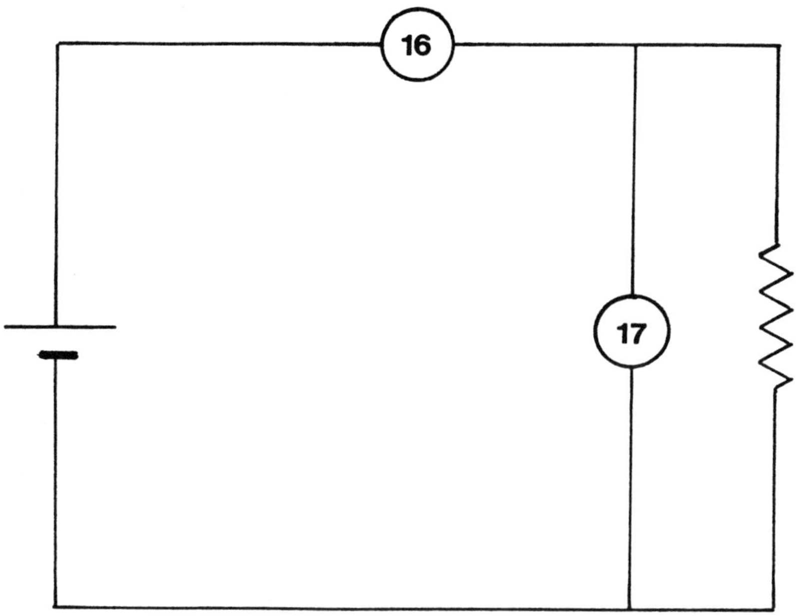

A. Ammeter
B. Voltmeter

16. Meter 16 is a __________.

17. Meter 17 is a __________.

18. A __________ can be used to store electrical charge.
A. Resistor
B. Ammeter
C. Voltmeter
D. Capacitor

Use for Problems 19–22

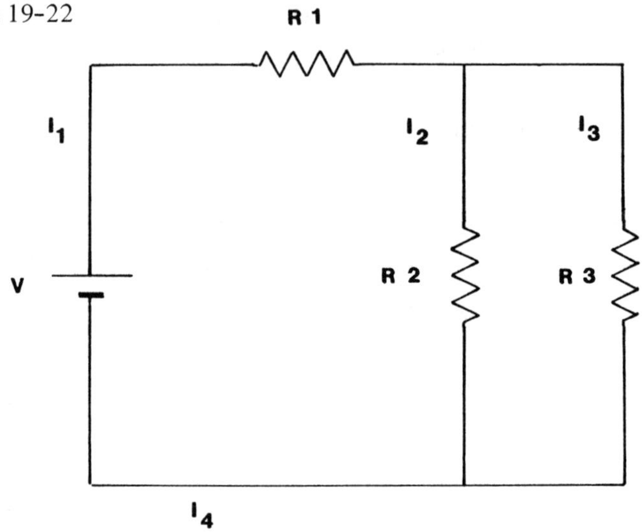

19. If V = 12 v and R_1 = 3 Ω, R_2 = 0, R_3 = 0, what is I_1?
    A. 9 amp
    B. 8 amp
    C. 4 amp
    D. 3 amp

20. If V = 12 v and R_1 = 3 Ω, R_2 = 0, R_3 = 0, what is I_4?
    A. 9 amp
    B. 8 amp
    C. 4 amp
    D. 3 amp

21. If V = 24 v and R_1 = 0, R_2 = 4 Ω and R_3 = 8 Ω, what is I_2?
    A. 9 amp
    B. 6 amp
    C. 4 amp
    D. 3 amp

22. If V = 24 v and R_1 = 0, R_2 = 4 Ω and R_3 = 8 Ω, what is I_3?
    A. 9 amp
    B. 8 amp
    C. 4 amp
    D. 3 amp

23. What is the power in a 3 Ω resistor with 5 amp flowing through it?

A. 15 watts
B. 25 watts
C. 45 watts
D. 75 watts

CHAPTER 4

ALTERNATING CURRENT AND ELECTRICAL CIRCUITS

Induced Currents

Electrical currents and magnetic fields are closely linked. When current flows in a conductor, a circular magnetic field is set up around the conductor. If a conductor moves in a magnetic field, the electrical charges in the conductor experience a force and a current can be induced in the moving conductor.

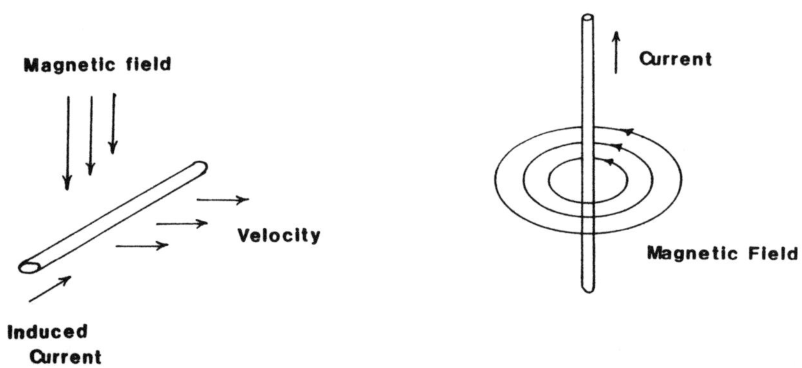

Figure 4.1. A conductor moving in a magnetic field B produces a current in the conductor. A current flowing in a conductor produces a magnetic field around the conductor.

A simple generator consists of a loop of wire rotating in a magnetic field. The current induced in the wire can be used to light a bulb, or operate a T.V. To increase the effect, the loop can be made of several coils of wire instead of only one turn. Figure 4.2 illustrates the operation of a simple generator.

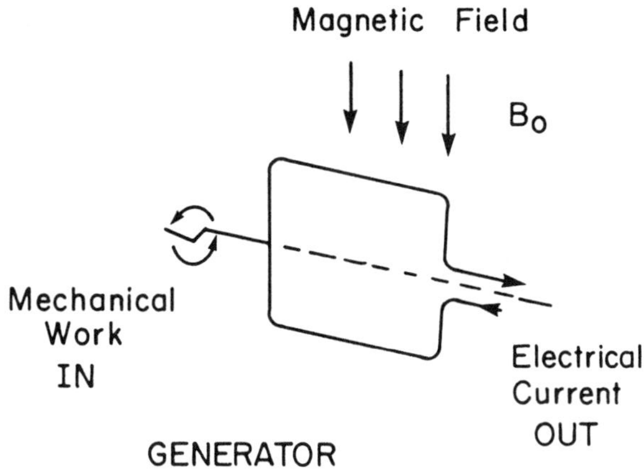

Figure 4.2. A conducting coil rotated in a magnetic field will produce a current. This is a generator.

A current-carrying-conductor in a magnetic field will experience a force and the conductor will move. This is how a motor works. A current-carrying loop of wire in a magnetic field will rotate and can do work. Figure 4.3 illustrates the operation of a simple motor.

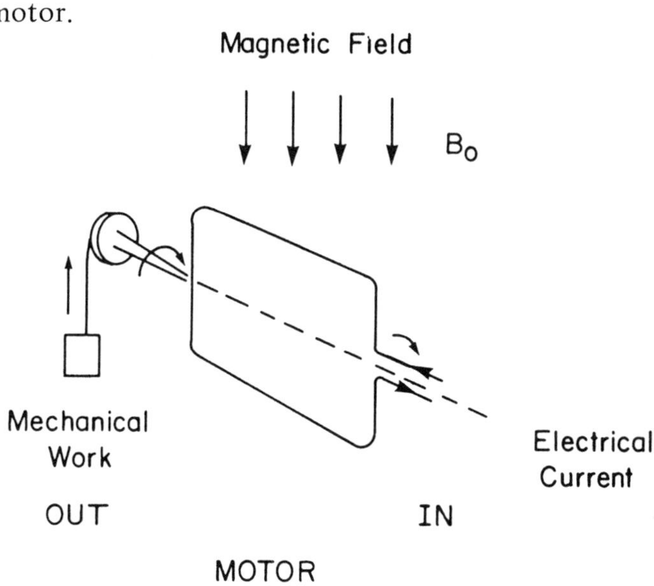

Figure 4.3. A current carrying coil in a magnetic field can do work. This is a motor.

The construction of a motor and generator can be identical. Mechanical energy is converted to electrical energy in a generator whereas electrical energy is converted to mechanical energy in a motor.

Alternating Current

When a conductor coil is rotated in a magnetic field, the induced current changes direction twice during each revolution. Figure 4.4 illustrates the resulting alternating current.

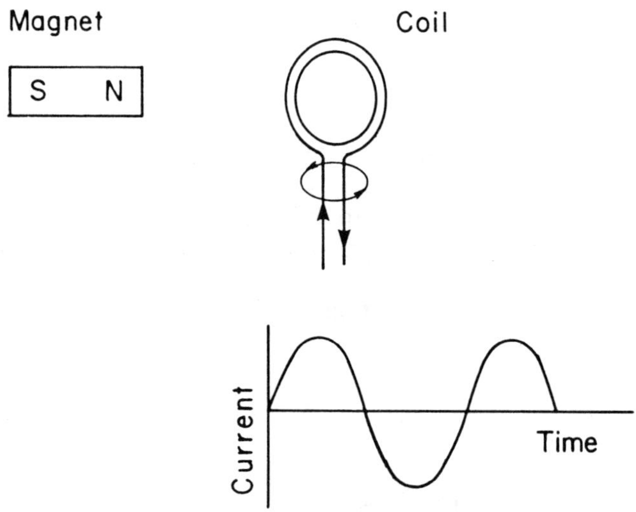

Figure 4.4 A conducting coil rotating in a magnetic field will produce AC current.

Efficiency

Efficiency is the work or power out of a device divided by the work or power into the device.

Example 4.1:
The electrical input to a motor is 1000 watts and the power output is 950 watts. What is the efficiency of this motor?

$$E = \frac{\text{Power Out}}{\text{Power In}} \quad 4.1$$

$$= \frac{950}{1000}$$

$$= 95\%$$

A stationary conductor in a stationary magnetic field has no current induced in the conductor. The magnetic field must be changing relative to the conductor.

In a practical motor, there are many turns of wire on the **armature** which rotates in the magnetic field which is provided by either permanent magnets or electromagnetic coils.

Transformers

All current-carrying wires set up a magnetic field around themselves. This field changes with the current. In an AC circuit the current (and associated magnetic field) drops to zero twice each cycle. An AC current in a coil of wire will set up or **induce** a current in a nearby coil.

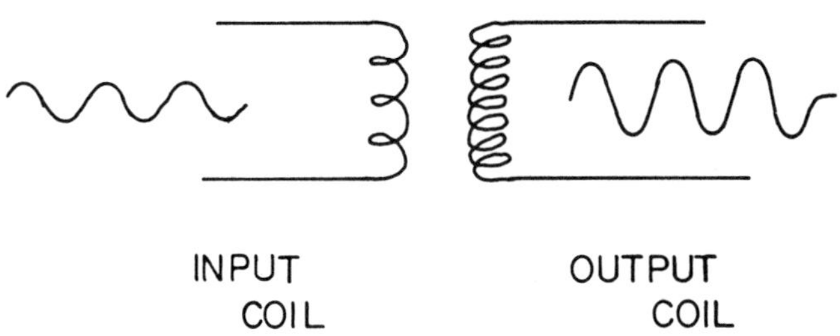

Figure 4.5. Input and output coils of a simple transformer.

This is the principle of a transformer.

Transformers usually have their coils linked and wound around an iron core to capture the magnetic field and concentrate it in the region of the coils. The induced voltage depends on the **turns ratio**:

$$N_s/N_p \quad 4.2$$

where N_s is the number of turns on the secondary and N_p is the number of turns on the primary. The transformer law:

$$V_s = \frac{N_s}{N_p} V_p \qquad 4.3$$

relates the secondary voltage V_s to the primary voltage, V_p, and the turns ratio N_s/N_p. The currents in the primary and secondary windings of a transformer are related by:

$$I_p N_p = I_s N_s \qquad 4.4$$

In a lossless transformer the **power in** (V_pI_p) equals the **power out** (V_sI_s).

Transformers can be either **step up** ($V_s > V_p$) or **step down** ($V_s < V_p$) depending on the application.

Rectifiers

Rectifiers are electronic devices which allow current to flow in only one direction. They are often called diodes because they have two electrical connections.

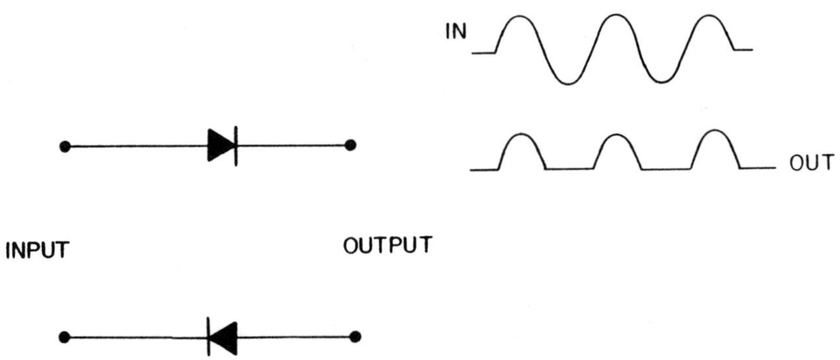

Figure 4.6. Halfwave rectifier circuit which changes AC input to DC output.

Figure 4.6 illustrates the action of a rectifier. Notice that only the positive portions of the voltage are allowed to pass through the rectifier.

For many circuits such as toasters and lightbulbs, it does not matter whether the current is flowing in one direction or the other. For other circuits such as battery chargers, television sets and x-ray machines, it is important that only positive voltage be applied to some parts of the circuit. Rectifiers are used to convert AC to DC current so that the polarity of the various portions of the circuit never changes.

A **halfwave rectified** circuit shown in Figure 4.6 is the simplest type of rectifier circuit but is also the most inefficient. Half the electrical energy is thrown away during every cycle.

By adding two additional diodes to a half wave rectified circuit, a full wave rectified circuit is produced. Figure 4.7 illustrates such a circuit.

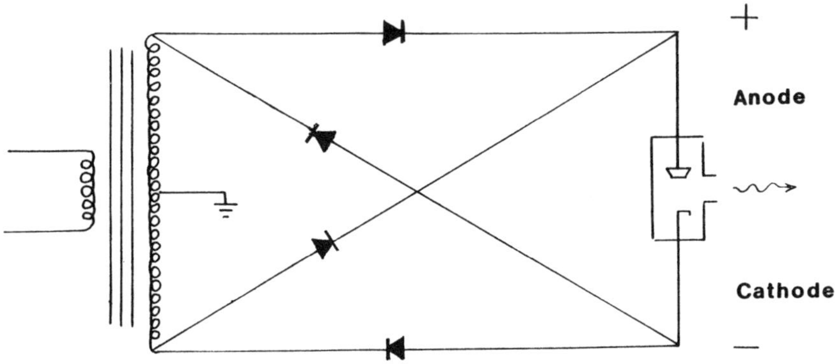

Figure 4.7. Full wave rectified x-ray circuit.

Notice that the positive side of the transformer is always connected to the anode of the x-ray tube and that the negative side of the transformer is always connected to the cathode of the x-ray tube. Figure 4.8 presents the same circuit drawn in the more conventional manner. This is known as a bridge rectifier circuit.

This arrangement of diodes is known as a "bridge circuit."

Three Phase AC

Three phase waves consist of a combination of three separate single phase waves which are 120° out of phase from each other. An example is shown in Figure 4.9.

The advantage of three phase circuits is that they permit motors and generators to operate much more efficiently and reduce the variation in the rectified DC voltage significantly and permit more efficient x-ray production.

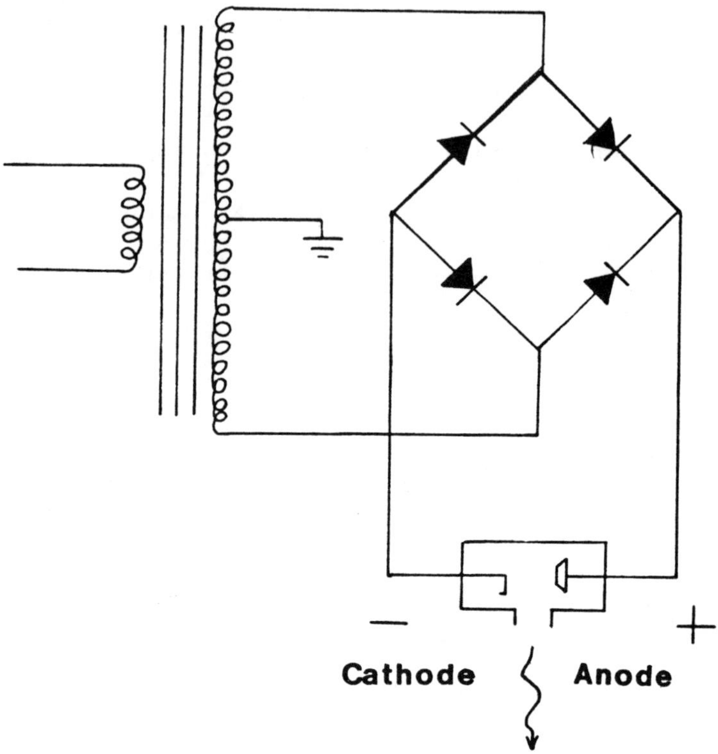

Figure 4.8. Full wave rectified bridge circuit.

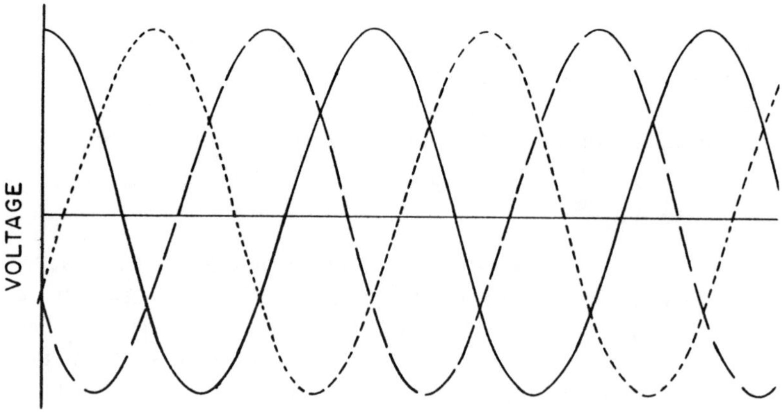

Figure 4.9. Three phase AC wave.

Three phase waves as illustrated in Figure 4.9 consist of three separate AC phases 120° apart. By connecting three separate bridge circuits to produce full wave rectified current from each of the three phases, we can obtain a six pulse three phase system. There are two ways to connect the three windings in the secondary of a three phase circuit. The two ways are called delta and wye. Figure 4.10 illustrates the delta and wye connection.

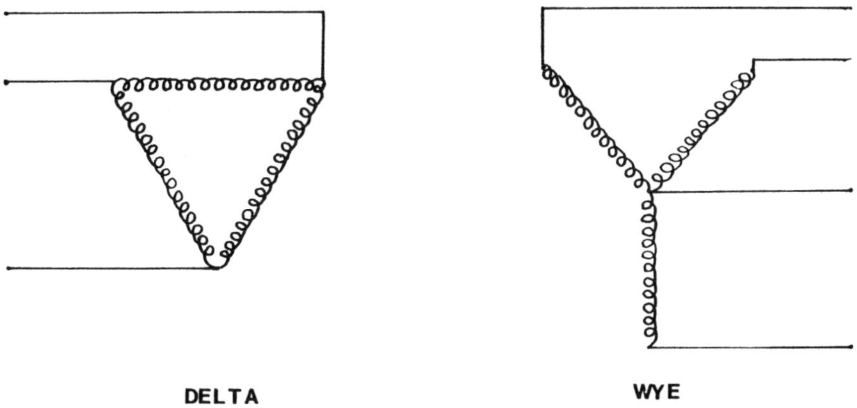

Figure 4.10. Three phase delta and wye connections.

The ratio of the turns between the primary and secondary still determines the output voltage. A schematic view of a full wave rectified three phase circuit is shown in Figure 4.11.

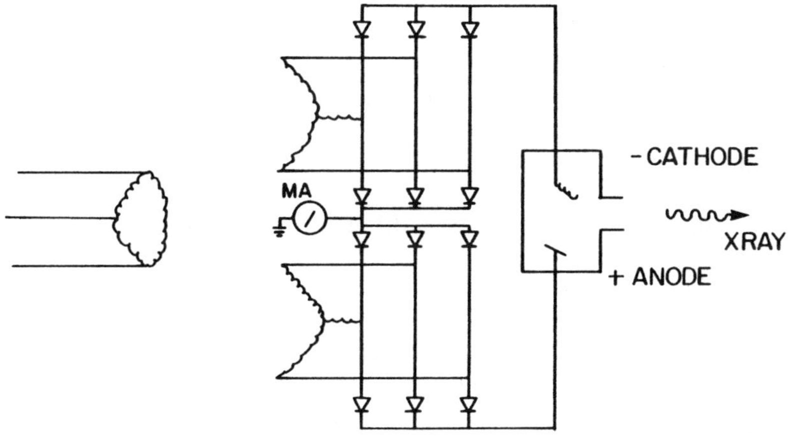

Figure 4.11. Three phase six pulse full wave rectified x-ray circuit.

The primary is connected in the delta configuration and the two secondary transformers are connected in the wye configuration. Two secondary transformers are used to provide center tap ground and to handle higher current loads. The circuits shown in Figure 4.11 would produce a three phase six pulse wave form shown in Figure 4.12.

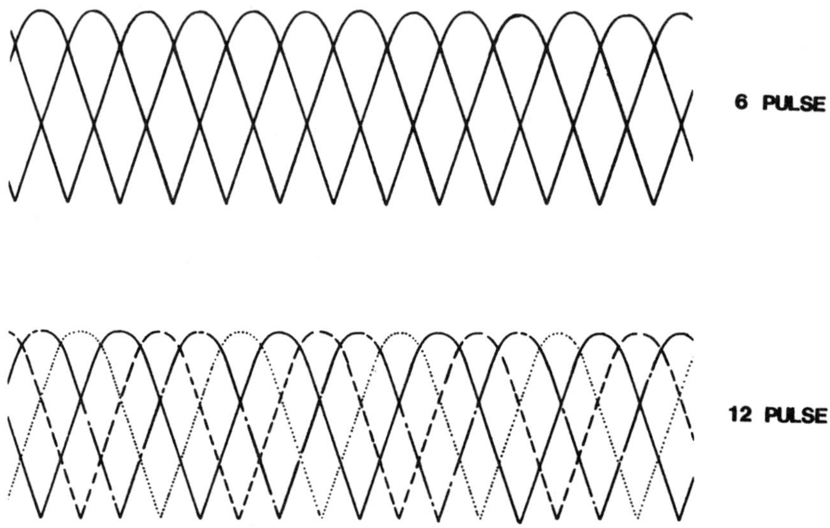

Figure 4.12. Three phase six pulse wave form and twelve pulse wave form.

If one of the wye transformers is replaced with a delta secondary transformer as shown in Figure 4.13, there will be a 30° shift between the delta and wye secondary output.

Ripple

Ripple is the change in voltage divided by the full applied voltage.

$$\text{Ripple} = \frac{\Delta V}{V} \qquad 4.5$$

Table 4.1 presents the percentage ripple for full wave rectified single phase, three phase and six pulse and three phase twelve pulse system.

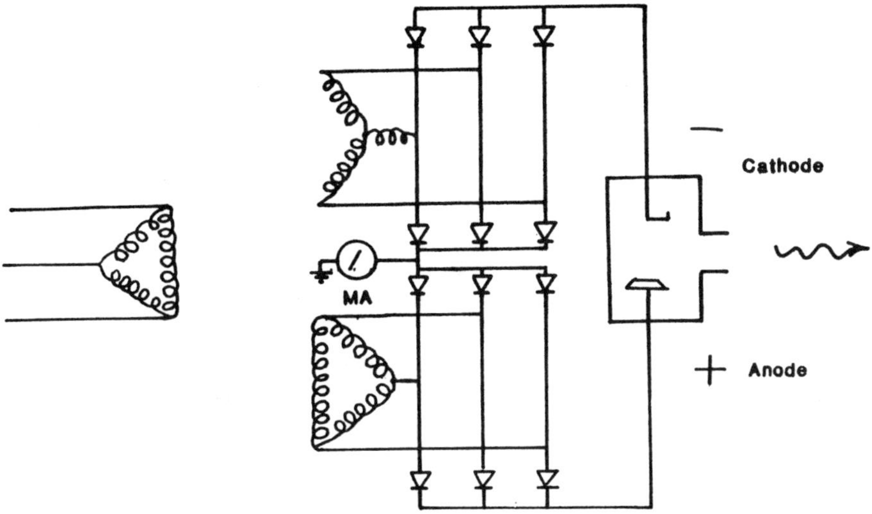

Figure 4.13. Three phase 12 pulse system. Note the delta - wye configuration of secondary circuit.

TABLE 4.1
PERCENTAGE RIPPLE

1 ϕ	Full wave	100%
3 ϕ	6 pulse	13%
3 ϕ	12 pulse	3%

CHAPTER 4 QUESTIONS

1. Which statement regarding conductors in a magnetic field is NOT correct?
   A. A moving conductor in a static magnetic field can generate a current.
   B. A stationary conductor in a static magnetic field can be used as a motor.
   C. A moving current carrying conductor in a static magnetic field can ge used as a motor.
   D. A current-carrying conductor in a moving magnetic field can be used as a motor.

2. Coils of wire are used in the armature of motors and generators
   A. to improve heat conduction.
   B. to improve cooling.
   C. to increase the effect of a single coil.
   D. to prevent generator-motor oversay.

3. A transformer has 300 input turns and 150,000 output turns. If the input voltage is 200 v, what is the output voltage?
   A. 10,000 v
   B. 30,000 v
   C. 60,000 v
   D. 100,000 v

4. A rectifier in an x-ray generator circuit
   A. prevents positive charge from reaching the anode.
   B. is used only in AC circuits.
   C. converts DC into AC.
   D. can be used with a step down transformer to reduce high voltage tension.

5. A current-carrying conductor
   A. is surrounded by a magnetic field.
   B. is surrounded by a primary transformer coil.
   C. is positive for only half the time.
   D. induces excess conductivity in a nearby coil.

6. A conductive coil rotating in a magnetic field
   A. can be either a motor or a generator.
   B. will generate a half wave rectified wave.
   C. will spin faster if the magnetic field is capacitor coupled to the coil.
   D. will continue to rotate as long as the magnetic field is present.

7. If the input to a motor is 500 watts and the output is 400 watts, the efficiency of the motor is
   A. 120%
   B. 50%
   C. 80%
   D. 40%

8. If the input to a motor is 800 watts and the output is 600 watts, the efficiency of the motor is
   A. 130%
   B. 80%
   C. 60%
   D. 75%

9. If the input to a transformer has 300 turns and the output has 150,000 turns, what is the turns ratio?
   A. 4.5×10^7
   B. 150300
   C. 500
   D. 2500

10. If the input to a transformer has 400 turns and the output has 160,000 turns, what is the turns ratio?
    A. 4.8×10^7
    B. 160400
    C. 6000
    D. 400

11. If the output current in a transformer with a turns ratio of 3000 is 300 mA, what is the input current?
    A. 90 amp
    B. 300 amp
    C. 600 amp
    D. 900 amp

12. A step down transformer
    A. has a secondary voltage less than the primary voltage.
    B. has a secondary current more than the primary current.
    C. has a turns ratio less than 1.
    D. All of the above.

13. A full wave rectifier requires at least ___________ rectifiers.
    A. 2
    B. 4
    C. 6
    D. 8

14. Three phase waves
    A. are made of three single phase waves differing in phase by 120°.
    B. are made of two single phase waves differing in phase by 120°.
    C. are made up of three single phase waves differing in phase by 180°.
    D. are made up of three single phase waves differing in phase by 360°.

CHAPTER 5

X-RAY GENERATORS

Figure 5.1 presents a schematic diagram of a typical x-ray circuit.

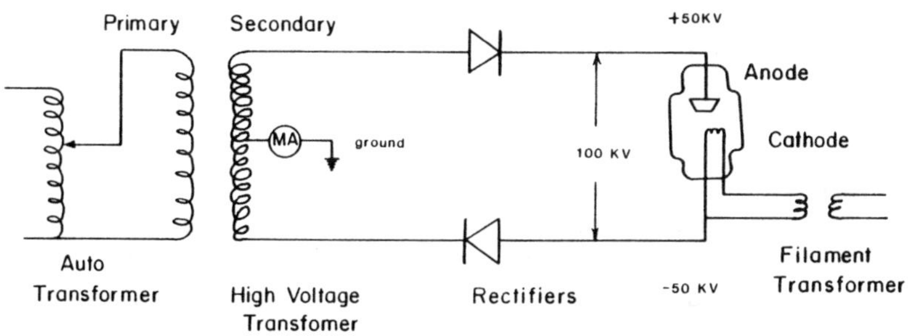

Figure 5.1. Schematic view of x-ray generator circuit. There is 100 kV applied across the x-ray tube. There is 10v applied across the filament which is at -50 kV potential. All voltages are measured relative to ground potential.

Auto Transformers

The auto transformer adjusts the input voltage to the primary windings of the high voltage transformer. The transformer secondary is connected with a center tap ground to the rectifiers which convert AC to DC voltages. Positive voltage is applied to the anode and negative voltage is applied to the cathode.

Figure 5.2 illustrates an auto transformer circuit used to change the primary voltage of the high voltage transformer.

High Voltage Transformer

The entire high voltage transformer is immersed in oil to provide both electrical insulation and cooling. All modern high voltage transformers have a center tap ground so that each end of

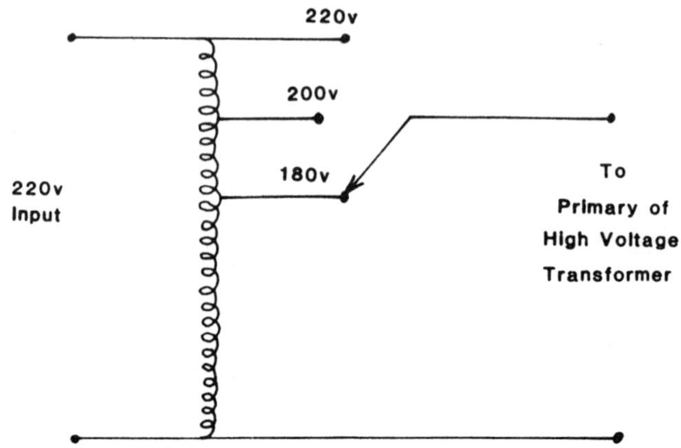

Figure 5.2. Autotransformer used to change the input voltage of high voltage transformer.

the transformer alternately reaches half the maximum voltage applied to the tube. Advantages of the center tap transformer include the fact that the current measuring (MA) meter can be placed at ground potential on the secondary side of the transformer and that the x-ray cables from the transformer to the x-ray tube need to withstand only half the voltage applied to the tube. As an example, if 150 kV is applied to the tube, the cables only have to withstand 75 kV.

Filament Transformer

The filament transformer provides the voltage across the filament (about 10v) as well as high voltage insulation. Figure 5.3 presents a schematic diagram of a typical filament transformer. The cathode contains the filament and is part of both the filament circuit and the high voltage circuit. The filament circuit applies 10v across the filament but is at large (40–75 kV) negative potential below ground potential. The filament transformer is a step down transformer which provides electrical insulation from the high voltage on the cathode.

Typical filament currents are 2–10 **amperes** (not milliamperes). Small changes in filament current or voltage will change the filament temperature and the number of electrons boiled off the cathode. This is how the tube current (MA) is adjusted. An

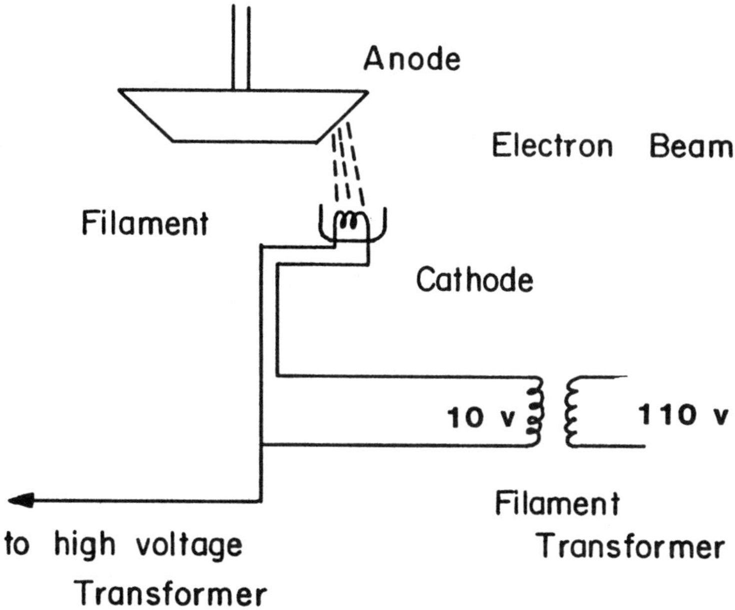

Figure 5.3. Filament transformer used to isolate the filament and step down the input voltage.

auto transformer is used to select different input values to the filament transformer. The steps of the filament auto transformer are marked in MA.

Rectifiers

The rectifiers pass current in only one direction. They are used to convert AC to DC. The rectifier symbols point in the direction of positive or conventional current flow. The rectifiers must be able to withstand the negative voltage trying to force current backwards.

Advantages and Disadvantages of Three Phase Circuits

In addition to having lower ripple, three phase (6 pulse) circuits have **higher** average voltage and current values than single phase (2 pulse) circuits. X-ray production is more efficient at higher voltages and so the higher average voltage of a three phase circuit yields more x-rays per MAS.

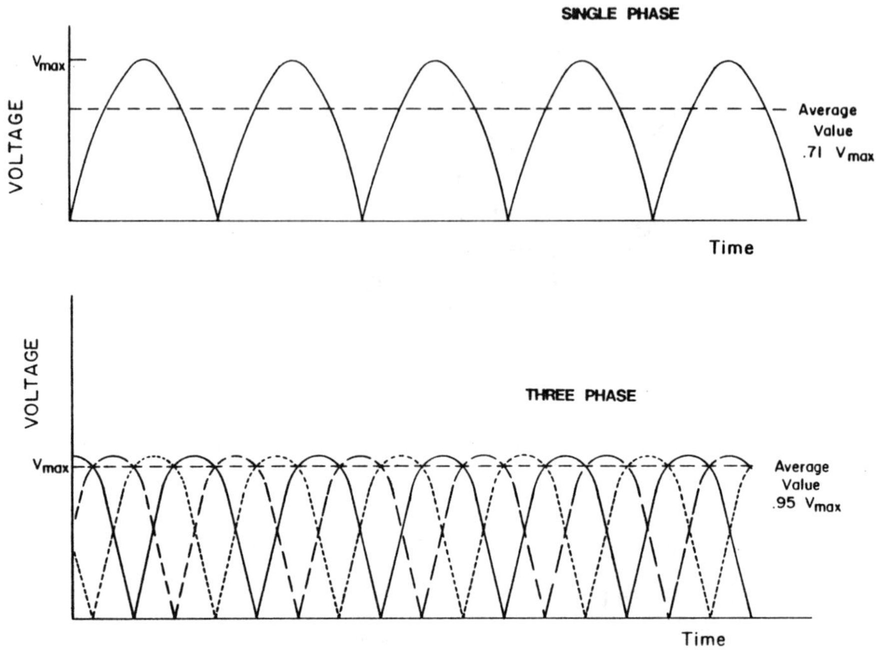

Figure 5.4. Average and maximum voltages for single and three phase wave forms.

The major disadvantages of three phase circuits is that they are more complex and hence are more expensive and more difficult to maintain.

Replacement of Single Phase by Three Phase Units

When a single phase unit is replaced by a three phase unit of the same peak kV, the average value of the maximum current and voltage will increase. Conversely, for the same average current, the peak current and voltage will decrease. Figure 5.5 illustrates how replacement of a single phase unit with a three phase unit results in a decreased tube current.

Generator Ratings

Generators are rated in terms of the amount of power they can supply measured in kilowatts (KW). By convention generators are rated by the MA supplied at a setting of 100 kV at 1/10 s.

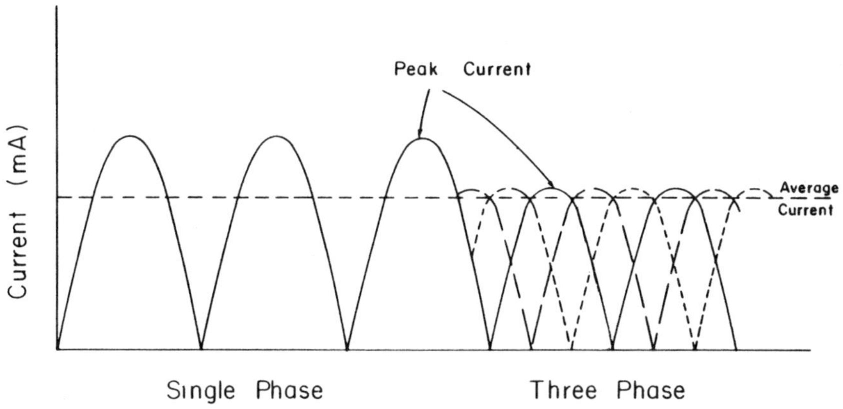

Figure 5.5. Comparison of peak current with single (two pulse) and three phase (six pulse) wave forms which yield the same average current.

Example 5.1:
What is the KW rating of a generator which can supply 300 MA at 100 kV and 1/10 s?

$$100 \text{ kV} \times 300 \text{ MA} = 30{,}000 \text{ watts}$$

This generator is rated at 30 KW.

Timing X-ray Exposures

Present day timing circuits use either silicon controlled rectifiers (SCRs) which can be turned on and off with electrical signals or thyraton gas filled switching tubes to terminate x-ray exposures.

Automatic Exposure Terminators - Phototimers

A phototimer is designed to measure the amount of radiation passing through the patient and striking the film screen cassette. For a particular film screen cassette combination, the phototimer detectors are adjusted to terminate the x-ray exposure when enough x-rays have passed through the patient to produce an acceptable radiograph.

Phototimer detectors are either scintillators which give off light when struck by x-rays or ion chambers which collect the

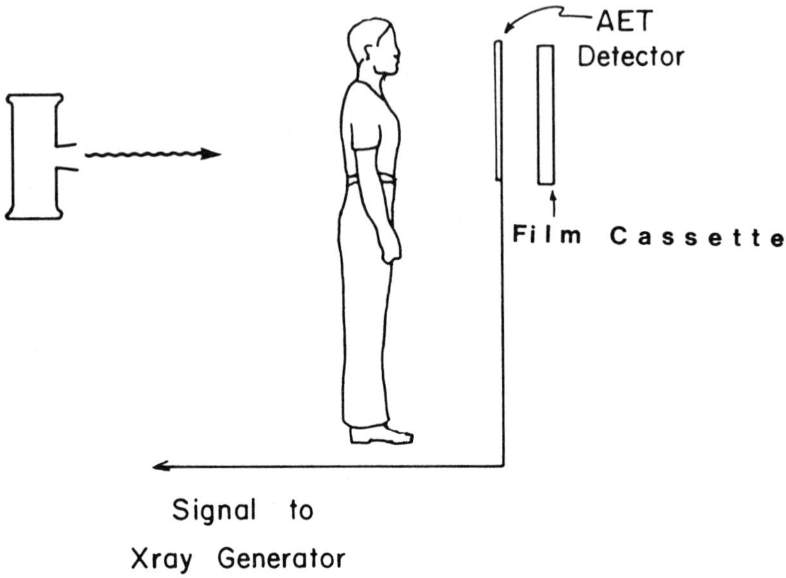

Figure 5.6. Automatic exposure termination circuits sense the radiation reaching the detector to terminate x-ray exposure when proper density is reached.

x–ray produced ionization. Phototimer generators have a density control to allow adjustment of the final film density.

Phototimer circuits are equipped with a safety circuit designed to cut off the exposure if the patient is too large or the phototiming circuit fails. Usually the circuit is set to terminate the exposure at 500 MAS.

Space Charge Compensation Circuits

As the filament is heated up, electrons are given enough thermal energy to leave the filament. If there is no voltage applied across the cathode–anode gap, no electrons will be attracted to the anode and a cloud of electrons will form near the filament. As the anode–cathode voltage is increased, more and more electrons will be attracted to the anode until eventually all electrons leaving the filament are attracted to the anode.

When the anode–cathode high voltage is increased, electrons near the surface of the filament can gain enough energy to leave the filament and strike the anode. This means that the tube current (MA) changes when the kVp is changed but the filament current is unchanged. This is undesirable because the kVp and MA should be controlled independently.

To counteract this **space charge** effect, a **space charge compensation** circuit is added to the filament circuit. The compensation circuit adds a small resistance to the filament circuit as the kVp is increased. The higher resistance results in a lower filament temperature which decreases the number of electrons boiled off the filament and compensates for the increased electron emission due to the high voltage increase.

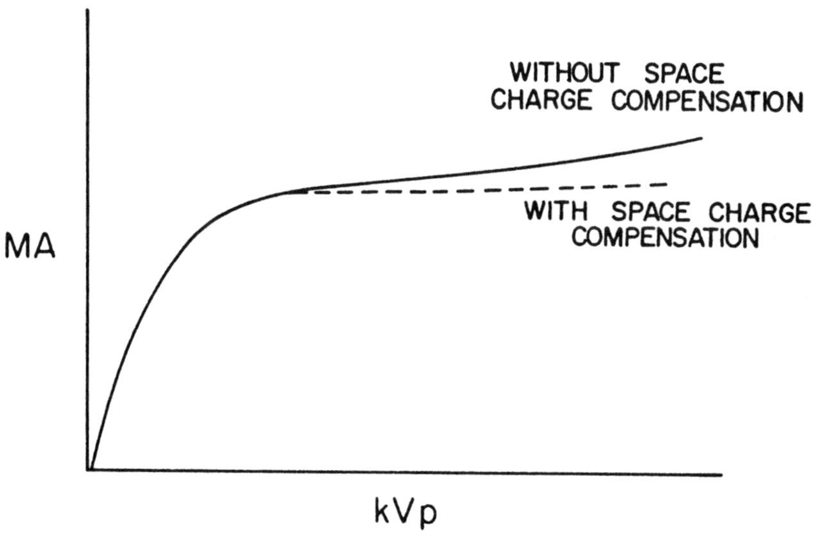

Figure 5.7. Variation of tube current (MA) as a function of applied kVp with and without a space charge compensation circuit.

Figure 5.7 illustrates the variation of tube current with applied kVp for circuits with and without space charge compensation.

Capacitive Discharge Units

Capacitive discharge units charge capacitors in parallel at relatively low voltages (2500v) and then connect the capacitors in series to place a high voltage across the x-ray tube. The advantage of capacitive discharge units is that they do not require elaborate

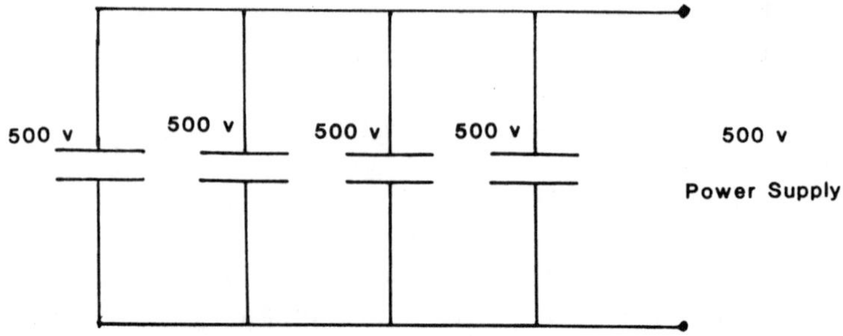

Figure 5.8. Capacitive discharge generator connected for charging.

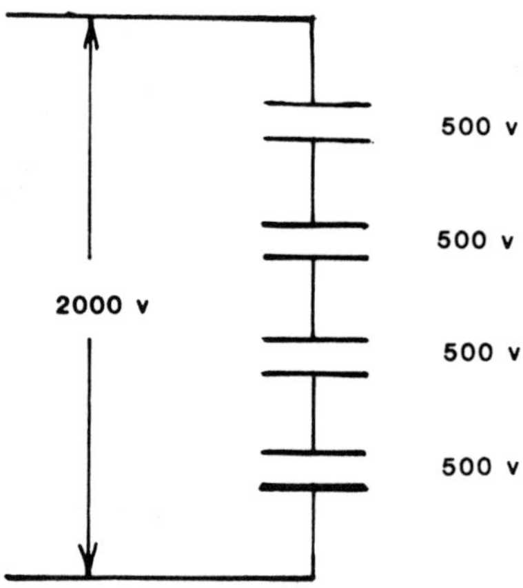

Figure 5.9. Capacitive discharge generator connected for x-ray exposure.

and heavy high voltage transformers so they can be made relatively light and portable. The disadvantage is that they require a significant, $\underset{\sim}{\sim}$ 30–75 sec., charging time before a second exposure can be made.

CHAPTER 5 QUESTIONS

1. The autotransformer in an x-ray generator
   - A. reduces ripple.
   - B. adjusts the input voltage of the high voltage transformer.
   - C. adjusts the output windings number in the high voltage transformer.
   - D. allows the MA meter to be placed at ground potential.

2. The rectifiers in an x-ray generator circuit
   - A. maintain constant current in the secondary windings of the HV transformer.
   - B. maintain constant voltage in the secondary windings of the HV transformer.
   - C. maintain constant current direction in the secondary windings of the HV transformer.
   - D. maintain constant current elevation in the primary windings of the HV transformer.

3-7, A for True, B for False

The filament transformer:

3. applies about 10 kV across the filament.
4. must provide insulation to withstand 50-75 kV.
5. is a step up transformer.
6. controls the anode cathode-voltage.
7. supplies 2-10 amperes to the filament.

8. High voltage transformers are immersed in oil
   1. to provide lubrication.
   2. to provide cooling.
   3. to provide negative conduction ground.
   4. to provide insulation.
   5. to provide three phase wave forms.

   A. 1 and 2
   B. 1 and 3
   C. 1 and 4
   D. 2 and 4

9. A center tap ground on the secondary of a high voltage transformer
   1. places the kVp meter at ground potential.
   2. places the MA meter at ground potential.
   3. allows for better cooling of the transformer.
   4. reduces the current carried in the HV cables.
   5. reduces the voltage applied to the HV cables.

   A. 2 and 5
   B. 2 and 4
   C. 2, 3 and 4
   D. 1, 3 and 5

10–14, A = increase, B = decrease

10. Ripple increases/decreases when a three phase generator is replaced by a single phase generator.

11. Ripple increases/decreases when a six pulse generator replaces a 12 pulse generator.

12. Ripple increases/decreases when a half wave rectified generator is replaced by a three phase generator.

13. For the same average current the peak current increases/decreases when a single phase generator is replaced by a 3 phase generator.

14. For the same average current the peak current increases/decreases when a 12 pulse generator replaces a 6 pulse generator.

15. The rating of a generator whose maximum MA is 450 MA at 100 kVp and 250 MA and 150 kVp is:

A. 67.5 kW
B. 112.5 kW
C. 45 kW
D. 37.5 kW

16. X-ray phototimers:

1. may use an ionization chamber to monitor film density.
2. terminate the exposure when sufficient x-rays have reached the detector.
3. use either a photodetector or an ionization chamber to monitor x-ray exposure.
4. must have a backup timer to limit exposure.

A. 1 and 2
B. 1, 2 and 3
C. 2, 3 and 4
D. 1, 2, 3 and 4

17. A space charge compensation circuit

A. reduces the kVp to compensate for changes in MA.
B. adjusts the tube current to compensate for changes in the filament current produced by kVp changes.
C. adjusts the filament current to compensate for MA changes produced by kVp changes.
D. adjusts the filament current to compensate for kVp changes produced by MA changes.

18. A capacitive discharge unit

A. can be used as a portable unit.
B. charges capacitors in parallel and discharges them in series.
C. requires 30–60 sec. to recharge the capacitors.
D. All of the above.

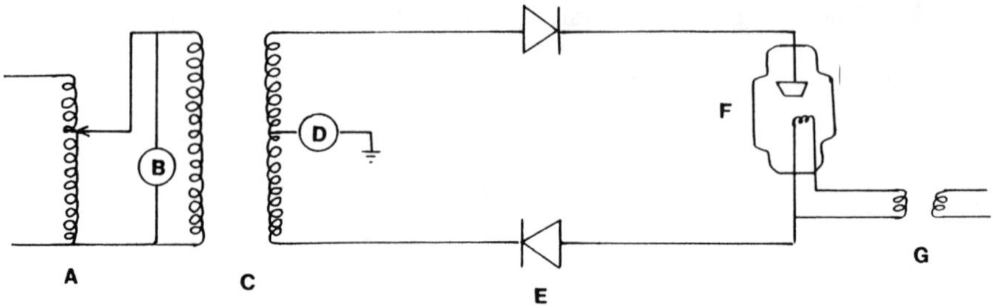

Identify the Components of the X-ray Circuit

19. X-ray Tube
20. High Voltage Transformer
21. Milliamp Meter
22. KVP Meter
23. Rectifier
24. Autotransformer
25. Filament Transformer

CHAPTER 6

X-RAY TUBES

X-ray Tube Design

Figure 6.1 is a photograph of a rotating anode x-ray tube. The anode and cathode assemblies are contained in an evacuated glass tube. The vacuum is necessary to allow the electrons free travel from the negative cathode to the positive anode without absorption of scattering and to withstand the high voltage applied between the cathode and anode.

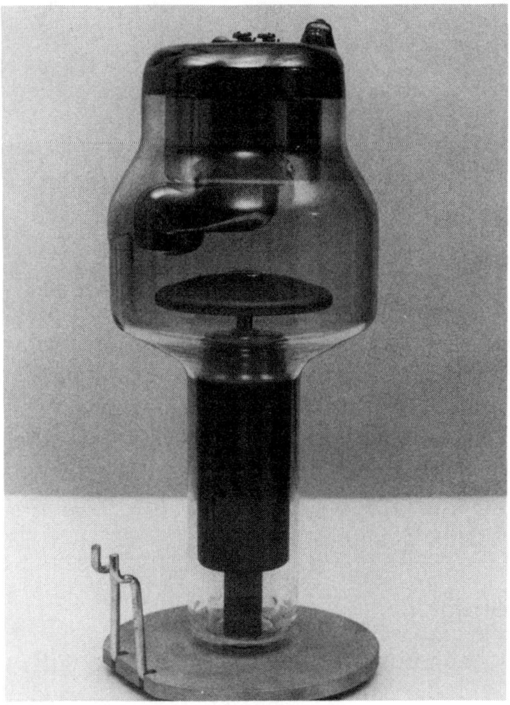

Figure 6.1. Rotating anode x-ray tube.

Electrons are boiled off a heated filament in the cathode and accelerated to the anode. When they strike the anode some of them produce x-rays.

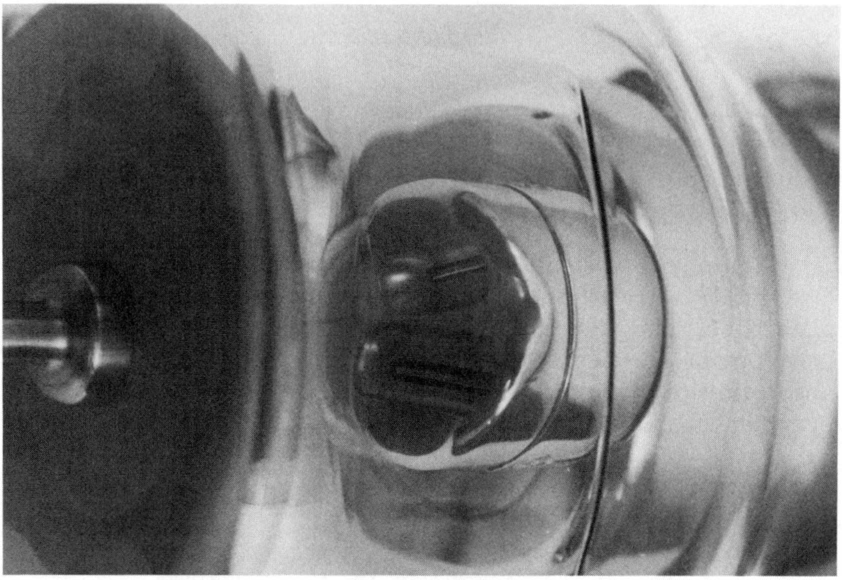

Figure 6.2. Cathode of modern x-ray tube showing dual filaments and focusing cup.

Cathode Assembly

Figure 6.2 illustrates a dual filament cathode assembly. The cathode consists of a metal cup containing two filaments. The different sized filaments produce different sized focal spots on the anode. The filaments are located at the bottom of a cup-shaped depression to focus the negatively charged electron beam on the positive anode focal spot. Without the focusing action of the cathode the mutual repulsion of the electrons would spread out the beam, resulting in an unacceptably large focal spot.

Focal Spot Blooming

The apparent increase in focal spot size with large tube currents is called focal spot blooming. It is caused by the mutual repulsion of the negative electrons. At high tube currents this repulsion counteracts the focusing effect of the cathode cup and spreads the electrons onto a larger area of the anode.

Electrons are boiled off when the tungsten (M.P. 3380°C) filament is heated to almost 3000°C. This process is known as **thermionic emission.** The tungsten is coated with thorium oxide to increase the number of electrons boiled off. The tube current is controlled by the temperature of the filament which depends on the current through the filament. The filament autotransformer is connected to the control panel push buttons to allow selection of desired tube current (MA).

There are two currents in an x-ray tube, the **filament current** which controls the temperature of the filament and the **tube current** which strikes the anode and produces x-rays. Filament currents are usually 2–10 **amperes.** The temperature of the filament controls the number of electrons boiled off the filament and attracted to the anode. These electrons make up the **tube current.** Tube currents are usually 50–500 **milliamperes.**

In normal operation, the filament transformer supplies a standby current of a few amperes to the filament. This is sufficient to keep the filament and cathode assembly warm but not hot. Just before the exposure, there is a slight (1 sec.) delay while anode rotation begins and a **filament boost voltage** is applied to bring the filament up to operating temperature. High voltage is then applied to the tube and x-ray emission begins. Holding the tube in the boost condition will significantly shorten its life because most filament evaporation occurs at the higher temperature.

Grid Controlled Tubes

In some tubes, the focusing cathode cup is insulated from the rest of the cathode. A negative voltage can be applied to this cup to prevent any electrons from leaving the cathode while the voltage is present. This voltage on the cup is called a grid voltage and can either turn the tube current on or off in a short time. The advantage of grid controlled tubes is their ability to form the short x-ray pulses needed in angiography and cineradiography.

Anode Design

Some mammographic and portable units have stationary anodes but most modern x-ray units employ rotating anode tubes.

Anode material selection, the line focus principle and the heel effect are the same for both stationary and rotating anodes.

Anode Material

X-ray production increases with increasing atomic number (Z). For this reason high Z materials are chosen for anode targets. Most of the electron energy is converted into heat in the anode, so anode materials must also have a high melting point. A layer of tungsten (Z=74, MP=3380°C) or molybdenum (Z= 42, MP= 2600°C) is usually bonded onto a base of copper (z=29, MP= 1083°C) to provide a high Z, high melting point target combined with a high conductivity substrate to distribute the heat.

Line Focus Principle

In order to spread the heat over a larger area, the target is inclined an angle θ to the x-ray beam. This is known as the line focus principle.

Figure 6.3 illustrates how the inclination of the anode surface spreads the heat over a larger area while maintaining a smaller apparent focal spot size. The electron beam from the cathode, and the heat is spread out from a to b, but the effective focal spot

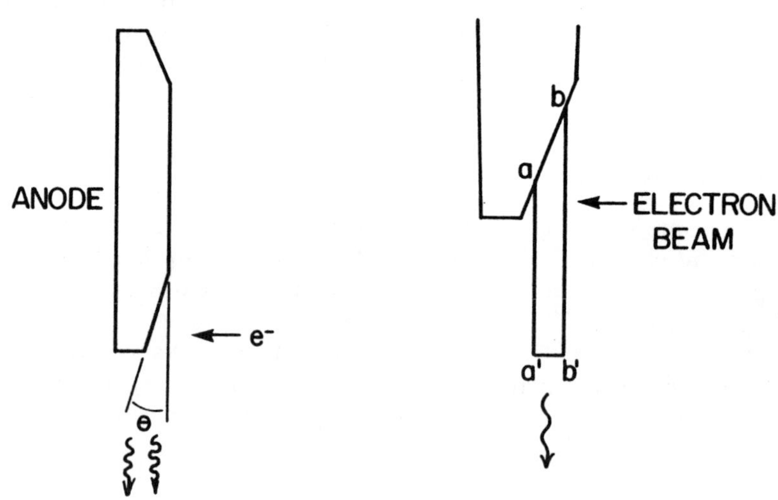

Figure 6.3. The line focus principle spreads the heat over a larger focal spot which appears smaller than actual size at the patient.

appears to extend only from a' to b'. As the target angle decreases, the heat capacity of the focal spot increases.

Table 6.1 presents the increase in area (actual/apparent focal spot size) for different target angles.

TABLE 6.1
CHANGE IN TARGET AREA WITH CHANGING TARGET ANGLES

Target Angle	*Relative Area*
7°	8.2
12°	4.8
17°	3.4

Focal spot sizes are always expressed in terms of the effective focal spot size.

The effective focal spot is given by:

$$\text{Effective area} = \text{Actual Area} \times \sin\theta \qquad 6.1$$

The anode angle θ is the angle between the anode surface and the x–ray beam direction. Smaller anode angles spread the heat over larger areas and result in larger heat capacities for the same **effective** focal spot. It is not possible to increase the heat capacity of the focal spot indefinately by making the anode target angle even smaller because the heel effect limits the useful size of the x–ray field.

Heel Effect

The **heel effect** produces a variation in intensity across the x–ray field.

The heel effect is caused by the fact that all of the x–rays are not produced on the surface of the anode. Some are produced by electrons which penetrate into the anode. X–rays produced inside the anode suffer different amounts of attenuation in leaving the anode depending on the angle of emission. Figure 6.4 illustrates how x–rays emitted toward the anode end of the tube are attenuated more than those emitted toward the cathode end of the tube.

Figure 6.5 presents a typical variation in intensity across the x–ray beam from anode to cathode side.

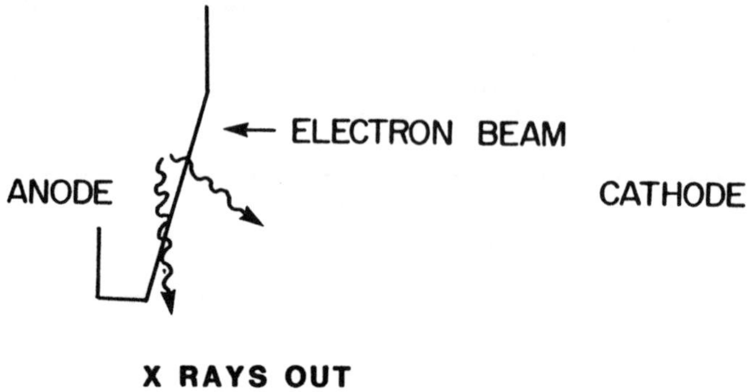

Figure 6.4. The heel effect attenuates x-rays emitted toward the anode end more than those emitted toward the cathode.

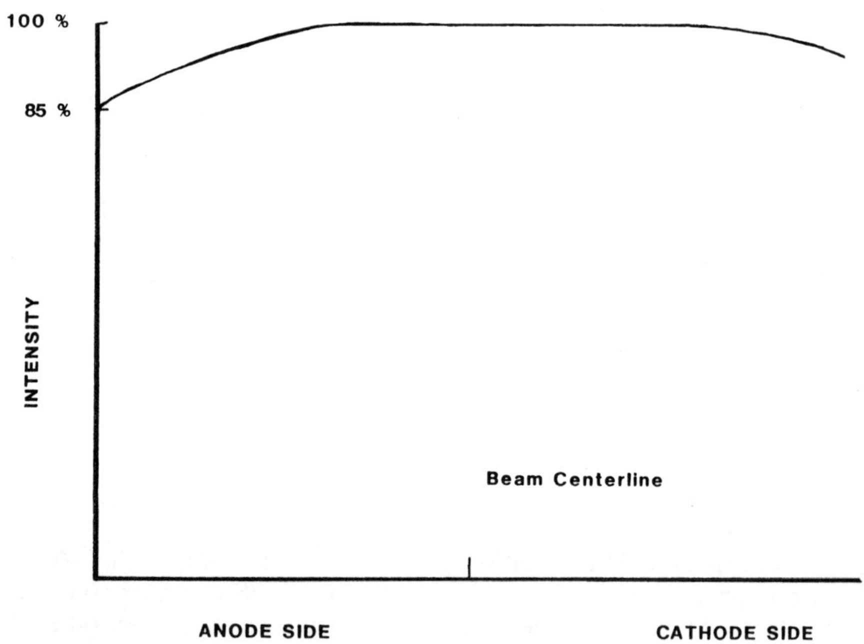

Figure 6.5. Intensity variation of x-rays across x-ray field due to heel effect.

The heel effect limits the size of the useful x-ray beam and is more pronounced with smaller angle anodes. Very small angle (6°) x-ray tubes are used in applications such as cardiac cineradiography which require very high instantaneous currents with a very limited field size.

Rotating Anode Tubes

Rotating anode tubes are used to spread the heat over a larger area than can be achieved with the line focus principle. Figure 6.6 illustrates how the target area heated by the electron beam is rotated away from the electron beam and replaced by a cool portion of the anode. The heat is spread over the entire circular track.

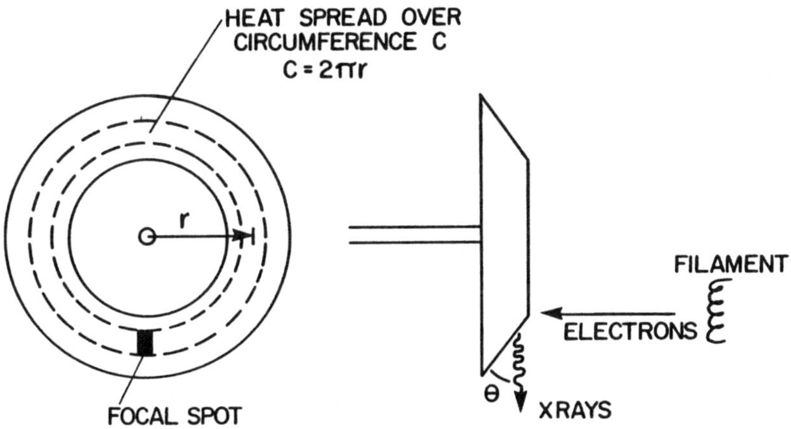

Figure 6.6. A rotating anode spreads the heat over the circumference of the anode.

The focal spot remains stationary but the heat is spread over the circumference of the circular anode. For an anode diameter of 5.0 cm the circumference is given by:

$$C = 2\pi r \qquad 6.2$$

or

$$C = D\pi$$

Because $D = 2r$

$$C = \pi \times 5$$

$$C = 15.7 \text{ cm}$$

Example 6.1:
What is the increase in effective focal spot area of a 1 mm x 1 mm effective focal spot when a 17° rotating anode (5 cm diameter) tube is substituted for a 17° stationary anode tube?

Actual area of stationary anode focal spot:

$$\text{Effective Area} = 1 \text{ mm} \times 1 \text{ mm}$$

$$\text{Effective Area} = \text{Actual} \times \sin 17°$$

$$1 \text{ mm}^2 = \text{Actual Area} \times \sin 17°$$

$$\text{Actual Area} = 1/\sin 17°$$

$$= 1/0.29$$

$$= 3.4 \text{ mm}^2$$

The heat is spread over 3.4 mm^2 in the stationary anode tube.

Area of Circular Ring

$$1 \text{ mm} \times \text{Circumference}$$

$$1 \text{ mm} \times \pi \times 50 \text{ mm} = 157 \text{ mm}^2$$

With the rotating anode the heat is spread over an area of 157 mm^2.

Increase in actual focal spot area:

$$\frac{157 \text{ mm}}{3.4 \text{ mm}^2} = 46 \text{ times as great}$$

Stators and Rotors

A magnetic induction motor is used to drive the rotating anode as shown in Figure 6.7. The anode disk is connected to the rotor by a molybdenum shaft. Molybdenum is a poor conductor so the heat is not conducted back to the rotor bearings.

The rotor is a combination of permanent magnets and conductors sealed inside the glass tube. The stator contains electromagnets which produce a rotating magnetic field at the rotor. Rotating anodes are driven at either 60 Hz with a rotation speed of about 3000 rpm (revolutions/min) or 180 Hz with a rotation speed of 9000 rpm.

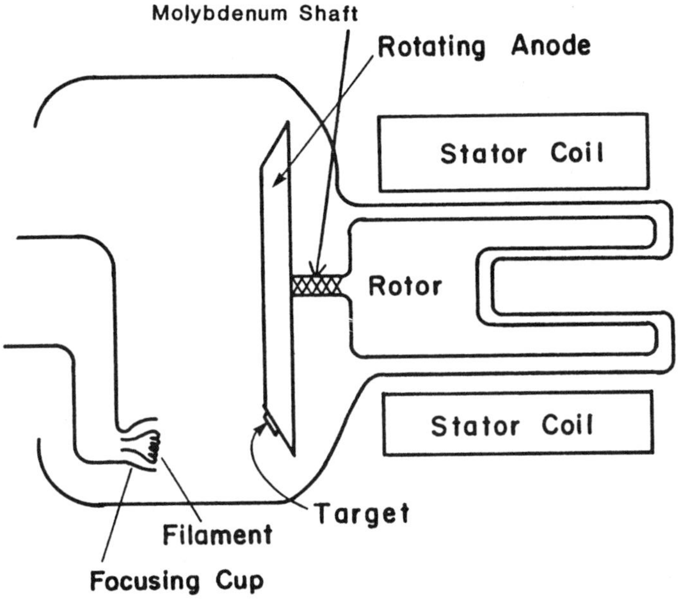

Figure 6.7. Schematic view of rotating anode x-ray tube.

When the exposure switch is first closed there is a 1 or 2 sec. delay while the anode is driven up to speed and the filament temperature is raised.

Anode Heat Storage, and Cooling

The major limitation on the operation of x-ray tubes is the heat produced during x-ray production. Over 99% of the energy in the electron beam bombarding the anode is converted to heat rather than x-rays. This heat must be removed from the x-ray tube and housing. There are three major heat limitations in the x-ray production process.

1. X-ray anode focal spot
2. Anode heat storage capacity
3. Tube housing heat capacity

The steps in heat dissipation in an x-ray tube are illustrated in Figure 6.8.

If the limits at any stage of this transfer process are exceeded, the tube will fail. This is considered undesirable.

X-RAY TUBE HEAT TRANSFER STEPS

Electron Beam	
↓	Heat Transfer Mechanism:
Focal Spot	
↓	Conduction
Anode	
↓	Radiation
Tube Housing	
↓	Convection
Room	

Figure 6.8. Steps in heat removal from an x-ray tube.

Heat Units

Heat deposited in the anode is expressed in terms of heat units (HU). For single phase wave form the heat units are given by

$$HU\ (1\phi) = (kVp) \times MAS \qquad 6.3$$

Example 6.2:
What are the heat units deposited in the anode from a 500 MA 1/10 sec exposure at 120 KVP?

$$HU = 120\ kVp \times 500\ ma \times 1/10\ sec$$

$$HU = 120 \times 500 \times \frac{1}{10}$$

$$HU = 6000\ HU$$

Equation 6.3 presents the relationship used to calculate heat units for single phase units. Because three phase current deposits more heat per milliamp than a single phase current with the same kVp and MAS, the HU for a three phase circuit must be multiplied by a wave form factor equal to 1.35. The heat units for a three phase unit are given by:

$$HU\ (3\phi) = 1.35 \times kVp \times MAS \qquad 6.4$$

Target Heat Limits

Focal spot heat limits are determined by the amount of heat the focal spot can safely withstand during a single exposure. With a rotating anode tube this occurs with high current, short time exposures. All modern x-ray generators have the target exposure limits programmed into the MAS setting switches so that it is not possible to produce a single exposure which exceeds the focal spot limit of the tube.

However, it is possible to damage the tube by making a series of repeated exposures each of which is within the acceptable focal spot limits.

Anode Heat Limits

Protection against repeated exposures, each less than the focal spot heat limit, is not possible by preprogramming the generator. Each tube manufacturer supplies a series of curves specifying the combinations of allowed exposure factors for each focal spot. Figures 6.9 and 6.10 present the heat limits for one mm focal spot for single phase (2 pulse and three phase (6 or 12 pulse) operation. If this tube is a dual focus tube there are another two curves for the other focal spot size.

Exposures below the curves are allowed, exposures above the curves are not allowed.

Example 6.3:
Using the data from Figure 6.9, determine whether a 1/2 s 120 kVp 1 ϕ 100 mA exposure is allowed.

From Figure 6.9, the 120 kVp curve intercepts the 100 mA line at 0.18 s. The 100 mA 1/2 s exposure point is above the 120 kVp curve. This exposure is not allowed.

Example 6.4:
Using the data from Figure 6.10, determine whether a 0.05 s 80 kVp 3 ϕ 200 mA exposure is allowed.

From Figure 6.10, the 80 kVp curve intercepts the 200 mA line at 0.07 s. The 200 mA .05 s exposure point is below the 80 kVp curve. This exposure is allowed.

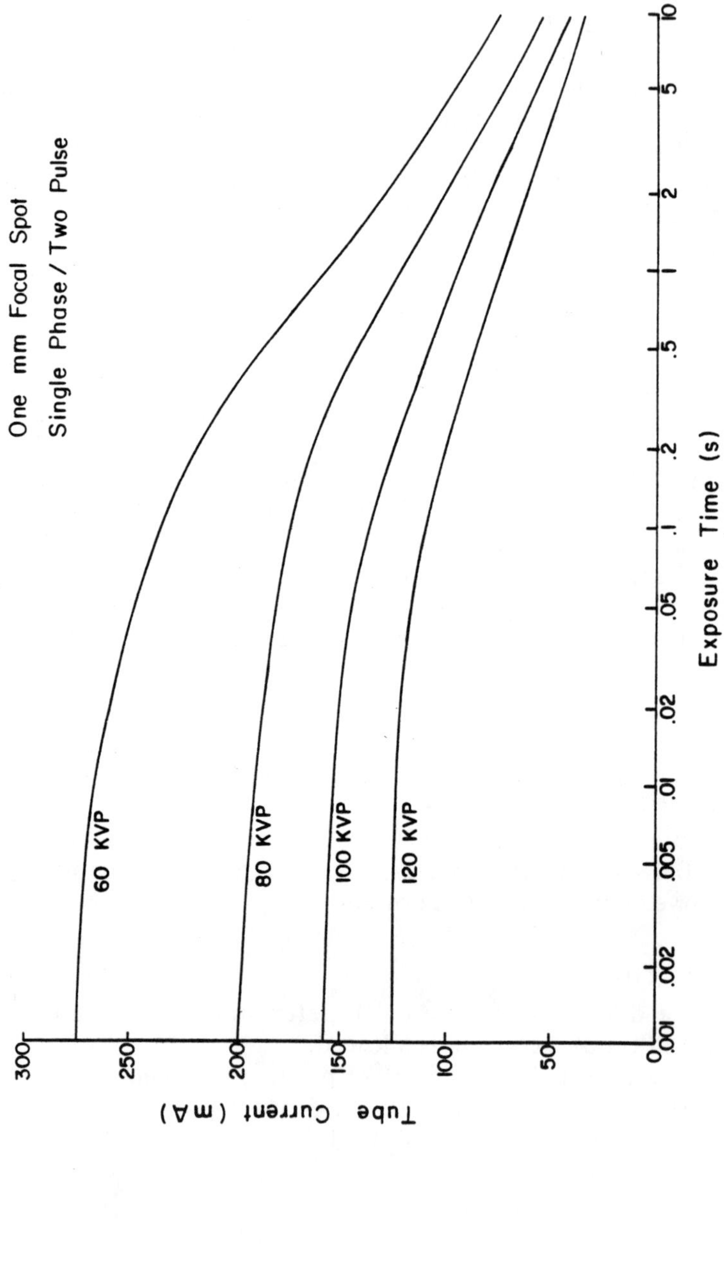

Figure 6.9. Focal spot heat limits for single phase (two pulse) operation.

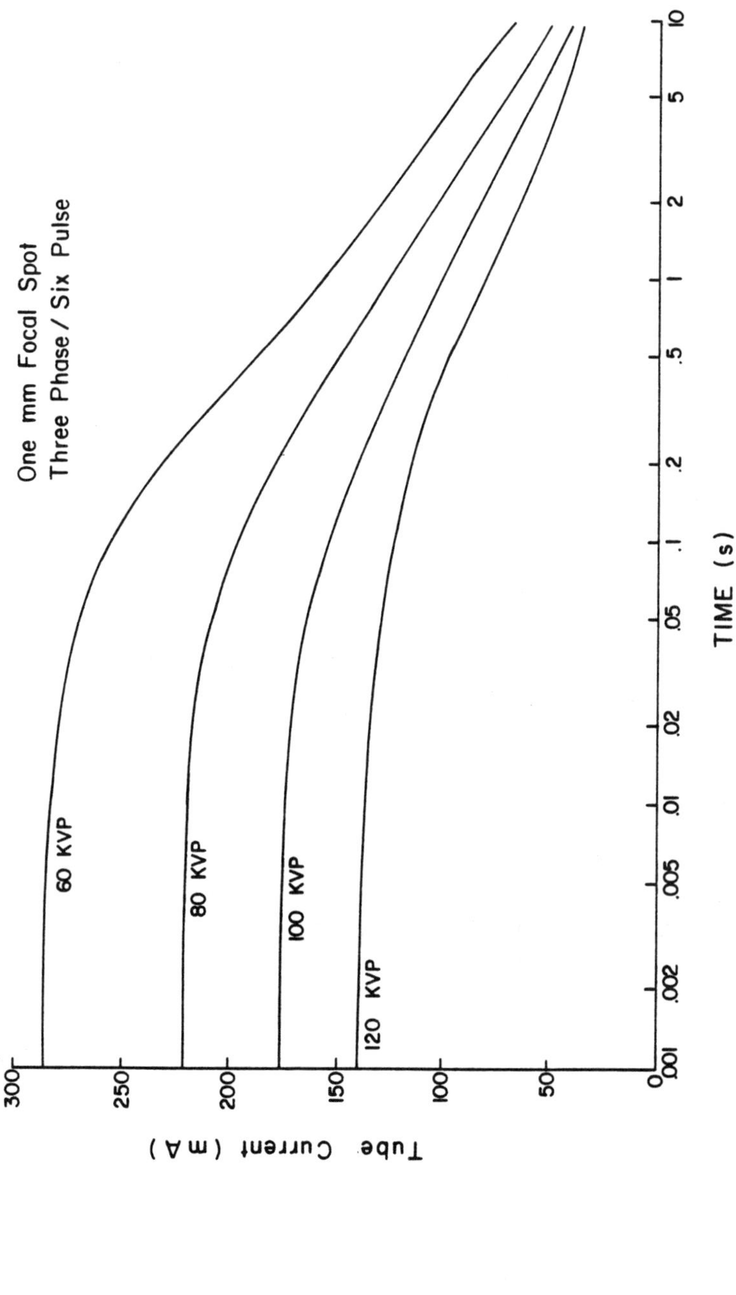

Figure 6.10. Focal spot limits for three phase (six or twelve pulse) operation.

In addition to the heat limits of the focal spot, the anode body also has a heat limit. Figure 6.11 presents the cooling curve for a 140,000 HU anode.

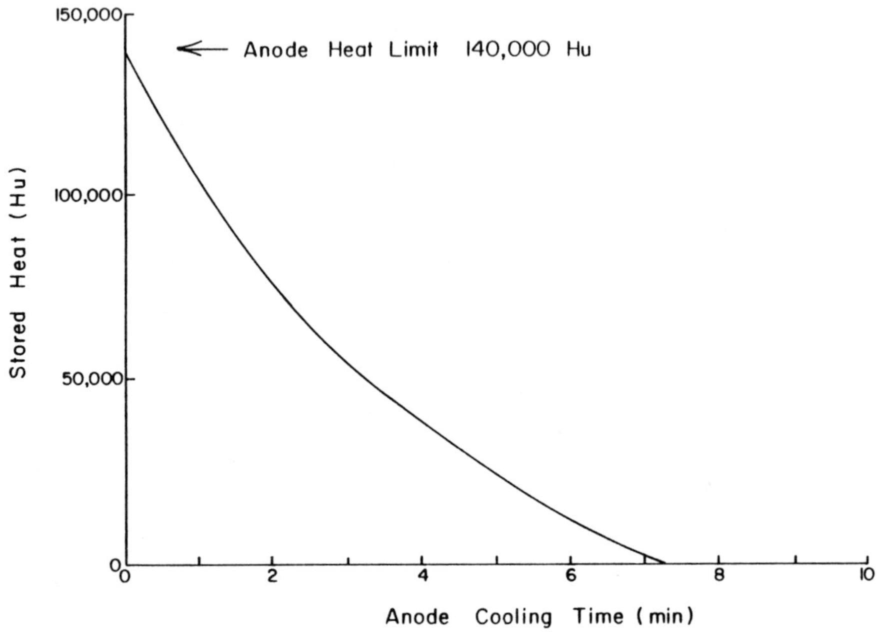

Figure 6.11. Anode cooling curve for a 140,000 HU tube.

Example 6.5:
How long after a series of exposures totaling 100,000 HU must we wait before another such series is allowed?

After the first series, the anode contains 100,000 HU. It must cool to 40,000 HU before the series can be repeated without exceeding the Anode Heat Limit.

From Figure 6.11, the time to cool from 100,000 HU to 40,000 HU is 2.8 min.

Example 6.6:
After the second 100,000 HU series, how long must the anode cool before a third series can begin?

Answer: The time to cool from 140,000 HU to 40,000 HU is 4 min.

Rotor Heat Load

The starting and stopping of the rotor will add 3000–4000 HU per exposure. This can become important in a series of many exposures.

Stereoradiographic Tubes

Stereoradiographic tubes have two separate cathode assemblies in the same glass housing.

X-rays from the two focal spots separated by about 12 cm can be used to form stereoradiographs.

Field Emission X-ray Tubes

Field emission or cold cathode x-ray tubes use a high voltage to pull electrons from the cathode. Instead of a hot filament, the cathode cylinder surrounding the anode contains many rows of sharp points. A high voltage (350 kV) pulse can pull electrons from the ends of the cathode spikes and accelerate them to the

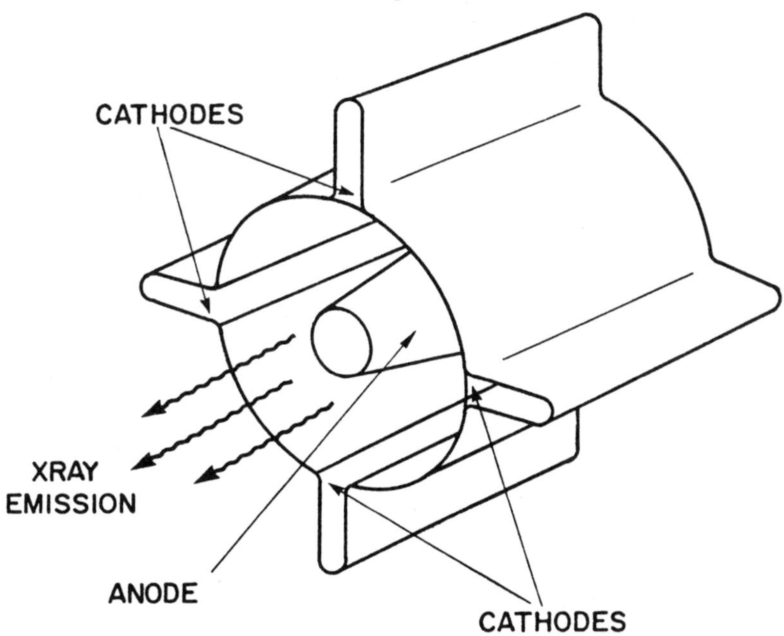

Figure 6.12. Field Emission x-ray tube with multiple cathodes and central anode.

anode. Field emission tubes have primarily been used for high kV (350KV) radiography. They produce low contrast wide latitude images. The chief disadvantage of the field emission tube is its large (3 cm) focal spot size. The major advantage is the very short exposure times.

Mammographic Tubes

Mammography is a special case of imaging low contrast structures in a relatively small volume. Very low energy x–rays are most suitable.

Special mammographic tubes with molybdenum anodes are used because molybdenum has characteristic x–ray energies of 17.5 and 19.5 KeV. If the output of a molybdenum anode tube is filtered with a 0.03 mm molybdenum filter, most of the Bremstrahlung radiation will be removed and the Mo characteristic x–rays will predominate. The average energy of an Mo filtered beam from an Mo anode tube is about 20 KeV and is almost independent of applied kVp below 30 kVp.

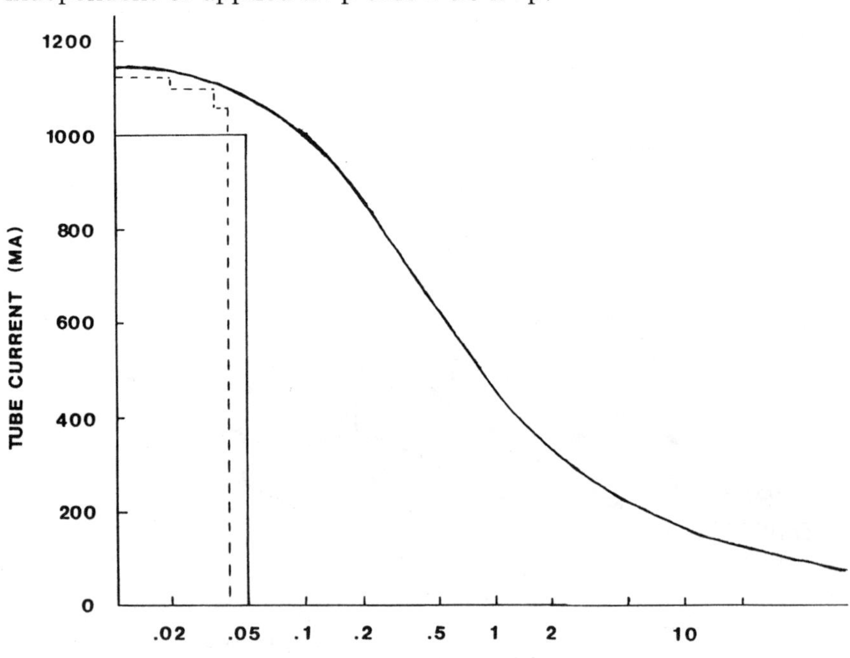

Figure 6.13. Falling load generator matches the tube current to the anode heat limits.

Falling Load Generators

Failing load generators adjust the tube current during the exposure to match the heat limit curve of the anode to obtain the shortest practical exposure time. Figure 6.13 illustrates how a 50 MAS exposure can be obtained either by a 50 ms exposure at a constant tube current of 1000 MA, or a falling load exposure of 45 ms.

Falling load generators are most useful in applications such as angiography where it is important to stop vessel motion with short exposures.

CHAPTER 6 QUESTIONS

1. X-ray tubes are evacuated to
   1. reduce photon scattering.
   2. reduce electron scattering.
   3. improve anode cooling.
   4. provide electrical insulation.
   5. reduce resistance of the rotating anode.

   A. 1 and 3
   B. 2 and 4
   C. 2 and 3
   D. 3 and 4
   E. 2, 3 and 5

2. The principle means of anode cooling is
   A. conduction.
   B. convection.
   C. radiation.

3. A rotating anode of Diameter D will spread the heat over a path length:
   A. πr^2
   B. $\pi D^2/4$
   C. πr
   D. πD

4. A molybdenum shaft is used to connect the anode to the rotor because
   A. molybdenum is a poor heat conductor.
   B. molybdenum is a good heat conductor.
   C. molybdenum has a high atomic number.
   D. molybdenum has 17.5 and 19.5 KeV characteristic x-rays.

5. Grid controlled tubes
   A. add a negative bias voltage to the anode.
   B. are used to produce short exposures.
   C. maintain a constant filament temperature.
   D. add a constant voltage to the cathode focusing cup.

6. The line focus principle
   A. makes the focal spot appear larger than it really is.
   B. makes use of a tilted cathode structure.
   C. produces x-ray lines.
   D. spreads the heat over a larger part of the anode.

7. The heel effect
   A. is caused because all x-rays are not produced at the surface of the cathode.
   B. is caused because x-rays produced beneath the surface of the cathode are attenuated more.
   C. limits the useful field size.
   D. A + B + C
   E. None of the above

8. Many x-ray tubes have two filaments because
   A. the second can be used when the first one burns out.
   B. to provide two focal spot sizes.
   C. to improve cooling by alternating exposures between the two.
   D. to reduce focal spot penumbra by sharing the exposures.

9. The boost current in a filament
   A. raises the filament temperature just before exposure.
   B. is used to improve the x-ray tube vacuum.
   C. maintains the filament at standby temperature.
   D. stops as soon as the anode reaches full rotation speed.

10. Filaments are coated with thorium oxide to
    A. improve filament cooling.
    B. increase filament temperature response.
    C. reduce filament outgassing.
    D. increase the number of electrons obtained at a given filament temperature.

11–13, A 12° anode angle tube is substituted for a 17° angle tube. A for increase, B for decrease, C remains the same.

11. The focal spot heat limits will ___________.
12. The useful field size at a given SID ___________.
13. The penetrating ability of the x-ray beam will ___________.

14. The heel effect is most pronounced at the ___________ end of the tube.
    A. anode
    B. cathode

15. The ___________ is inside the vacuum tube of a rotating anode tube.
    A. stator
    B. rotor

16–18, A for True, B for False

Increasing the ___________ will ___________ the heat capacity of a tube.

16. tube angle, increase
17. anode diameter, increase
18. rotation speed, increase

19. What are the heat units for a three phase (six pulse) 80 kVp 200 MA 500 ms exposure?
    A. 8×10^6 HU
    B. 1.08×10^7 HU
    C. 8000 HU
    D. 10800 HU

20. What are the heat units for a single phase (2 pulse) 70 kVp 150 MA 300 ms exposure?
    A. 3.15×10^6 HU
    B. 4.25×10^6 HU
    C. 3150 HU
    D. 4252 HU

21. What are the heat units for a three phase (six pulse) 110 kVP 75 MA 50 ms exposure?

A. 412500 HU
B. 556875 HU
C. 472 HU
D. 557 HU

Use Figures 6.9, 6.10 and 6.11 for Problems 22-28

Can the following exposures be made? A for Allowed, B for Not Allowed.

22.	1 mm focal spot	1 ϕ	150mA	1/2 sec.	100 kVp
23.	1 mm focal spot	3 ϕ	300 mA	1/20 sec.	60 kVp
24.	1 mm focal spot	1 ϕ	250 mA	1/20 sec.	80 kVp
25.	1 mm focal spot	1 ϕ	200 mA	1/10 sec.	110 kVp
26.	1 mm focal spot	1 ϕ	150 mA	1/5 sec.	100 kVp

One series of 20 films each has been run using factors of 110 kVp 400 mA 1/10 3 ϕ.

27. What is heat load of HU?

A. 69,000
B. 80,000
C. 110,000
D. 119,000

28. How long must we wait until another such series can be repeated?

A. 2 min.
B. 4 min.
C. 6 min.
D. 8 min.

29. Focal spot size depends on

A. the cathode angle.
B. the kVp selected.
C. the filament selected.
D. the filament transformer turns ratio.

CHAPTER 7

X-RAY PRODUCTION

X-rays are produced when electrons accelerated from the cathode strike the anode.

Two processes contribute to x-ray production:
a. Bremsstrahlung
b. Characteristic x-ray production

Bremsstrahlung is the German word for "braking radiation." A moving electron gives off this radiation whenever it stops. When an electron is stopped by the nuclei in the anode, some of the electron energy is converted to x-rays and most is converted to heat. At diagnostic energies about 99% of the electron energy is converted to heat and only 1% of the energy appears as x-rays.

X-ray Energies

Even though all electrons striking the anode have the same energy, the Bremsstrahlung process produces x-rays with many different energies. Figure 7.1 presents a typical x-ray spectrum produced by Bremsstrahlung. The x-ray intensity is plotted against the x-ray energy E.

Bremsstrahlung x-rays range in energy from zero to a maximum energy equal to the energy of the bombarding electrons. X-ray production via the Bremsstrahlung process increases with increasing energy of the bombarding electron beam as well as increasing Z of the target. Most of the low energy photons cannot penetrate the walls of the x-ray tube. The dotted curve illustrates an x-ray spectrum produced at the anode. The solid curve illustrates the x-ray spectra emitted from an x-ray tube.

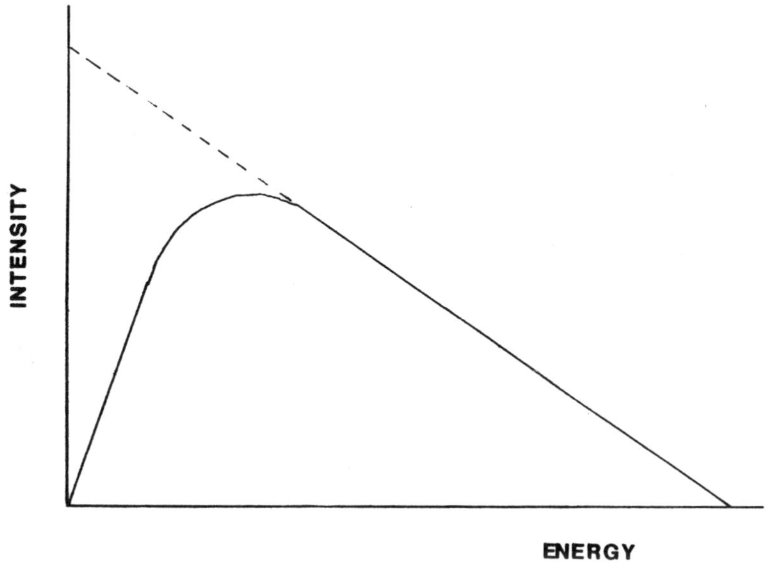

Figure 7.1. Energy spectrum of x-rays produced by Bremsstrahlung.

Minimum Wavelength

The minimum wavelength photons correspond to photons with energies equal to the maximum applied voltage. The minimum wavelength is given by:

$$\lambda_{min} = \frac{12.4}{kVp} \times 10^{-10} \text{ m} \qquad 7.1$$

Example 7.1:
What is the minimum wavelength of x-rays produced by an 80 kVp generator?

$$\lambda_{min} = \frac{12.4}{80} \times 10^{-10}$$

$$\lambda_{min} = .155 \times 10^{-10} \text{ m}$$

Characteristic X-rays

Characteristic x-rays are produced by transitions between electron orbits. The difference in the binding energies of the two orbits is released as an x–ray photon. Because these orbital energies are unique for each atom, the x–rays are characteristic of the particular atoms. Figure 7.2 illustrates the energy levels of tungsten.

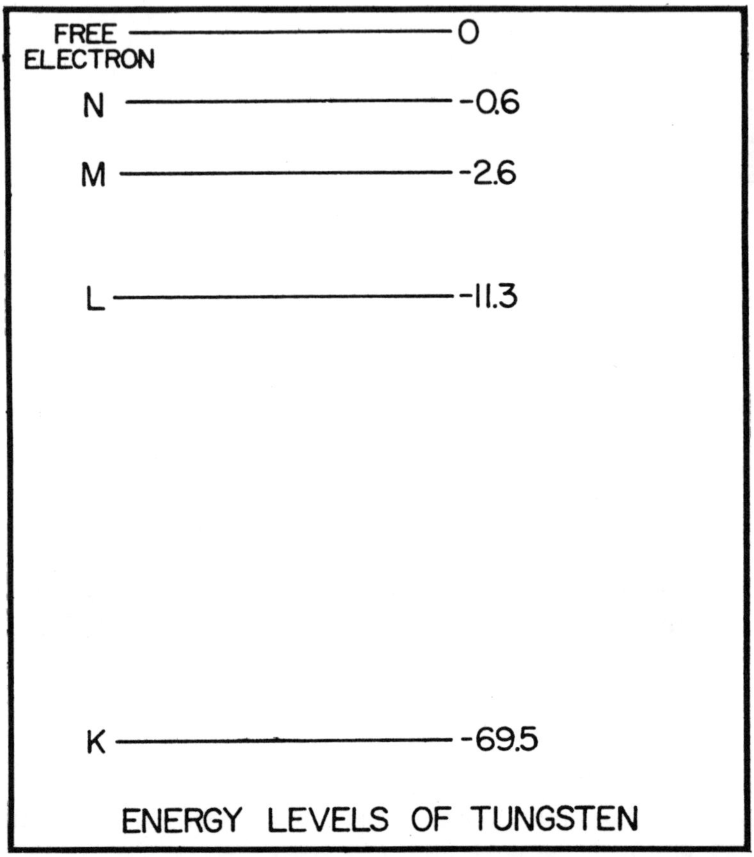

Figure 7.2. Energy levels of tungsten.

Table 7.1 presents the possible transitions together with the resulting characteristic x–ray energies when tungsten is bombarded with a 70 KeV electron beam. If tungsten is bombarded with a 69 KeV electron beam, the K shell orbital electrons cannot be removed and there will be no K shell vacancies and no transitions to the K shell. Figure 7.3 presents an x–ray spectra obtained from the bombardment of a tungsten target with 100 KeV electrons.

The lines produced by the characteristic transition are superimposed on the Bremsstrahlung spectra. The relative number of photons produced by the Bremsstrahlung and characteristic processes depends on the bombarding energy of the electron beams. Table 7.2 presents the distributions of the x-rays between the two production processes.

TABLE 7.1
POSSIBLE TRANSITIONS FOLLOWING 70 KeV ELECTRON BOMBARDMENT OF TUNGSTEN

Orbital Transition	*Energy*
L - K	58.2
M - K	66.9
N - K	68.9
Free - K	69.5

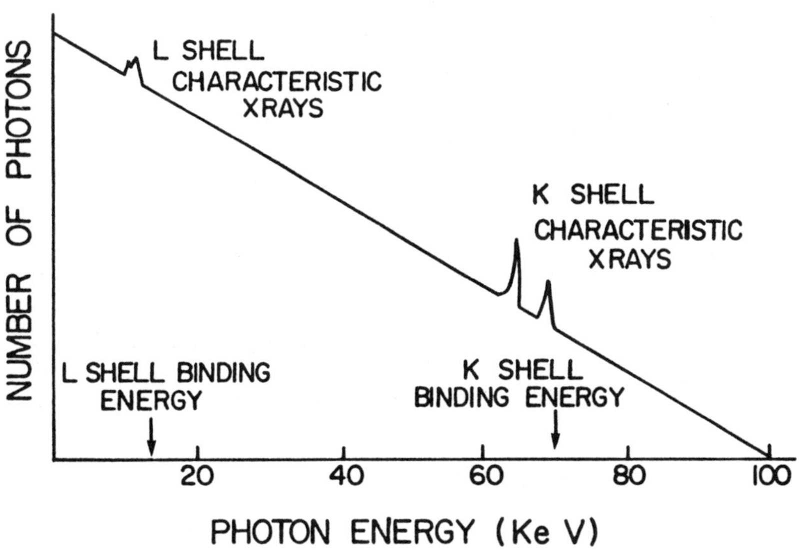

Figure 7.3. Energy spectra produced by 100 KeV electrons on tungsten.

TABLE 7.2
PERCENT X-RAY PRODUCTION BY

KVP	*Characteristic*	*Bremsstrahlung*
80	10	90
100	20	80
120	25	75

Variation of X-ray Output with MA

Changes in the number of electrons bombarding the anode (MA) changes only the **number** of x-rays **not** the **energy distribution** (shape of x-ray spectrum) nor the maximum energy x-rays. Figure 7.4 illustrates the change in x-ray spectrum with MA.

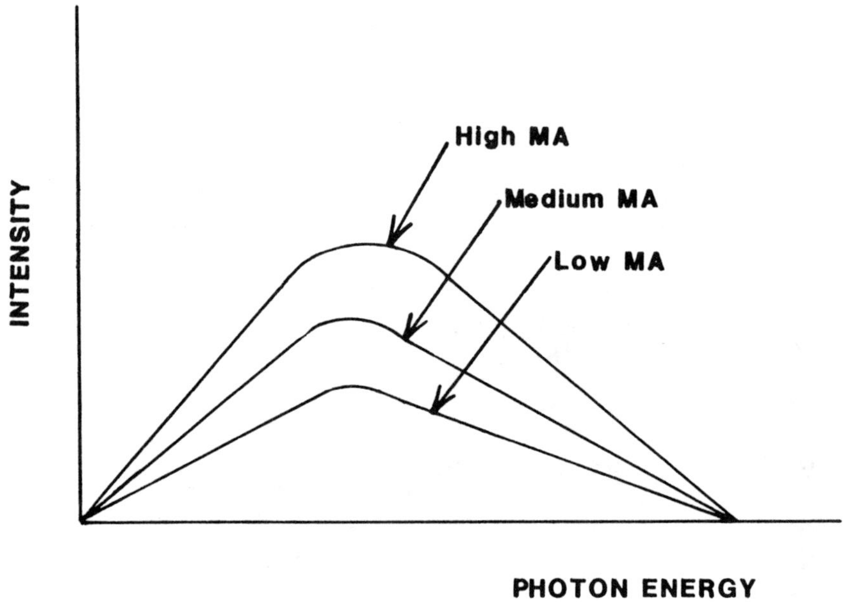

Figure 7.4. Variation of intensity with changes in MA.

Variation of Intensity with kVp

At the anode, the intensity of x-ray production varies as $(KV)^2$. Many of the low energy x-rays are filtered out of the beam by the tube walls. What is important is how many x-rays pass through the patient and reach the detector.

The intensity I of the x-ray beam **at the detector** varies approximately as:

$$I = k Z \ (kVp)^3 \qquad 7.2$$

Where k is a proportionality constant, Z is the atomic number of the anode material and kVp is the applied voltage.

A rule of thumb is that in the diagnostic energy range a **15% change in kVp is equivalent to a factor of two change in MAS.**

Example 7.2:
An exposure of 100 kVp 150 MAS has acceptable density but too little contrast so the applied voltage is dropped to 85 kVp. What MAS value should be selected?

100 kVp to 85 kVp is a 15 kVp change

$$\frac{15}{100} = 15\% \text{ change}$$

A 15% change in kVp corresponds to a factor of two change in MAS. The kVp was decreased so the MAS must be increased.

$$150 \text{ MAS} \times 2 = 300 \text{ MAS}$$

The final exposure factors should be:

85 kVp and 300 MAS

Figure 7.5 illustrates the effect of changing the kVp on the intensity of the x–rays emitted from the tube. As the kVp is increased, both the energy of the highest energy photons and the number of photons at all energies increases. Notice that very few of the x–ray photons in the beam have energies equal to the applied kVp. **The "average" energy of the x–ray beam is about 1/3 to 1/2 the applied kVp.**

Effective Filtration on the Beam

Figure 7.6 illustrates the effect of added filtration on the x–ray beam. The dotted line indicates the x–ray spectrum produced at the anode. Most of the very low energy x–rays are removed from the beam by the **inherent filtration** of the x–ray tube walls and collimator. The inherent filtration of most x–ray collimator–tube systems is equivalent to at least 1 mm aluminum. Adding filtration reduces the number of photons at all energies but the lower energy photons are reduced proportionately more than higher energy photons. Most of the low energy photons contribute nothing to the diagnosis because they are absorbed in the

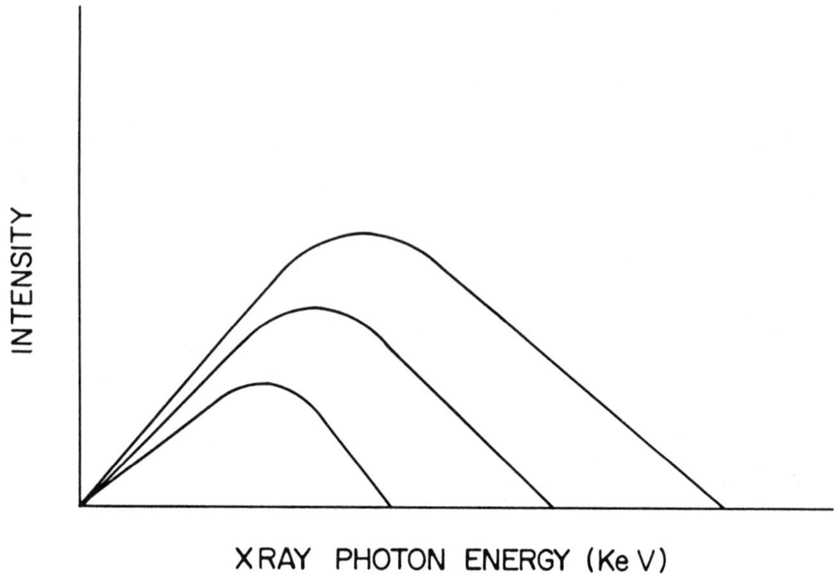

Figure 7.5. Effect of changing kVp on x-ray spectra.

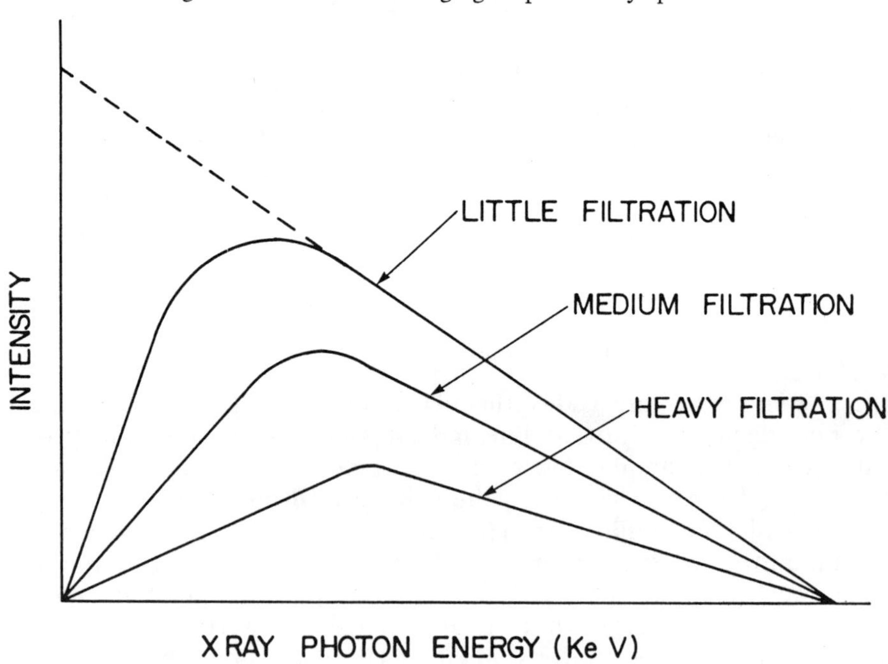

Figure 7.6. Effect of changing filtration on x-ray spectra.

patient. By adding filtration, the penetrating ability of the x-ray beam is increased and patient dose is reduced. State and Federal regulations require at least 1.5 mm Al filtration for 70 kVp x-ray beams and at least 2.5 mm aluminum filtration for x-ray beam energies greater than 90 kVp.

X-ray Production as Part of Electrical Cycle

Because x-ray production is so dependent on KV, almost all useful x-rays are produced only when the applied voltage is near maximum. Figure 7.7 compares a full wave rectified electrical cycle with the x-ray production cycle.

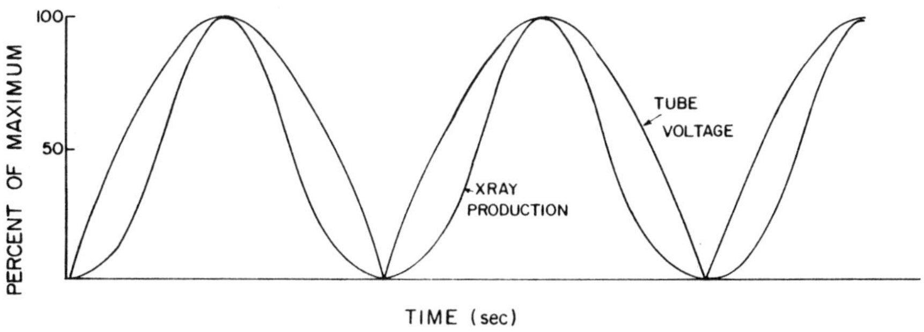

Figure 7.7. X-ray production as a function of tube voltage. Note that most of the x-rays are produced when the tube voltage is near a maximum.

Comparison of Single and Three Phase Circuits

When a three phase (6 pulse) unit is substituted for a single phase (2 pulse) unit, the average energy deposited in the anode for a given kVp and MAS setting increases by a factor of 1.35. However, the average energy applied across the x-ray tube is higher so the x-ray intensity and the penetration of the x-ray beam is higher. A rule of thumb is that three phase equipment produces a 12% increase in radiation reaching the detector compared to single phase equipment. In addition, the average tube current is higher with three phase than with single phase current. The focal spot is limited to a **maximum** current and not the **average** current on the anode. Figure 5.5 illustrates why larger three phase average currents are permitted without exceeding the maximum focal spot temperature limit.

CHAPTER 7 QUESTIONS

1. A Bremsstrahlung x-ray spectra
   A. consists of discrete photon energies.
   B. consists of continuous photon energies.
   C. has a maximum wavelength.
   D. is produced by orbital transitions.

2. Characteristic x-rays
   A. consist of discrete photon energies.
   B. consist of continuous photon energies.
   C. are produced by orbital transitions.
   D. A and C
   E. A, B and C

3. At 100 kVp _____% of the x-ray production is due to characteristic x-ray production.
   A. 5
   B. 10
   C. 15
   D. 20

4-12, A for True, B for False

4. A change in MA does change the number of x-rays produced.

5. A change in MA does change the maximum energy of the x-ray beam.

6. A change in MA does change the minimum wavelength of an x-ray beam.

7. A change in kVp does change the number of x-rays produced.

8. A change in kVp does change the maximum energy of the x-ray beam.

9. A change in the kVp does change the minimum wavelength of an x-ray beam.

10. A change in filtration does change the number of photons in an x-ray beam.

11. A change in filtration does change the maximum energy of an x-ray beam.

12. A change in filtration does change the minimum wavelength of an x-x-ray beam.

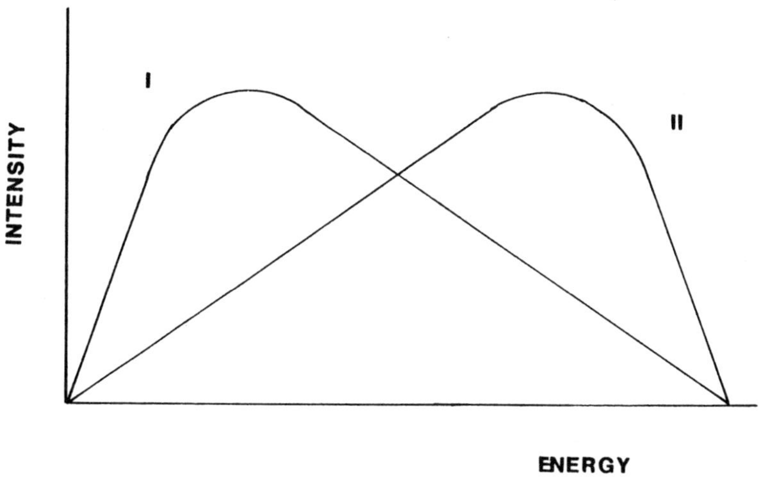

13. The technical factors are changed from condition I to condition II producing the change in spectra shown: Select the correct factors

A. Increase MA, Increase kVp
B. Increase MA, Increase Filtration
C. Increase kVp, Decrease Filtration
D. Increase MA Decrease Filtration

14. An exposure at 200 MA 90 kVp 0.1 sec would produce the same density as a 200 MA, 0.2 sec exposure at

A. 83 kVp
B. 80 kVp
C. 77 kVp
D. 73 kVp

15. An exposure at 85 kVp 100 MAS would produce the same density as a 50 MAS exposure at

A. 94 kVp
B. 98 kVp
C. 112 kVp
D. 120 kVp

16. An exposure at 85 kVp 100 MAS 40" SID will produce the same exposure as an 80" SID 100 MAS exposure at

A. 94 kVp
B. 98 kVp
C. 112 kVp
D. 120 kVp

17. The effective energy of an x-ray beam is approximately _____ times the applied kVp.

A. .3
B. .3%
C. equal to
D. 3

18. Three phase (6 pulse) wave forms permit higher average currents than single phase (2 pulse) wave forms because

A. x-rays are produced more efficiently near the voltage maximum.
B. the average current is closer to the maximum current.
C. the average current is more easily rectified.
D. the cooling between wave pulses is more efficient.

19. 100 kilovolts is applied to an x-ray tube.

1. the anode is bombarded with 100 KeV electrons.
2. Most of the x-rays will have energies of 100 KeV.
3. The minimum wavelength will be $.124 \times 10^{-10}$m.
4. The average energy of the x-ray beam is about 35 KeV.

A. 1, 2, 3 and 4
B. 1, 2 and 3
C. 2, 3 and 4
D. 1, 3 and 4

20. An x-ray beam from a three phase (6 pulse) generator will differ from a beam from a single phase generator of the same kVp and MAS in that it:

A. is less penetrating.
B. has fewer photons.
C. has a longer minimum wavelength.
D. None of the above.

21. Filters are added to an x-ray beam to

A. add short wavelength photons.
B. remove short wavelength photons.
C. add long wavelength photons.
D. decrease long wavelength photons.

22. For the same film density and applied kVp, if a three phase (6 pulse) unit is substituted for a single phase (2 pulse) unit

A. the kVp must be decreased.
B. the MAS must be decreased.
C. the number of photons will increase.
D. the ripple will increase.
E. there will be no change.

CHAPTER 8

X-RAY INTERACTIONS

The intensity of an x-ray beam passing through a layer of attenuating material depends on the thickness and type of material. If successive layers of attenuating material are added to the beam as shown schematically in Figure 8.1, and the transmitted beam intensity is measured, we find (for a monoenergetic beam) that the fractional intensity change $\Delta I/I$ is a constant for a constant added thickness Δx.

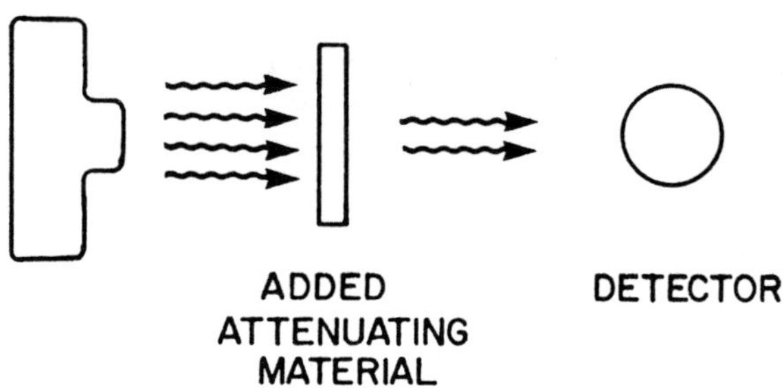

Figure 8.1 Simple attenuation experiment.

That is:

$$\Delta I = -I\mu\Delta x$$

$$\frac{\Delta I}{I} = -\mu\Delta x \qquad 8.1$$

$$= \text{Constant if } \Delta x \text{ is a constant}$$

Where ΔI is the change in intensity, I is the intensity, μ is the "linear attenuation coefficient" and Δx is the added thickness of material. The minus sign indicates a decrease in intensity. Figure 8.2 presents the transmitted intensity as a function of added thickness for a monoenergetic beam. The linear attentuation coefficient, μ, is measured in units of /cm (pronounced "per centimeter"). This equation can be integrated to give

$$I = I_o e^{-\mu x} \qquad 8.2$$

The linear attentuation coefficient gives the **fractional reduction of x-ray intensity per cm of attenuating material.**

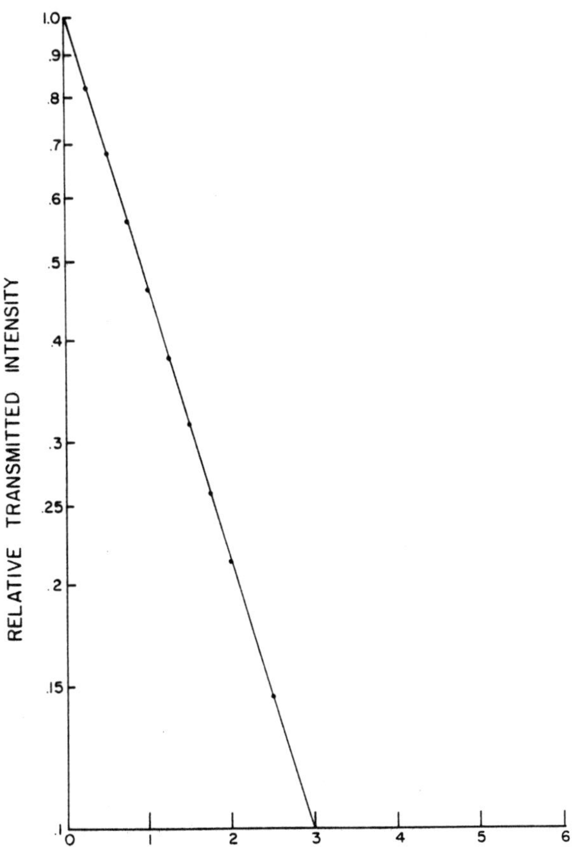

Figure 8.2 Transmitted intensity of a monoenergetic (single energy) x-ray beam as a function of added thickness of aluminum.

Mass Attenuation Coefficients

Consider a series of measurements to determine the linear attenuation coefficients of water, ice, and steam. These measurements yield the linear attenuation coefficients given in Table 8.1.

TABLE 8.1
LINEAR ATTENUATION COEFFICIENTS OF WATER, ICE AND STEAM

Material	*Linear Attenuation Coefficient*
Water	.18/cm
Ice	.16/cm
Steam	.0002/cm

It didn't take very long before the person making these measurements realized that the H_2O molecules producing the attenuation were the same under all three conditions. The only thing different was the density ρ measured in grams per cubic centimeter. The linear attenuation coefficient divided by the density of the material ρ produces the mass attenuation coefficient μ_m.

$$\mu_m = \mu/\rho \qquad 8.3$$

Example 8.1:
The linear attenuation coefficient of bone (density $\rho = 1.65$ g/cm^3) for a 50 kVp x-ray beam is 3.63/cm. What is the mass attenuation coefficient of bone for this beam energy?

$$\mu_m = \mu/\rho$$

$$= 3.63/\text{cm.} \times \frac{1\ \text{cm}^3}{1.65\ \text{g}}$$

$$\mu_m = 2.2\ \text{cm}^2/\text{gm}$$

Half-Value Layer

The half-value layer (HVL) is defined as the amount of material which must be added to the x-ray beam to reduce the original intensity by a factor of 2. The half-value layer can be expressed in terms of the attenuation coefficient as:

$$I = \frac{I_o}{2} \qquad 8.4$$

$$\frac{I_o}{2} = I_o e^{-\mu(HVL)}$$

The I_o terms cancel and:

$$\frac{1}{2} = e^{-\mu(HVL)}$$

but $$e^{-.693} = \frac{1}{2}$$

because $$.693 = \ln 2$$

The exponents are equal to each other. Hence:

$$(\mu)\,(HVL) = .693 \qquad 8.5$$

or $$\mu = \frac{.693}{HVL}$$

or $$HVL = \frac{.693}{\mu}$$

First and Second Half-Value Layer Measurements

The half-value layer of an x-ray beam is defined as the amount of material required to attenuate the original intensity, I_o, of the beam to one half its original value ($I_o/2$). The second half-value layer is defined as the amount of material required to reduce the beam intensity by an additional factor of two (i.e., to $I_o/4$). If all the x-rays have the same energy, then the first and second HVL's are the same as shown in Figure 8.2.

If the x-ray beam contains a **mixture** of x-ray energies, the first and second HVL's will be different. When an x-ray beam passes through the body more low energy, "softer" x-rays are absorbed by body tissues than higher energy x-rays. The penetrating ability of the beam **increases** as it passes through more tissue because relatively more of the lower energy photons are removed from the x-ray beam. The second half-value layer is always greater than the first HVL for diagnostic x-ray beams. Only with a monoenergetic (single energy) beam are the first and second HVL's equal.

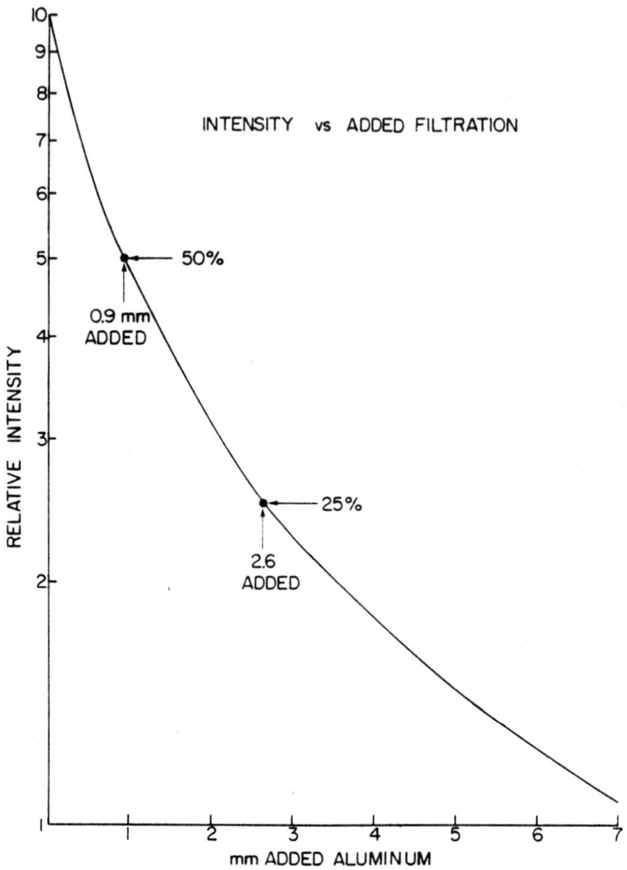

Figure 8.3. Transmitted intensity of a heterogeneous (multi-energy) x-ray beam as a function of added aluminum thickness.

Figure 8.3 presents a plot of intensity as a function of added material (Al) for a heterogeneous (multienergy) x-ray beam. In this case, the first half-value layer is 0.9 millimeters of aluminum. If additional aluminum is added, we find that the second half-value layer is 1.7 millimeters of aluminum.

The second half-value layer is calculated as follows:

Example 8.2:
Thickness of material required to reduce original intensity to one half the original value (first HVL) = 0.9 mm Al.

Total thickness of material to reduce beam intensity to 25% of original value = 2.6 mm Al.

Difference = (second HVL) = 2.6 - .9 = 1.7 mm Al

Tissue Half-Value Layer

The half-value layer in tissue of most diagnostic x-ray beams is between 4 and 6 centimeters. This means that a change in patient thickness of 5 cm requires an MAS change by about a factor of 2. With an average patient, only about one percent of the incident x-rays emerge from the patient.

X-ray Interactions in Matter

There are five ways in which x-rays can interact with matter. They are:

1. Coherent Scattering
2. Photoelectric Interactions
3. Compton Scattering
4. Pair Production Interactions
5. Photodisintegration Interactions

The total attenuation coefficient μ_{Tot} is a combination of these interactions

$$\mu_{\text{Coherent}} + \mu_{\text{Photo Electric}} + \mu_{\text{Compton}} + \mu_{\text{Pair Production}} + \mu_{\text{Photo Disintegration}} \qquad 8.6$$

μ pair production and μ photodisintegration are zero below 1 MeV and so do not participate in interactions at diagnostic energies.

Coherent Scattering

Coherent scattering, also called Classical or Thompson scattering, is important only at low energies. There is no energy transfer in coherent scattering, only a change in photon direction. It has little importance in diagnostic radiology except for a slight blurring of edges.

Photoelectric Absorption

In a photoelectric interaction shown schematically in Figure 8.4, the x–ray photon is completely absorbed by the atom. This interaction usually results in the emission of a K or L shell electron. The ejected electron leaves a vacancy in the orbit. This vacancy is filled by an electron from an outer orbit. The inner orbit has a higher binding energy so the electron releases its excess energy. The released energy appears as a characteristic x–ray.

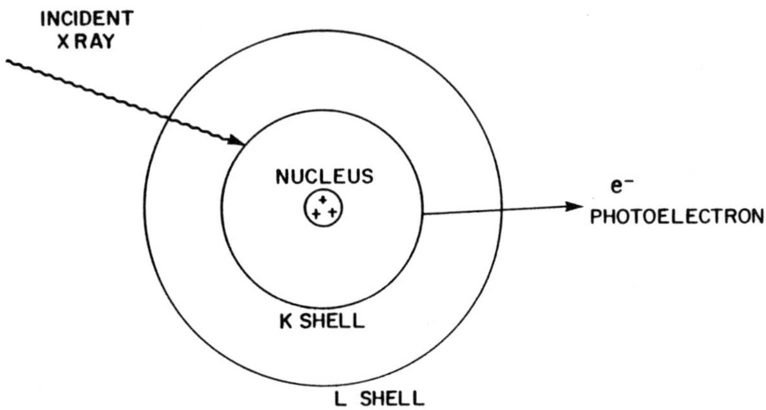

Figure 8.4. Photoelectric absorption process.

The energy of the orbital electron ejected from the atom, the photoelectron, is given by:

$$E_e = h\nu - E_b \qquad 8.7$$

In equation 8.7, E_e is the kinetic energy of the photoelectron, $h\nu$ is the energy of the incident x–ray and E_B is the binding energy of the orbital electron.

Example 8.3:
What is the photoelectron energy if a K shell electron (binding energy = 37 KeV) is ejected following the photoelectric absorption of a 55 KeV photon?

$$E_e = h\nu - E_b$$

$$= 55 - 37$$

$$= 18 \text{ KeV}$$

Ranges of Photoelectrons and Characteristic X-rays

The range of photoelectrons in tissue is less than 1 mm. The range of the characteristic radiation depends on the type of atom undergoing the photoelectric absorption and the energy of the characteristic x-rays. In tissue, the binding energy of normal tissue materials is a few ev so the ranges of the characteristic x-rays are a fraction of 1 mm. Table 8.2 lists the K-shell binding energies and Atomic number of elements in tissue and contrast materials.

TABLE 8.2
ATOMIC NUMBERS AND K-SHELL BINDING ENERGIES OF ELEMENTS IN TISSUE AND CONTRAST MATERIALS

Element	*Z*	*K-shell Binding Energy (KeV)*
H	1	.014
C	12	.28
N	14	.40
O	16	.53
Ca	20	4.0
I	53	33.2
Ba	56	37.4

As the x-ray energy is increased from less than the K-shell binding energy to more than the K-shell binding energy, the attenuation coefficient μ increases significantly. This increase is known as the **K absorption edge** and occurs when the x-ray energy is equal to the K-shell binding energy.

Figure 8.5 presents a plot of the attenuation coefficient of iodine as a function of photon energy. The K absorption edge for iodine occurs as 33.2 KeV. Notice that photon energy (keV) is plotted and **not** the voltage applied to the x-ray tube (kVp).

Energy Dependence of Photoelectric Absorption

Except in the region near the binding energy of the orbital shells, the photoelectric mass attenuation coefficient decreases with energy as $1/E^3$. That is, if the photon energy is doubled, the photoelectric interaction will be reduced by 1/8. Mammography uses low ($\sim$ 30 kVp) energy x-ray beams to take advantage of the increased photoelectric absorption to enhance the small differences between breast tissue and tumor tissue.

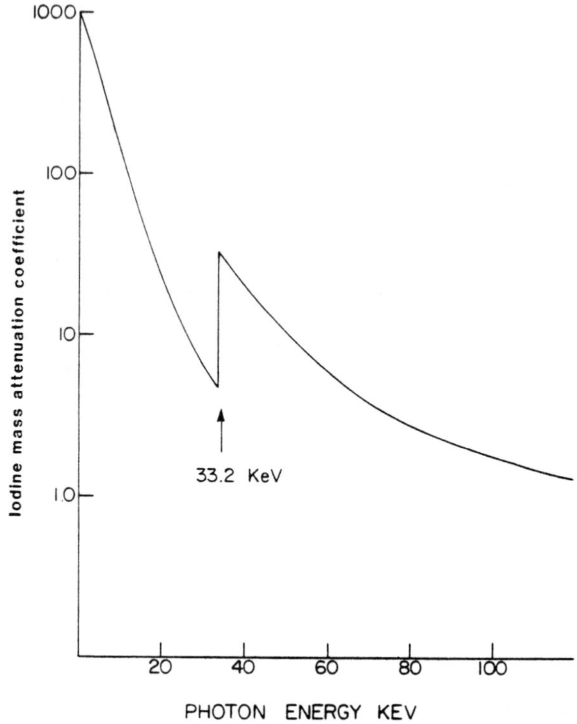

Figure 8.5. Mass attenuation coefficient of iodine as a function of photon energy.

Variation of Photoelectric Effect With Attenuating Material Z

The photoelectric effect mass attenuation coefficient increases with the increasing Z of the attenuating material. This dependence is proportional to Z^3.

In summary, the photoelectron mass absorption coefficient dependence on Z and photon energy is given by Equation 8.8

$$\mu_m = kZ^3/E^3 \qquad 8.8$$

where k is a proprotionality constant.

The energy in equation 8.8 is the **photon energy** (KeV) and not the voltage applied to the x-ray tube (kVp).

Photoelectric absorption is responsible for the major difference in radiographic appearance (contrast) between bone and soft tissue.

Compton Scattering

In Compton scattering, the x–ray photon interacts with a loosely bound outer shell orbital electron as illustrated schematically in Figure 8.6.

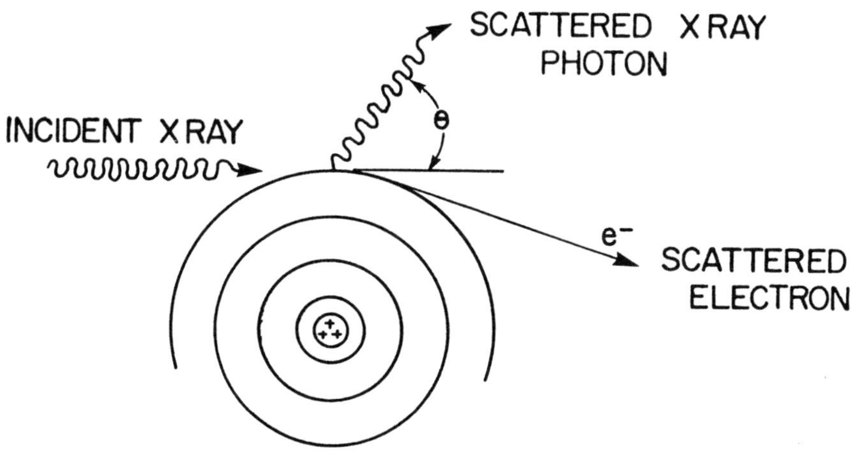

Figure 8.6. Comptom scattering process.

The photon transfers some energy to the electron in the scattering process and proceeds in a different direction with a reduced energy. The binding energy of an orbital electron is so small (a few ev) that it can be ignored compared to the photon energy (KeV). The wavelength of the Compton scattered photon is related to its scattering angle as given in equation 8.9

$$\Delta\lambda = \lambda' - \lambda = .024\,(1 - \cos\theta)\ \text{Å} \qquad 8.9$$

where $1\text{Å} = 10^{-10}$m and $\Delta\lambda$ is the change in wavelength.

The relation between photon energy and wavelength is given by:

$$E = \frac{12.4}{\lambda} \qquad 8.10$$

where E is in KeV and λ is the wavelength in Angstrom (1Å = 10^{-10}m). The change in wavelength (and energy) depends only on the scattering angle. The scattered electrons have ranges in tissue of a fraction of a mm.

Energy Dependence of the Compton Scattering Process

The mass energy absorption coefficient for Compton scattering is linearly dependent on the incident photon energy and is almost completely independent of Z. This is because all materials (except hydrogen) have about the same number of electrons per gram and so the number of orbital outer electrons available for Compton interactions is approximately the same for all materials. Equation 8.11 summarizes the energy dependence of Compton scattering

$$\mu_m = (\mu/\rho)_{Compton} = K/E \qquad 8.11$$

where K is a proportionality constant.

Pair Production

Pair production interactions occur when a high energy photon interacts in the neighborhood of an atomic nucleus to produce a positive electron and a negative electron. The nucleus acts in a manner similar to a catalyst in a chemical reaction. In order for a pair production interaction to occur, the incident photon must have at least twice the rest mass of an electron (0.511MeV). The variation of mass attenuation coefficient for pair production is given by equation 8.12

$$\mu_m = (\mu/\rho)_{Pair\ Production} = K(E-1.02\ MeV) \qquad 8.12$$

where K is a proportionality constant.

Tissue Attenuation

Figure 8.7 presents the photoelectric, Compton and total mass attentuation coefficients for tissue as a function of energy.

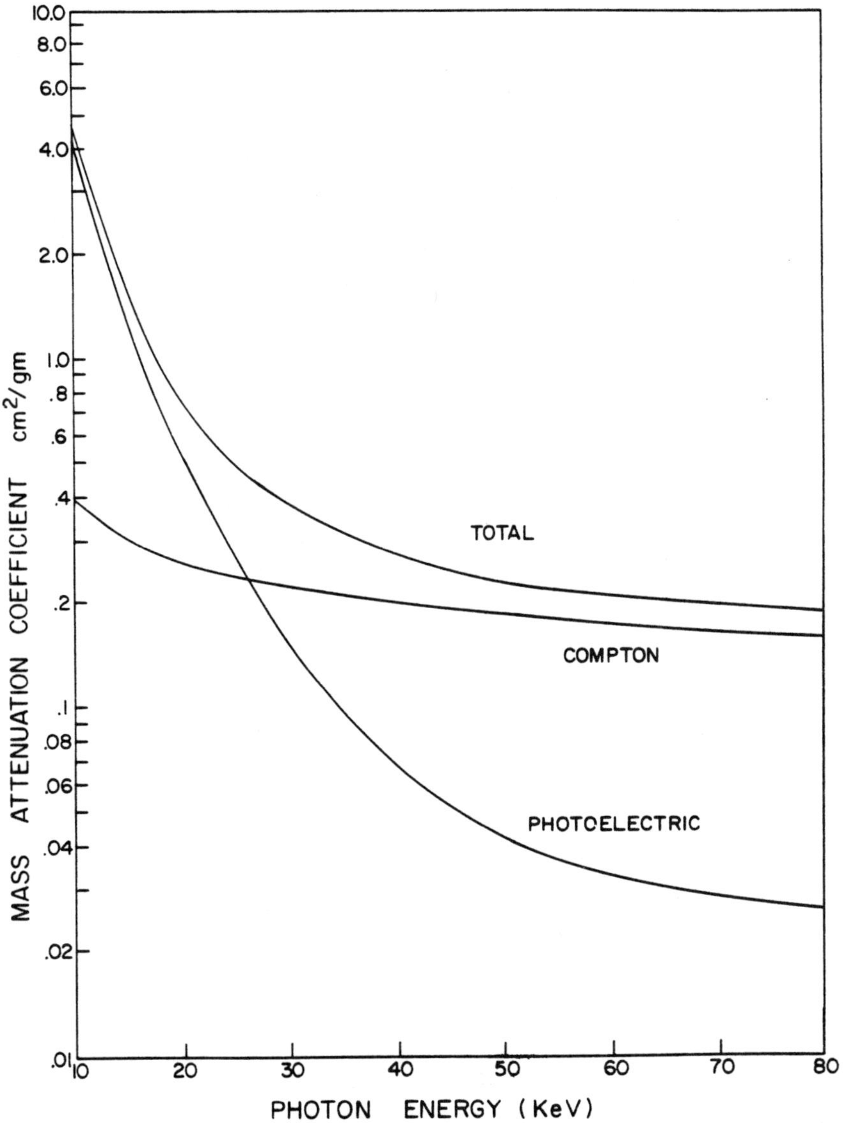

Figure 8.7. Photoelectric, Compton and total mass attenuation coefficients for tissue as a function of energy.

Relative Importance

The relative importance of the photoelectric and Compton interactions can be considered in two ways.

1. The number of interactions
2. The energy transferred in the interactions.

For soft tissue, the relative importance of the photoelectric and Compton interactions is given in Figure 8.8 in terms of the **number oi interactions.** The number of photoelectric and Compton interactions is equal at 26 KeV. The average Z of fat is less than muscle so the **number** of Compton and photoelectric interactions is equal at 20 KeV. For bone with a higher average Z, the **number** of Compton and photoelectric interactions is equal at 40 KeV.

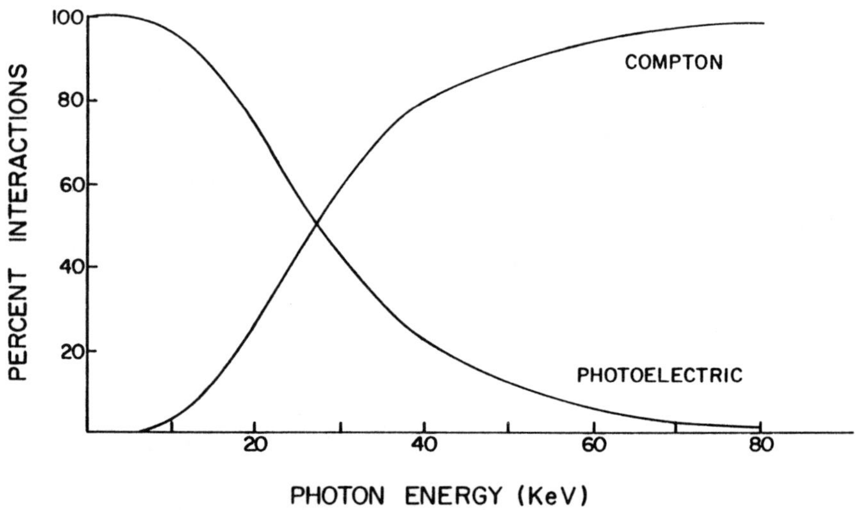

Figure 8.8. Comparison of the number of photoelectric and Compton interactions as a function of photon energy.

The relative importance between Compton and photoelectric interactions in terms of the **energy deposited** is different because a photoelectric interaction absorbs all the incident photon energy. Figure 8.9 presents the relative importance of photoelectric and Compton interactions in energy transfer as a function of photon

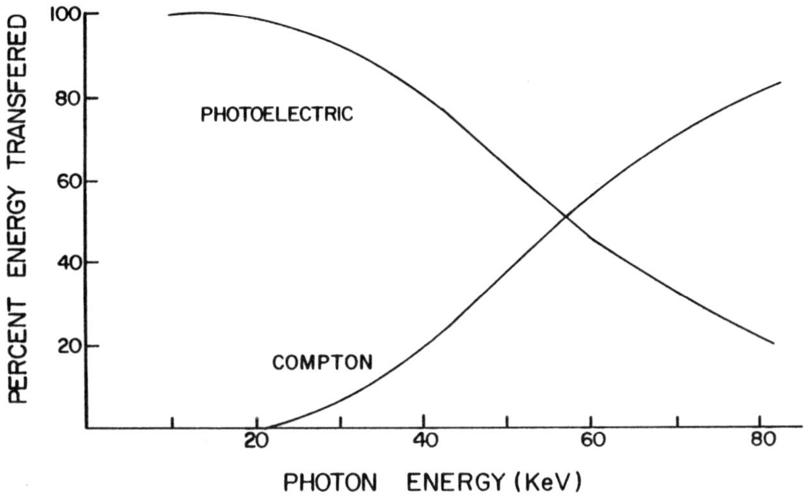

Figure 8.9. Relative energy transferred as a function of photon energy for the photoelectric and Compton interactions.

energy. Note that the energies plotted in Figures 8.8 and 8.9 are photon energies, the corresponding kVp would be between two and three times greater.

Below 50 KeV, the photoelectric process is predominant. Between 50 and 90 KeV, the photoelectric and Compton interactions are both important. Between 100 KeV and 10 MeV, the Compton interaction is predominant. Above 20 MeV pair production interaction is predominant.

Relation Between Exposure and Dose

When an x-ray beam passes through a patient, different tissues absorb different amounts of energy even though they are exposed to the same x-ray beam. This difference in absorption is due to differences in average atomic number and mass attenuation coefficiencies. The **f factor** or rad to roentgen factor shown in Figure 8.10 relates the dose to exposure for different materials. Contrast media such as iodine and barium absorb much more than bone because of their high Z values.

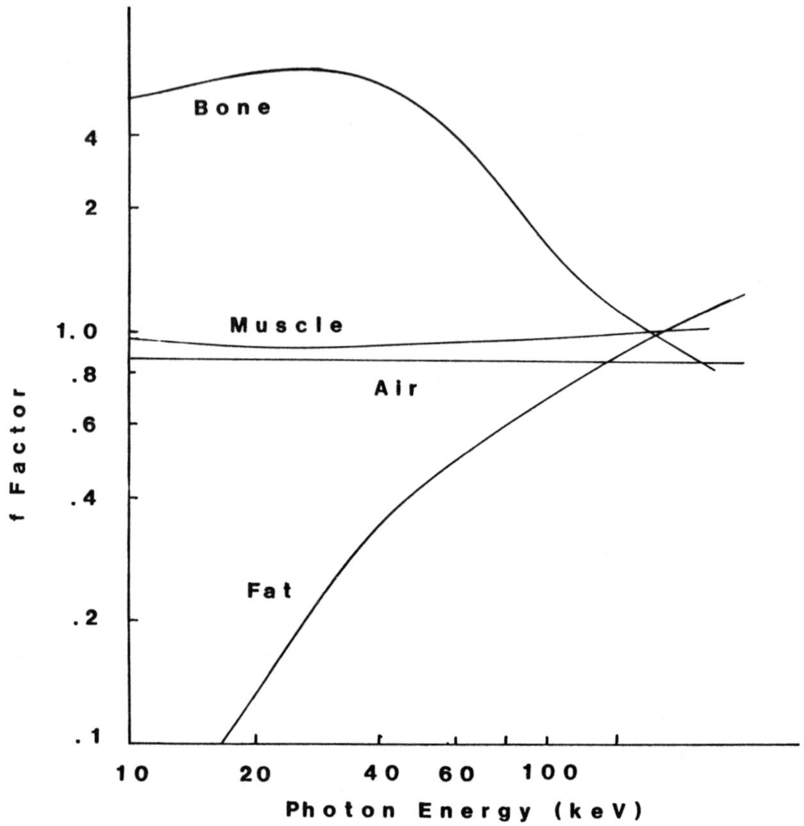

Figure 8.10. The "f" factor which relates dose to exposure as a function of energy for different tissues.

CHAPTER 8 QUESTIONS

1-5, A for True, B for False:

1. Compton scattering is independent of energy.
2. The binding energy of the orbital electron can be neglected in Compton scattering.
3. The energy of the orbital electron cannot be neglected in photoelectric interactions.
4. Photoelectric interactions depend more strongly on Z than Compton interactions.
5. Photoelectric interactions depend more strongly on E than Compton interactions.

6. The second half-value layer in tissue is greater than the first HVL because
   A. the attenuation increases with tissue depth.
   B. the mass attenuation coefficient is constant with tissue depth.
   C. Compton scattering is more important with increasing depth.
   D. the incident beam is heterogeneous.

7. What is the energy of a photoelectron ejected by a 65 KeV photon from a K-shell whose binding energy is 33 KeV?
   A. 95 KeV
   B. 9.5 KeV
   C. 3.2 KeV
   D. 32 KeV

8. The range of a Compton scattered electron in tissue due to a diagnostic x-ray is:
   A. .01 mm
   B. 0.1 mm
   C. 1.0 mm
   D. 10 mm
   E. 100 mm

9. The K edge absorption of iodine (K-shell binding energy 33.2 KeV) will appear

   A. at photon energies of 33.2 KeV and above.
   B. at energies of 33.2 KeV and below.
   C. only at 33.2 KeV energy.
   D. only at energies above 69.5 KeV.

10. The number of Compton and photoelectric interactions in muscle tissue are equal at

    A. 15 KeV
    B. 25 KeV
    C. 35 KeV
    D. 45 KeV
    E. 55 KeV

11. The energy transferred by photoelectric and Compton interactions is equal in muscle at

    A. 25 KeV
    B. 35 KeV
    C. 45 KeV
    D. 55 KeV

12 Compton scattering

   A. involves scattering from inner shell electrons.
   B. involves scattering from outer shell electrons.
   C. involves complete absorption of the incident photon.
   D. involves a change in direction with no change in energy.

13. The energy and Z dependence of Compton scattering can be written as

    A. E
    B. 1/E
    C. Z/E
    D. Z^3/E^3

14. K shell absorption

A. occurs only at energies equal to and below the K shell binding energy.
B. occurs only at energies equal to and above the K shell binding energy.
C. excludes photoelectric interactions.
D. includes Compton interactions.

15. Photoelectric interactions vary as

A. Z^2/E^3
B. E^3/Z^3
C. Z^3/E^2
D. Z^3/E^3

16. Place in order of descending absorbed dose from a 100 kVp exposure.

1. Air
2. Bone
3. Fat
4. Muscle

A. 1, 2, 3, 4
B. 2, 4, 1, 3
C. 2, 1, 4, 3
D. 2, 4, 3, 1

17. What is the first and second HVL of the x-ray beam whose attenuation curve is shown below?

A. 1.0 and 2.5 mm
B. 0.9 and 0.9 mm
C. 0.9 and 1.6 mm
D. 0.9 and 2.5 mm

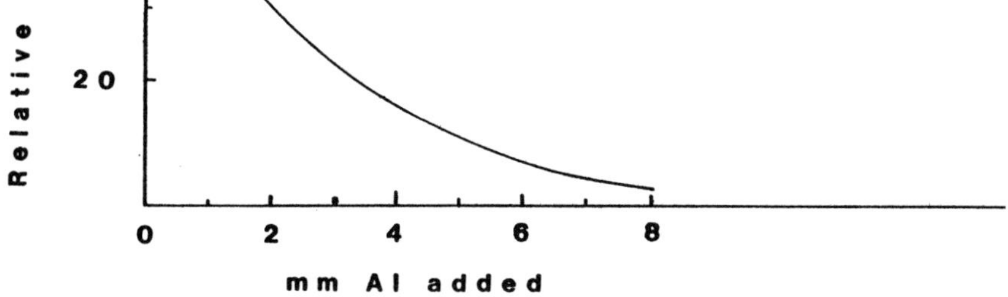

18. Coherent scattering

A. is important at large scattering angles.
B. involves no transfer of energy.
C. involves a change of direction and energy.
D. is important at high energies.

19. Photoelectric absorption

A. involves a change in energy and direction of the incident photon.
B. involves complete absorption of the photoelectron.
C. involves complete absorption of the incident photon.
D. involves ejection of a Compton electron.

20. If the linear attenuation coefficient of a material is 0.2/cm, what is the half-value layer of the material?

A. (0.2) ln 2
B. 0.2/ln 2
C. ln 2/0.2
D. Not enough information given

21. If the mass attenuation coefficient of a material is 0.11 cm^2/gm and the density is 2.7 gm/cm^3, what is the linear attenuation coefficient?

A. 0.297/cm
B. 6.3/cm
C. 24.5/cm
D. 0.041/cm

22. In an x-ray attenuation experiment successive layers of constant thickness x are added to a monoenergetic x-ray beam:

A. The attenuation is constant as the successive thicknesses are added.
B. The transmission is a constant as the successive thicknesses are added.
C. The fractional attenuation is a constant as successive thicknesses are added.
D. The fractional attenuation decreases exponentially as successive thicknesses are added.

23. The second HVL is greater than the first HVL
   A. only for monoenergetic beams
   B. because more long wavelength photons are absorbed in the patient.
   C. because more material must be added to the beam.
   D. because scattered radiation contributes more to the 2nd HVL.

24-25, Adding Al to an x-ray beam produces the following results

Added AL (mm)	Intensity
0	100%
0.5	50%
1.0	40%
2.0	27%
3.0	22%

24. The first HVL is
   A. 0.5
   B. 1.0
   C. 2.5
   D. 2.0

25. The second HVL is
   A. 0.5
   B. 1.0
   C. 2.5
   D. 2.0

26. A material of density 2 gm/cm^3 has a mass attentuation coefficient of 0.3 cm^2/gm. Its linear attentuation coefficient is
   A. 0.6/cm
   B. 0.15/cm
   C. 6.67/cm
   D. 0.693/cm

27. The HVL of the material in problem 26 is
   A. 4.62 cm
   B. 1.16 cm
   C. 0.104 cm
   D. 1.0 cm

28. The photoelectric mass attenuation coefficient of water is 0.004 cm^2/gm. What is the photoelectric mass attenuation coefficient for lead at the same energy if Z water = 8 and Z lead = 82?

A. 400
B. 40
C. 4
D. .4
E. .04

29. A monoenergetic x-ray beam has an absorption of 5% per cm in water. The half-value layer of this beam in water is:

A. 5 cm
B. 6.93 cm
C. 10 cm
D. 13.8 cm

30-32, Identify the particles in the photoelectric interaction.

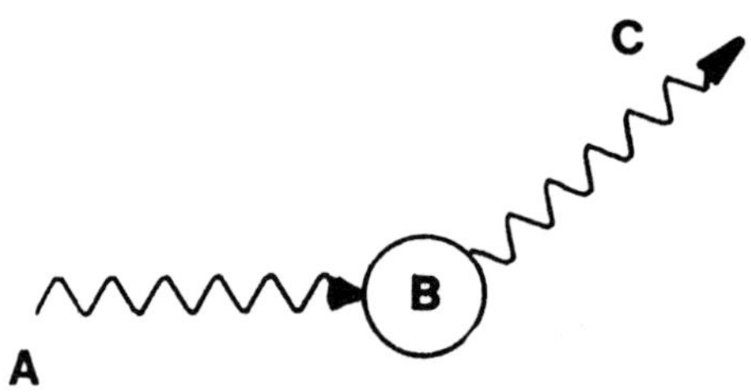

30. Characteristic Radiation
31. Atom
32. Incident Photon

33-36, Identify the radiation and particles in the Compton interaction.

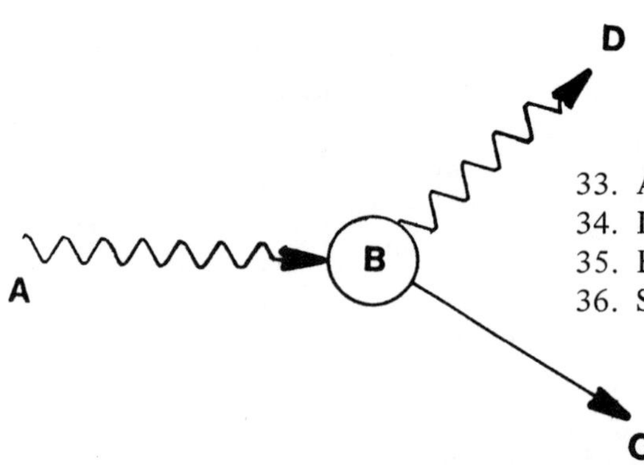

33. Atom
34. Incident Photon
35. Electron
36. Scattered Photon

37–41, Identify the particles and radiation in the pair production interaction.

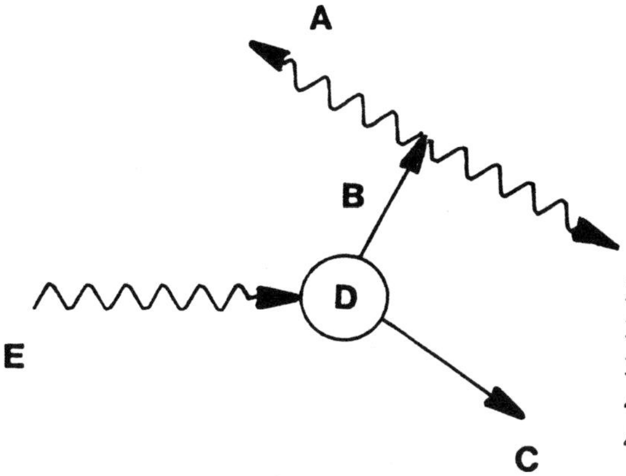

37. Incident Photon
38. Nucleus
39. Electron
40. Positron
41. Annihilation Radiation

CHAPTER 9

STATISTICS

Random Nature of X-rays

If an image intensifier is irradiated with a uniform beam of x-rays and the front face of the image intensifier is divided into a regular arrangement (a matrix) of equal area picture elements (pixels), the number of photons collected in each pixel will not be exactly the same. The number of photons detected follows random statistics. When the exposure is repeated, the number of photons collected in any pixel will be different but the **average** number of photons per pixel will remain the same.

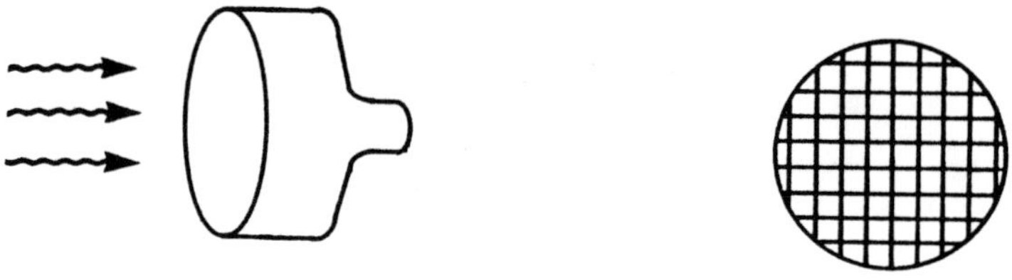

Figure 9.1. Uniform x-ray beam irradiating a detector divided into a matrix of picture elements.

The average value for the number of photons per pixel is obtained by adding up the individual pixel values and dividing by the number of pixels. The **mean** or average value, $\overline{N}$, is given by equation 9.1

$$(N_1 + N_2 + N_3 + N_4 + N_5) / 5 = \overline{N} \qquad 9.1$$

The **modal** value is the most common value. The **median** value is the central value, there are as many numbers greater than the median value as there are less than the median value.

Figure 9.2 shows the **Gaussian** or **Normal** distribution of values from a random process. The number of pixels with **n** counts

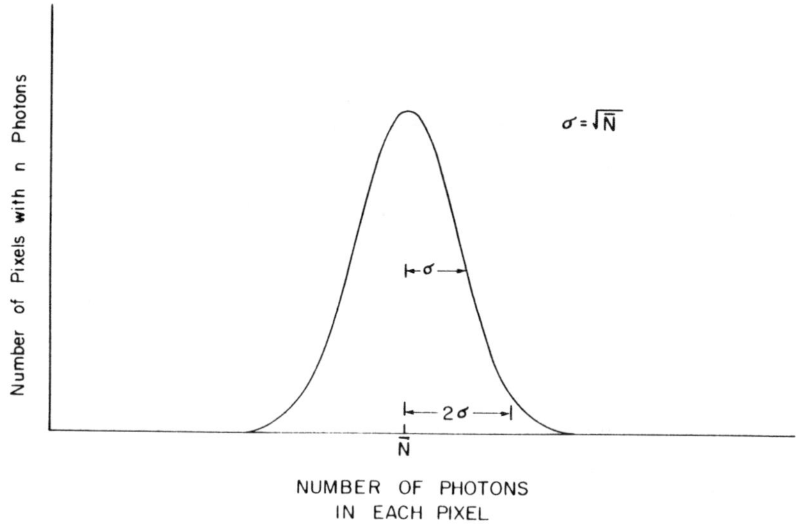

Figure 9.2. Random distribution of photons per pixel.

is plotted as a function of n. All random distributions of photons in Radiology are Gaussian distributions.

If there were no statistical fluctuations, the image intensifier image would be perfectly uniform and it would be easy to see small differences in intensity. Statistical fluctuations, which are always present, mask the signal and make detection tasks more difficult.

The standard deviation σ measures the difference between a particular value, n, and the average value, $\overline{N}$.

The standard deviation σ is given by:

$$\sigma = \sqrt{\overline{N}} \qquad 9.2$$

σ is a way of describing the shape or "fatness" of the distribution curve. Usually, we don't bother measuring enough numbers to find the average value. We assume the first, or only, measurement is the average value. Under this assumption the standard deviation can be approximated by:

$$\sigma = \sqrt{n} \qquad 9.3$$

That is, the number of counts, n, collected in a pixel is assumed to be the average value $\overline{N}$.

In repeated trials of random events the distribution of results is well established. Table 9.1 presents the percentage of measurements which will lie within the various ranges of $\overline{N}$.

TABLE 9.1

PERCENTAGE OF MEASURES WHICH LIE IN SPECIFIED RANGE FOR AN AVERAGE VALUE $\overline{N}$ AND A STANDARD DEVIATION σ

Range	*Measurements Which Lie Within the Range*
$\overline{N} \pm \sigma$	68%
$\overline{N} \pm 2\sigma$	95%
$\overline{N} \pm 3\sigma$	99%

As an example consider a situation where an average of 1,000 counts are recorded. This might be the number of gamma rays emitted in a specific time period, it might be the number of photons collected per detector or the number of photons per pixel in one exposure.

What number will be collected on the next try? It's not possible to predict the number exactly but 68% of the time the next number will lie in the range between 968 and 1,032; 95% of the time it will lie in the range between 937 and 1,063 and 99% of the time it will lie between 905 and 1,095. Although we cannot predict exactly what the next value will be we can make a good estimate of its probable value, or at least the range it will lie in.

Percent Standard Deviation

It's common to use not only the standard deviation but the percentage standard deviation in discussing image noise. The percent standard deviation is given by:

$$\%\sigma = \frac{\sigma}{n} \times 100 \qquad 9.4$$

$$\%\sigma = \frac{\sqrt{n}}{n} \times 100$$

This variation of the number of photons collected is called the **quantum noise** or the **statistical noise** of the system. It is caused by the random fluctuations in x–ray emission and detection.

Example 9.1:
What is the standard deviation and percent standard deviation if 6,400 counts are collected?

The standard deviation is given by:

$$\sigma = \sqrt{6400}$$

$$\sigma = \pm 80$$

The percent standard deviation is given by:

$$\%\sigma = \frac{\sigma}{6400} \times 100$$

$$\%\sigma = \frac{80}{6400} \times 100$$

$$\%\sigma = 1.25\%$$

Example 9.2:
What is the percent noise in an imaging system where an average of 1500 counts per pixel per exposure are collected?

$$\sigma = \sqrt{1500}$$

$$\sigma = 38.7$$

$$\%\sigma = \frac{38.7}{1500} \times 100$$

$$\%\sigma = 2.6\%$$

As more counts are collected the standard deviation increases but the percentage standard deviation or statistical noise decreases and the reliability of the measure improves. Table 9.2 indicates how the standard deviation increases and the percentage standard deviation or statistical noise decreases as more counts are collected.

Number of Counts Required for a Given Noise Level

It is possible to calculate how many counts must be collected to achieve a certain noise level.

TABLE 9.2

VARIATION OF σ AND $\%\sigma$ WITH TOTAL NUMBER n OF COUNTS COLLECTED

n	σ	$\%\sigma$
100	10	10%
1,000	30	3%
2,500	50	2%
10,000	100	1%

Example 9.3:
How many counts must be collected per pixel per exposure to achieve a 5% statistical uncertainty (noise level) at the 95% confidence level?

5% noise at the 68% confidence level would be:

$$\frac{\sigma}{n} = .05$$

For 95% confidence level, we have (from Table 9.1):

$$\frac{2\sigma}{n} = .05$$

then

$$\frac{2\sqrt{n}}{n} = .05$$

$$\frac{2}{\sqrt{n}} = .05$$

$$\sqrt{n} = 2/.05$$

$$\sqrt{n} = 40$$

$$n = 1600 \text{ counts}$$

Combination of Uncertainties

A common application of digital imaging is Digital Subtraction Angiography (DSA) where a mask image of the patient is stored, followed by contrast image storage after the contrast has been introduced into the patient. The two images are subtracted pixel by pixel and the difference image is displayed. The subtraction image will contain more uncertainty (noise) than either the mask or the contrast images.

If the Mask image contains m photons per pixel

and

the Contrast image contains c photons per pixel

the subtraction image will have

$$s = m - c \text{ photons/pixel} \tag{9.5}$$

the uncertainty in c is

$$\sigma_c = \sqrt{c}$$

and the uncertainty in m is

$$\sigma_m = \sqrt{m}$$

and the uncertainty in the subtraction image s is given by:

$$\sigma_s = \sqrt{\sigma_c^2 + \sigma_m^2} \tag{9.6}$$

and the percentage uncertainty in s is:

$$\%\sigma_s = \frac{\sigma_s}{s} \times 100$$

Note that if

$$C = A + B$$

or

$$C = A - B$$

then

$$\sigma_C = \sqrt{\sigma_A^2 + \sigma_B^2} \tag{9.7}$$

Note that the uncertainty, σ, is always formed as the square root of the **sum** of the two measured values.

Example 9.4:
What is the average number of photons per pixel value and the noise level (percentage uncertainty σ) in the subtracted image if the mask image has 1600 photons/pixel and the contrast image has 1100 photons/pixel?

$$s = 1600 - 1100$$

$$s = 500$$

$$\sigma_s = \sqrt{\sigma_m{}^2 + \sigma_c{}^2}$$

$$\sigma_s = \sqrt{1600 + 1100}$$

$$\sigma_s = 52$$

$$\text{Noise Level} = \%\sigma_s$$

$$\%\sigma = \frac{\sigma_s}{s}$$

$$\%\sigma = \frac{52}{500} \times 100$$

$$\%\sigma_s = 10\%$$

Example 9.5:
What is the value of the net counts, the uncertainty and the percentage uncertainty in the net counts if 7000 gross counts are collected and the background is 2300 counts?

The Net count value is:

$$N = 7000 - 2300$$

$$N = 4700 \text{ counts}$$

The uncertainty, σ, is:

$$\sigma = \sqrt{7000 + 2300}$$

$$\sigma = 96.4$$

and the Percentage Uncertainty is

$$\%\sigma = \frac{96.4}{4700} \times 100$$

$$\%\sigma = 2.05\%$$

Uncertainty in Count Rates

The statistical uncertainty in count rate experiments is calculated assuming there is no random uncertainty in the time measurement. The count rate R is given by:

$$R = N/t \tag{9.8}$$

where N is the total number of counts collected in time t. The uncertainty in the count rate is given by:

$$\sigma_{cr} = \sqrt{\frac{R}{t}} \tag{9.9}$$

Note that both R and t are under the square root sign.

Example 9.6:
What is the Net Count Rate and the uncertainty in the Net Count Rate if 15,000 counts are collected in 10 minutes and 4500 background counts are collected in 20 minutes?

$$\text{Gross Count Rate G} = \frac{15{,}000}{10} = 1500 \text{ counts/min}$$

$$\text{Background Count Rate B} = \frac{4500}{20} = 225 \text{ counts/min}$$

$$\text{Net Count Rate cr} = 1500 - 225$$

$$cr = 1275 \text{ counts/min}$$

$$\sigma_{cr} = \sqrt{\sigma_G{}^2 + \sigma_B{}^2}$$

$$\sigma_{cr} = \sqrt{\frac{1500}{10} + \frac{225}{20}}$$

$$\sigma_{cr} = \sqrt{150 + 11}$$

$$\sigma_{cr} = \sqrt{161}$$

$$\sigma_{cr} = 12.7$$

Thus the net count rate and associated uncertainty is:

$$R_{net} = 1275 \pm 13$$

The percentage uncertainty is:

$$\%\sigma_{cr} = \frac{12.7}{1275} \text{ x } 100 = 1\%$$

Time to Count

Equation 9.8 can be used to calculate the time required to collect enough counts to achieve a given noise level.

Example 9.7:
What counting time is required to determine a count rate of 1800 cpm to within ± 1.5% at the 95% confidence level?

For 68% confidence level:

$$\frac{\sigma}{R} = .015$$

$$\sigma = .015 \text{ x } 1800$$

$$\sigma = 27$$

For 95% confidence level:

$$\frac{2\sigma}{R} = .015$$

$$2\sigma = 1800 \text{ x } .015$$

$$2\sigma = 27$$

and

$$\sigma = 13.5$$

For count rates:

$$\sigma = \sqrt{\frac{R}{t}}$$

or

$$\sigma = \sqrt{\frac{1800}{t}}$$

$$13.5 = \sqrt{\frac{1800}{t}}$$

Squaring both sides we have:

$$182.25 = 1800/t$$

or

$$t = 1800/182.25$$

$$t = 9.9 \text{ min}$$

That is, we would have to count for 9.9 minutes to measure a count rate of 1800 cpm to 1.5% uncertainty at the 95% confidence level.

CHAPTER 9 QUESTIONS

Find the standard deviation of the following number of counts:

1. 100
2. 1000
3. 3000
4. 960
5. 10,000
6. 200
7. 22
8. 850
9. 5800
10. 22,000

Find the percent standard deviation of the following number of counts:

11. 100
12. 1000
13. 10,000
14. 960
15. 3000
16. 200
17. 22,000
18. 800
19. 650
20. 1700

Find the count rate and standard deviation:

21. 6000 counts in 2 min
22. 8000 counts in 3 min
23. 10,000 counts in 5 min
24. 1600 counts in 0.8 min
25. 10,000 counts in 2 min
26. 100,000 counts in 5 min
27. 14,000 counts in 10 min
28. 7500 counts in 1.5 min
29. 41,900 counts in 3 min
30. 2200 counts in 1.5 min

Find the net counts and percent uncertainty for:

31. 5000 gross and 1300 background counts
32. 10,000 gross and 3000 background counts
33. 7500 gross and 2700 background counts
34. 12,800 gross and 5500 background counts
35. 1400 gross and 460 background counts

36. How long must we count to determine a count rate of approximately 2500 cpm to 3% uncertainty?

37. How long must we count to determine a count rate of approximately 3000 cpm to 1.5% uncertainty at the 95% confidence level?

38. How long must we count to determine a count rate of approximately 1200 cpm to 2% uncertainty at the 99% confidence level?

39. How long must we count to determine a count rate of approximately 1200 cpm to an uncertainty of 2% at the 95% confidence level?

40. How long must we count to determine a count rate of approximately 1200 cpm to an uncertainty of 2%?

41. The mean value is

A. formed by dividing the sum of the individual values by the number of values.
B. formed by dividing the number of values by their sum.
C. the most common value.
D. the central value.

42. The modal value is

A. formed by dividing the sum of the individual values by the number of values.
B. formed by dividing the number of values by their sum.
C. the most common value.
D. The central value.

43. The median value is

A. formed by dividing the sum of the individual values by the number of values.
B. formed by dividing the number of values by their sum.
C. the most common value.
D. the central value.

44. If N counts are collected the standard deviation is given by:

A. $\sqrt{N}$
B. $\sqrt{N}/N$
C. N^2
D. $\sqrt{N^2}/N$

45. In a series of measurements 95% will lie in the range:

A. $N \pm \sigma$
B. $N \pm 2\sigma$
C. $N \pm 3\sigma$
D. $N \pm 1/\sigma$

46. If N counts are collected, the percent standard deviation is:

A. $N^2 \times 100$
B. $N \times 100$
C. $(\sqrt{N}/N) \times 100$
D. $(\sqrt{N^2}/N) \times 100$

47. What is the percent noise in a system where 1800 counts/pixel are collected?

A. 42.4
B. 42.4%
C. 0.24%
D. 2.4%

CHAPTER 10

CONTRAST AND IMAGE FORMATION

Image quality is a measure of the ability of an image to provide diagnostic information to a trained observer. Image quality is determined by:

I. Contrast
II. Resolution

Image Contrast

Image contrast, also called **Radiographic Contrast** depends on:

1. Subject contrast
2. Scatter
3. Display contrast

Subject Contrast

The x–ray image is formed because of differences in x–ray transmission through various parts of the object.

The **Subject Contrast** is defined as the absolute value of the difference between the intensity of the x–ray beam passing through an object (I_o) and the surrounding material (I_b) divided by the intensity of the beam passing through the surrounding material; (I_b). Subject contrast can be calculated using Equation 10.1.

$$C = \left| \frac{I_o - I_b}{I_b} \right| \times 100 \qquad 10.1$$

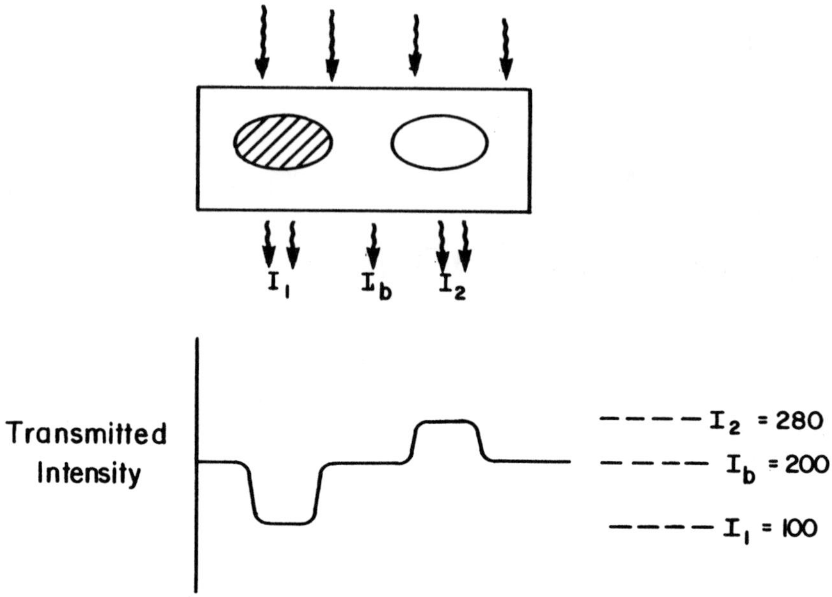

Figure 10.1. Subject contrast.

Example 10.1:
In the example shown in Figure 10.1, the contrast of object 1 can be calculated as:

$$C_1 = \left| \frac{200 - 100}{200} \right| \times 100$$

$$C_1 = 50\%$$

and the contrast of object 2 is given as:

$$C_2 = \left| \frac{280 - 200}{200} \right| \times 100$$

$$C_2 = 40\%$$

Subject contrast depends on:

1. Thickness
2. Density
3. Material
4. kVp and Beam Filtration

Thickness

Thicker objects have greater contrast than thinner objects of the same composition.

Density

Objects with greater density have greater contrast than less dense objects with the same composition.

Material

Objects with a higher atomic number (Z) have a higher contrast than objects with a lower atomic number. How much difference will depend on the kVp and filtration of the x-ray beam. In many cases, it is possible to improve subject contrast by adding contrast material. Table 10.1 lists the average atomic number (Z) and the density of some common tissue and contrast materials.

TABLE 10.1

AVERAGE ATOMIC NUMBER AND DENSITY FOR TISSUE AND CONTRAST MATERIALS

Material	*Average Atomic Number*	*Density, g/cm^3*
Fat	5.9	0.91
Muscle	7.4	1.0
Water	7.4	1.0
Air	7.6	0.0013
Bone	13.8	1.8
Iodine	53	4.9
Barium	56	3.5

Variation of Subject Contrast with kVp

Subject contrast decreases with increased kVp.

Higher kVp x-rays have greater penetrating ability because the absorption coefficient decreases with increasing energy. With higher kVp, the differences in absorption are smaller and there are more Compton than photoelectric interactions. Figure 10.2 illustrates the decrease in subject contrast with increased kVp for the same number of photons incident on the detector.

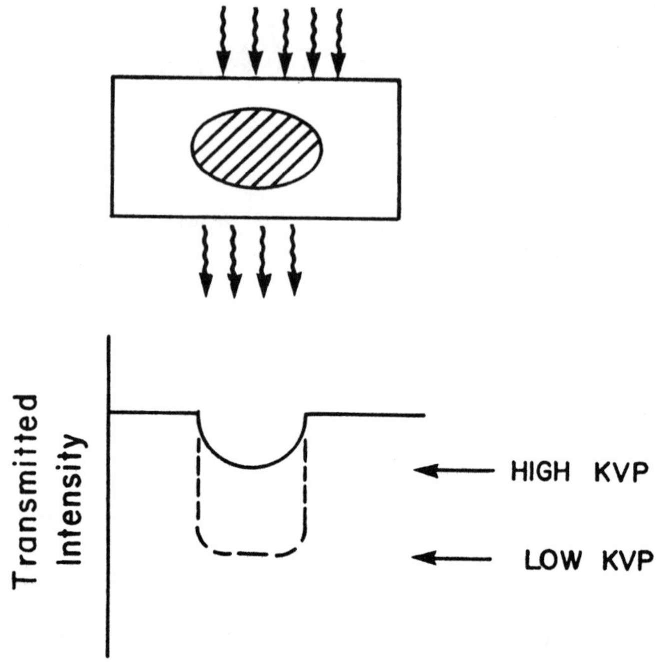

Figure 10.2 Contrast with high and low kVp techniques.

Long and Short Contrast Scales

Figure 10.3 illustrates the penetration of an aluminum step wedge at 70 and 120 kVp. Notice that the low kVp technique produces high contrast over a few number of steps. This is known as **short scale** radiography because there are few steps between black and white. Higher kVp techniques result in less contrast between steps but include more steps in the useful density range. This is known as **long scale** radiography. Long scale radiography is more "forgiving" because the technical factors do not have to be exactly correct to produce an acceptable radiograph. Long scale radiography has a greater latitude. Figures 10.4 A and B present two chest radiographs taken at 70 and 120 kVp. Note the greater contrast in the 70 kVp radiograph. The sternum and heart shadows are completely white and the apices of the lungs are black. The 120 kVp radiograph shows some spinal structures and the lung apices are not completely black.

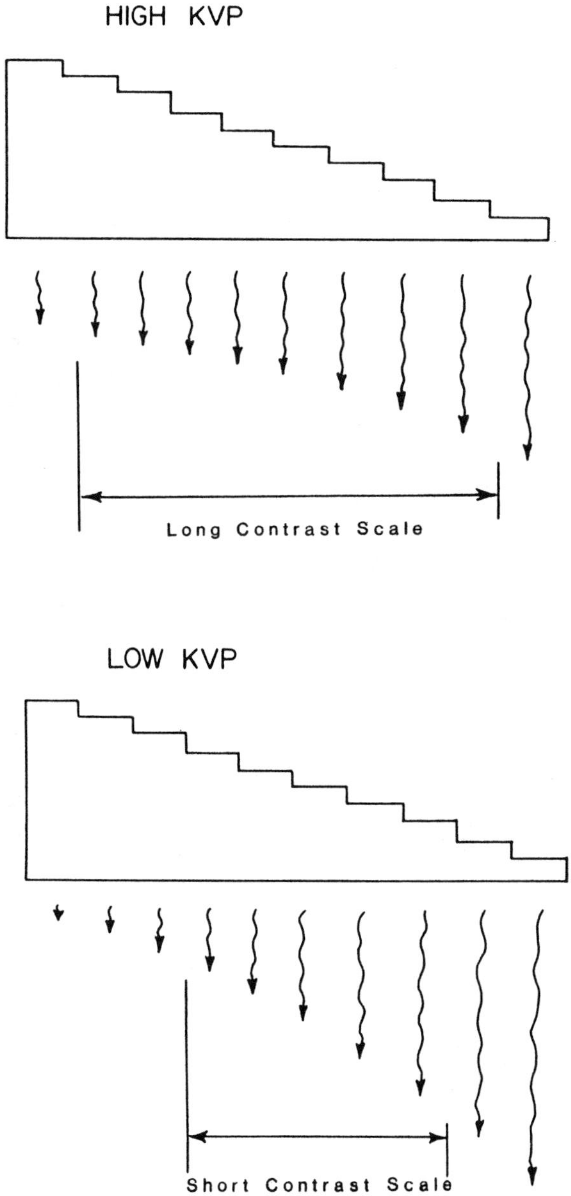

Figure 10.3. High and low kVp exposures of a step wedge produce long and short scale radiographs.

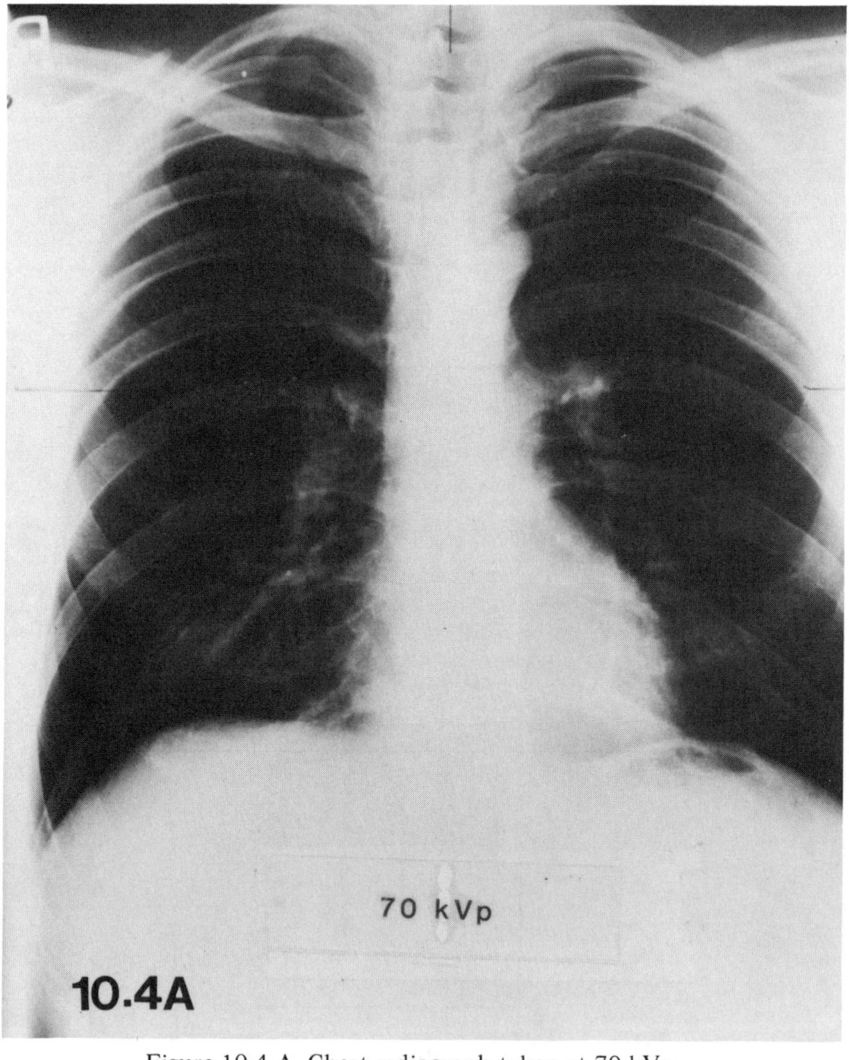

Figure 10.4.A. Chest radiograph taken at 70 kVp.

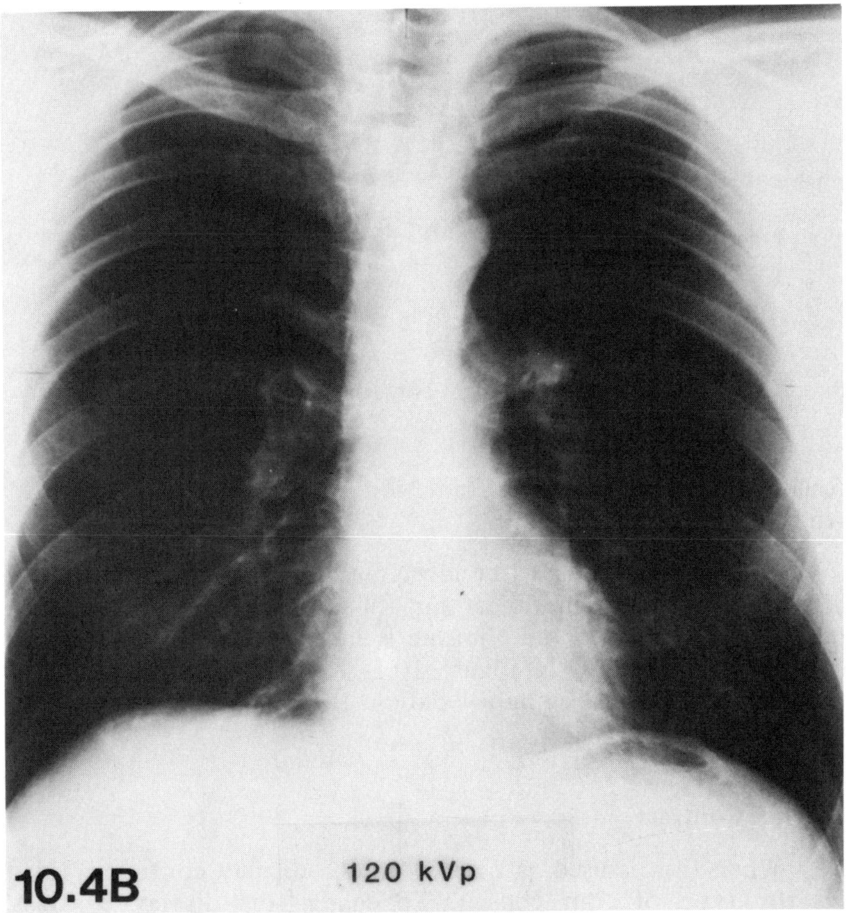

Figure 10.4.B. Chest radiography taken at 120 kVp.

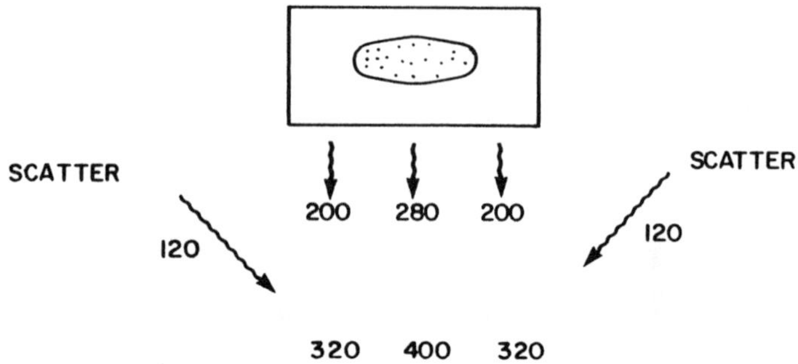

Without Scatter

$$C = \left| \frac{280 - 200}{200} \right| \times 100$$

$$C = 40\%$$

With Scatter

$$C = \left| \frac{400 - 320}{320} \right| \times 100$$

$$C = 25\%$$

Figure 10.5. Effect of scatter on contrast

Relation Between Scattered Radiation And Image Contrast

The presence of scatter always reduces image contrast. The difference between the object and the surround remains the same but the total number of photons is increased. This reduction in contrast is illustrated in Figure 10.5. If 60% scatter is added to the radiation beam leaving the patient the contrast decreases from 40% to 25%.

Display Contrast

When film is used as a detector, the display contrast is fixed by the type of film chosen. To change the display contrast, another film type must be used. With CT and Digital imaging the detection and display functions are completely separate. The display can be modified at any time after the image data have been collected.

All video display systems are limited by the number of brightness steps between light and dark. Two controls are used to alter the display within this range – the **level** and **window** controls.

Level Control

The level control selects the x-ray transmission value to be displayed as black. All transmission values less than the selected value are also displayed as black.

Window Control

The window control determines how many transmission values are required to change the display from black to white. The window control alters the display contrast scale or latitude. Figure 10.6 illustrates how changes in level and window controls modify the appearance of the final image.

Spatial Resolution

Spatial resolution of an imaging system is defined as the separation at which two objects can just be distinguished as two distinct objects rather than one. Spatial resolution is measured in line pairs/mm (lp/mm). In any actual imaging system, a point will be imaged as a spot because of **unsharpness** or **blur** in the imaging system.

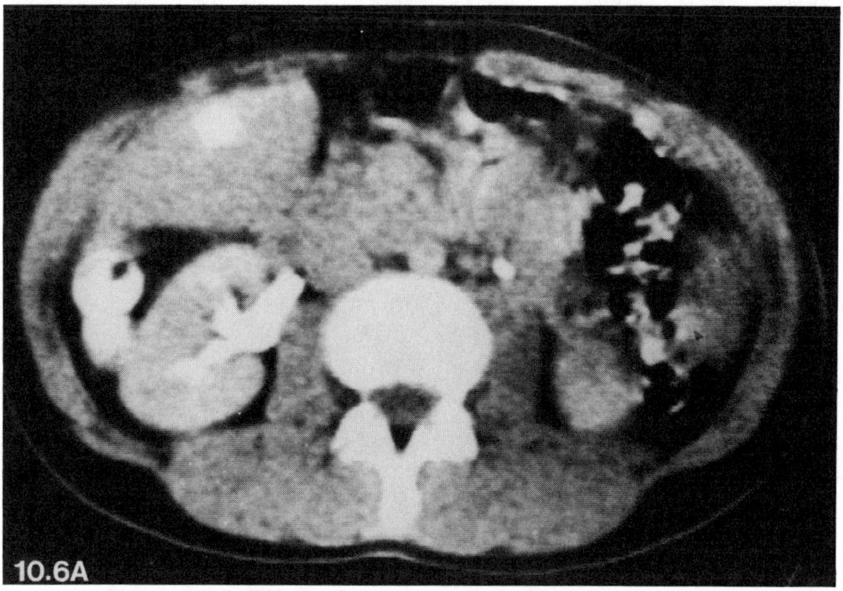

Figure 10.6. Effect of changing window and level controls.

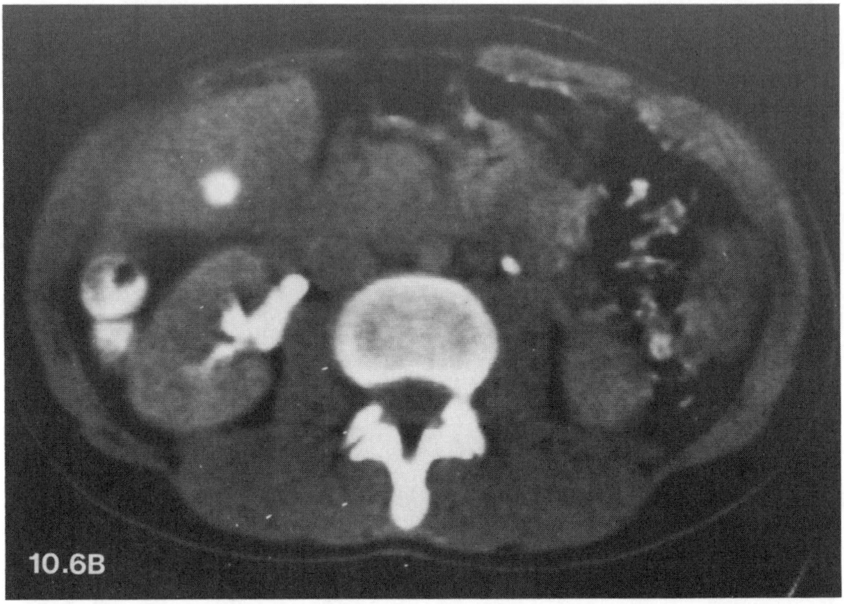
10.6B

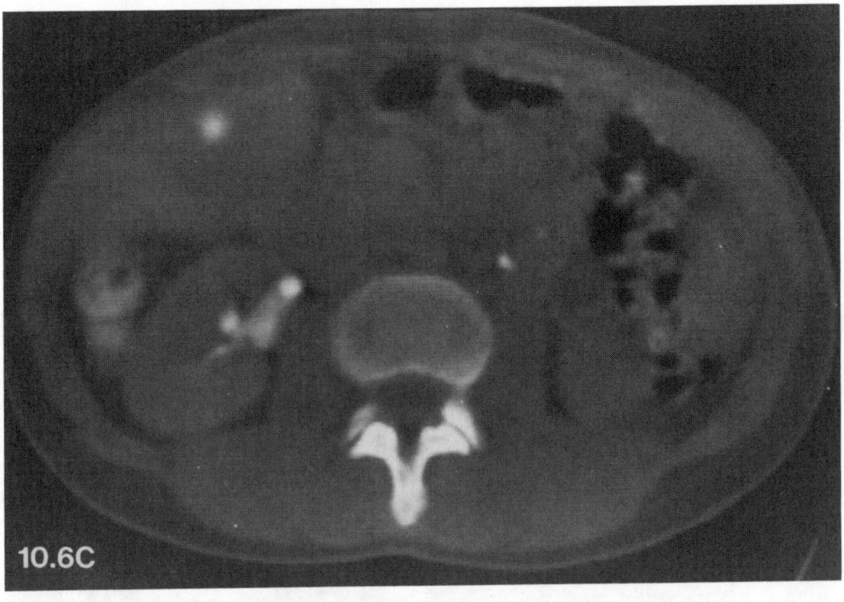
10.6C

Figure 10.7 illustrates the image formation of two adjacent objects under an ideal and an actual imaging system. Notice that blurring spreads out the edges so that the image is wider than the object and blurring also reduces the contrast.

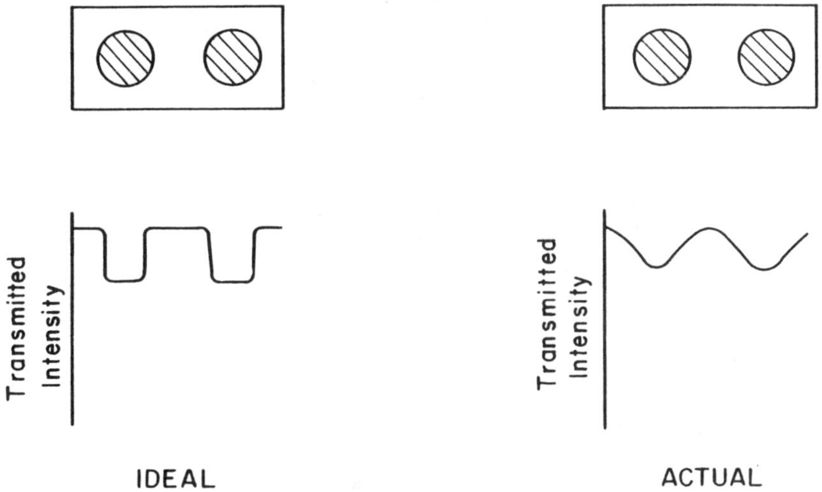

Figure 10.7. Ideal and actual transmission intensities.

The resolution of an imaging system can be measured by radiographing a test object whose lines are varying distances apart and determining how many line pairs per millimeter can be seen. Figure 10.8 is a radiograph of a typical test object constructed of lead strips so that the image is a high contrast image.

One line pair consists of one dark and one light line. Two objects separated by a distance equal to half the reciprocal (one over) of the resolution in lp/mm can just be resolved as two objects. Table 10.2 gives some resolutions in lp/mm and minimum separation distances.

Sources of Unsharpness

There are four major sources of unsharpness in radiography.

1. focal spot penumbra
2. absorption blur
3. motion blur
4. detector blur

Figure 10.8. Resolution bar pattern.

TABLE 10.2

Resolution 1p/mm	*Minimum Separation Distance mm*
0.25	2.0
0.5	1.0
1	0.5
2	0.25
5	0.1

Focal Spot Penumbra

Focal spot penumbra blurs the edges of objects to be imaged.

Figure 10.9 illustrates how the edge of an object is blurred out because of the finite size of the focal spot. A smaller focal spot produces a smaller penumbra and is required to image smaller objects.

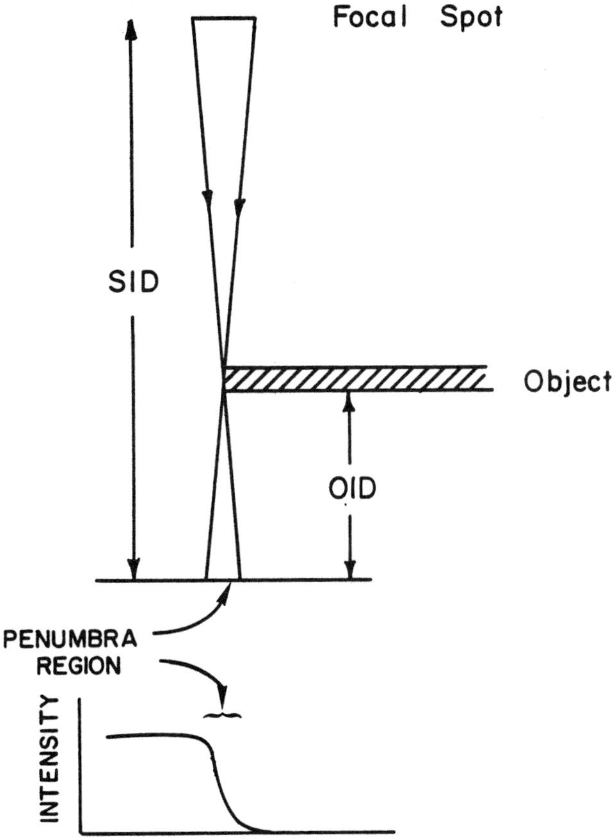

Figure 10.9. Relation between the size of penumbra blur, and focal spot size, source image distance and object image distance.

The size of the penumbra P is given by:

$$P = f \times \frac{OID}{SID - OID} \qquad 10.2$$

where P is the size of the penumbra in mm, f is the focal spot size in mm, SID is the Source-Image-Distance and OID is the Object-Image-distance. Smaller focal spots are required for small penumbra.

Example 10.2:
What is the size of the penumbra blur in a radiograph taken with

a 2 mm focal spot if the SID is 40" (102 cm) and the object is 10" (25 cm) from the film?

$$P = 2 \times \frac{10}{30} = 0.67 \text{ cm}$$

Absorption Blurring

Figure 10.10 illustrates how the edges of a circular or elliptical object are blurred because of decreased absorption near the thinner edges.

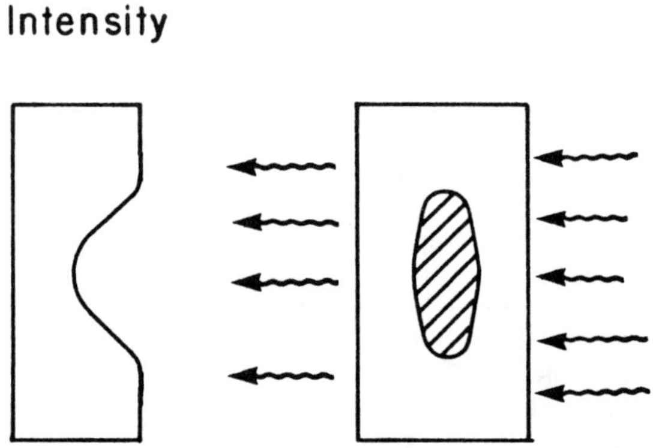

Figure 10.10 Absorption blurring is produced by different object thickness near the edges.

Motion Blur

Motion blur occurs due to motion of the object being imaged. Some motions such as cardiac and peristalic motion are impossible to stop. Motion blur is reduced by decreasing the exposure time. Motion blur is equal to the velocity of the object times the exposure time.

$$B = V \times t \qquad 10.3$$

Example 10.3:
What is the blurring of a cardiac image if the heart wall moves with a velocity of 15 cm/s and the exposure time is 0.1 seconds?

$$\text{Blur} = 15 \frac{\text{cm}}{\text{s}} \times 0.1 \text{ s} = 1.5 \text{ cm}$$

Chest radiographs should be taken with exposure times of 0.030 s or less to eliminate cardiac motion blurring.

Detector Blur

Detector blur is produced by spaces between the detectors or by diffusion of light from the intensifying screens. In either case, it may be impossible to resolve two nearby objects of detector limitations.

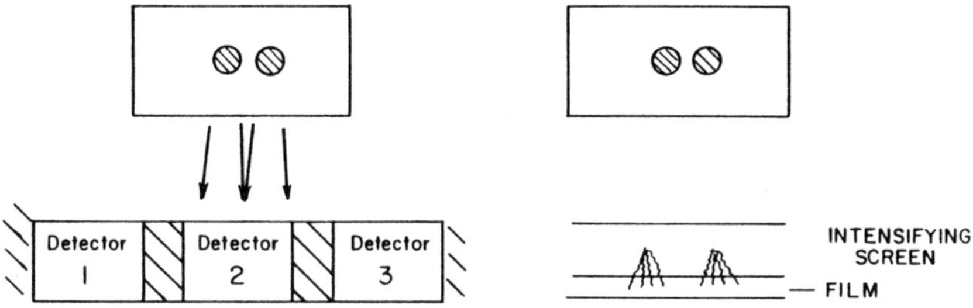

Figure 10.11. Detector blurring produced either by interdetector spaces of diffusion of light from intensifying screens.

Image Quality

The quality of an imaging system can be measured by forming an image of a thin line in a lead plate. With no blurring, the image would be a line. The image will be blurred as shown in Figure 10.12 by all the blurring factors.

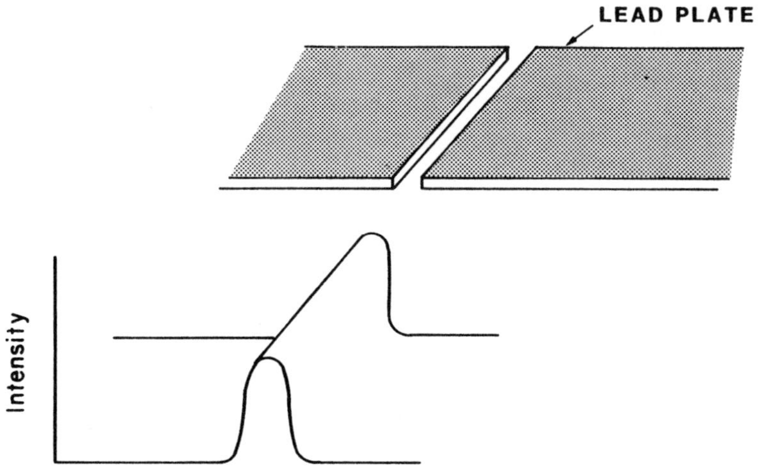

Figure 10.12. Transmission of x-rays through a thin line in a lead plate to form a blurred image of the line.

By measuring the amount of blurring the **Line Spread Function** can be used to calculate the **Modulation Transfer Function.**

Modulation Transfer Function

The imaging characteristics of a system can be described by the modulation transfer function (MTF). This describes the ability of the imaging system to transfer the input signal characteristics (the modulation) to the output signal.

The MTF of an imaging system is analogous to the frequency response curve of an audio system. The **MTF** is expressed in terms of **spatial frequencies** and has units of line pairs/mm.

The output (image) depends not only on the object being radiographed but on the imaging system used. The imaging system may be able to faithfully reproduce the large (low frequency) parts of the object but may not be able to reproduce the fine detail (high spatial frequency) parts of the object. The characteristics of the output depend on the frequency (lp/mm) response of the imaging system.

Figure 10.13 illustrates a typical MTF curve for an image detector. 100% MTF means that the modulation is transferred

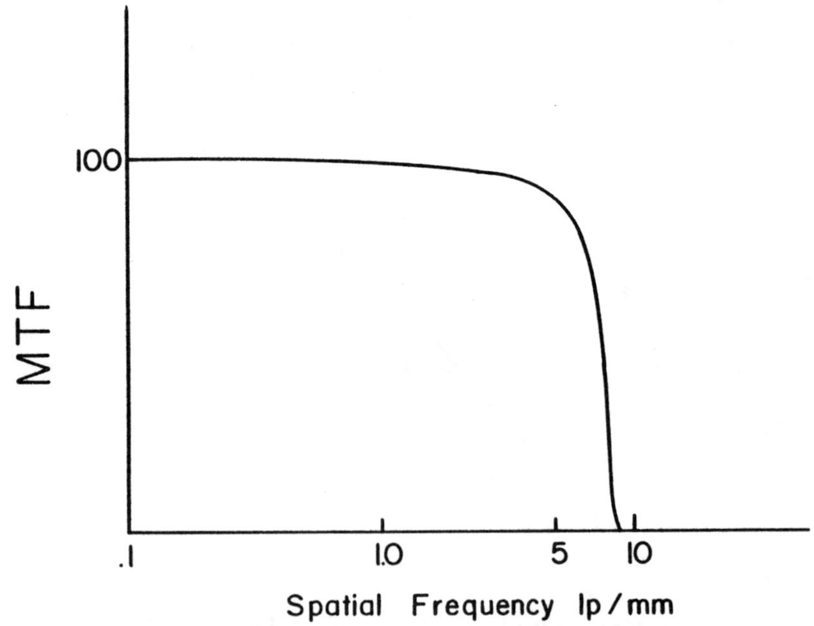

Figure 10.13. Modulation transfer function of a detector.

from the input to the output with 100% amplitude. 50% MTF at 7 lp/mm means that the output amplitude of a 7 lp/mm signal will be 50% of the input amplitude. With the system shown in Figure 10.13, all information at frequencies below 5 lp/mm is reproduced faithfully in the output. The response begins to fall off above 5 lp/mm and no information is transferred above 10 lp/mm. Essentially, no information is transferred at MTF values lower than 0.1.

Combination of MTF Values

The advantage of the MTF is that individual MTF's of the components in an imaging system can be individually measured. The final MTF of the overall system can be obtained by multiplying the MTF of the various components together. Figure 10.14 illustrates the combination of MTF values of the electron optics and input and output phosphors to obtain a final MTF value for a typical fluoroscopic image intensifier system.

Inspection of Figure 10.14 indicates that improvements in the electron optics or output phosphor would not be noticeable in the overall performance of the image intensifier. Any significant improvements in performance could come only through improving the characteristics of the input phosphor.

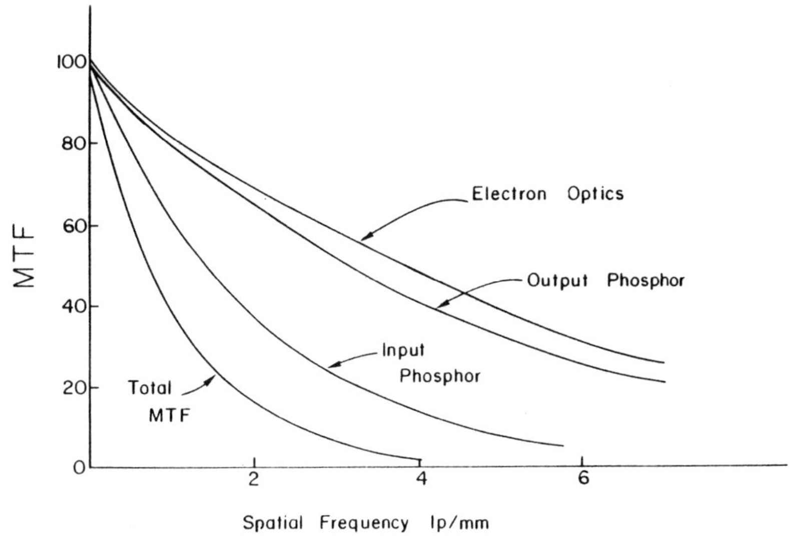

Figure 10.14. MTF of an image intensifier system.

Observer Performance Measures of Image Quality

Regardless of how many physical measures of the image quality are made, the most important property of the image is how well it conveys diagnostic information to the Radiologist. There are two important observei performance measures of image quality:

Contrast Detail Tests
ROC Tests

Contrast Detail Tests

Contrast detail tests consist of asking observers to indicate the smallest diameter (detail) which can be seen at a given contrast. Figure 10.15 illustrates a typical contrast detail test pattern.

The different groups of data have different patterns. The test pattern is imaged with two different imaging systems and the images are presented to a group of observers. Figure 10.16 presents the results of one comparison of two systems.

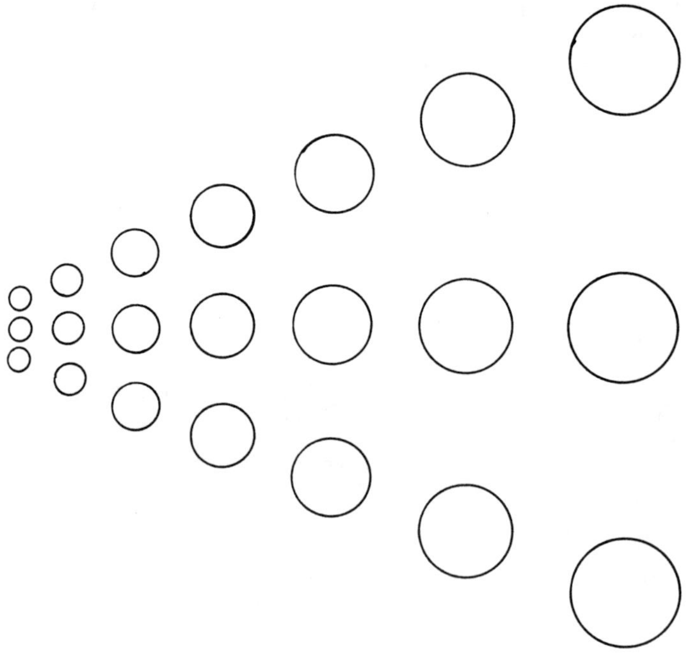

Figure 10.15. Contrast detail test pattern.

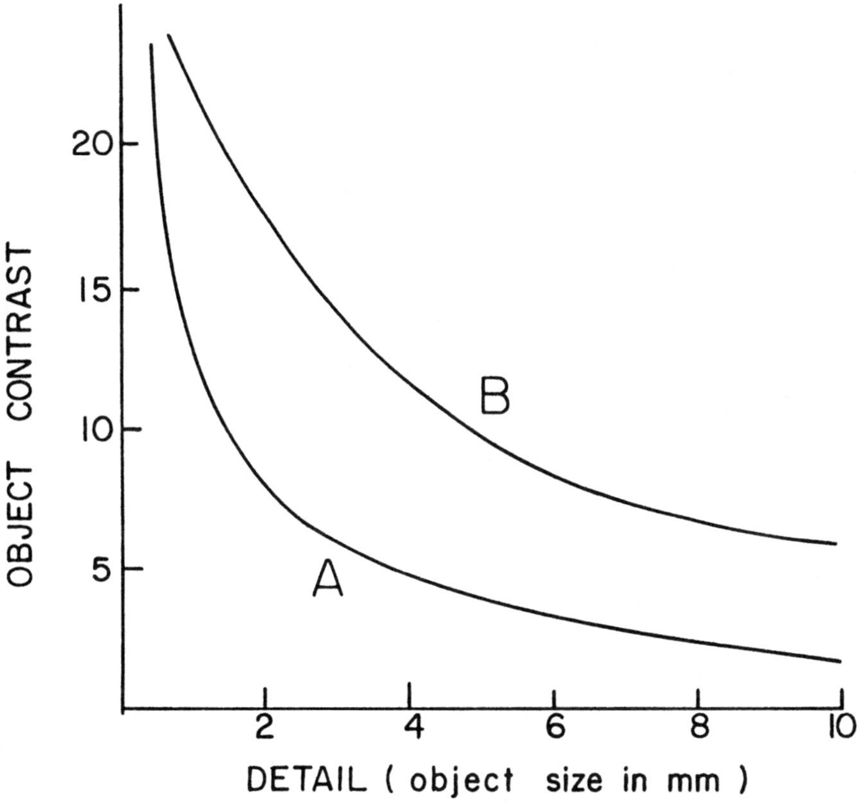

Figure 10.16. Results of contrast detail test comparing system A with System B.

System "A" has better performance than system "B." Contrast detail tests are simple and rapid to conduct but do not provide any information on false positive or false negative rates. For this reason, contrast detail tests are most suited for relative ranking of different imaging systems.

Receiver Operating Characteristic (ROC) Tests

ROC tests are useful in evaluating imaging systems because they allow an evaluation of the trade-offs between true-positive, and false-positive responses. Table 10.3 presents all possible observer responses.

TABLE 10.3
POSSIBLE RESPONSES
OBSERVER RESPONSE

		Yes	*No*
Signal Present? i.e., Does the patient have the disease?	Yes	True Positive TP	False Negative FN
	No	False Positive FP	True Negative TN

The **Sensitivity** is the **True Positive Fraction (TPF)** which is defined as:

$$TPF = \frac{TP}{TP + FN} \qquad 10.4$$

That is, the TPF is the number of true positive responses divided by the number of positive cases.

The **Specificity** is the **True Negative Fraction (TNF)**

$$TNF = \frac{TN}{FP + TN} \qquad 10.5$$

The accuracy is the fraction of corrent responses.

$$\text{Accuracy} = \frac{TP + TN}{TP + FN + FP + TN} \qquad 10.6$$

Note that:

$$TPF + FNF = 1$$

and

$$FPF + TNF = 1$$

where TPF is the true positive fraction, FPF is the false positive fraction, FNF is the false negative fraction and TNF is the true negative fraction.

Decision Criteria and Threshold Values

Detection theory says the observer makes judgements on whether or not the signal is present on the basis of two distributions as shown in Figure 10.17.

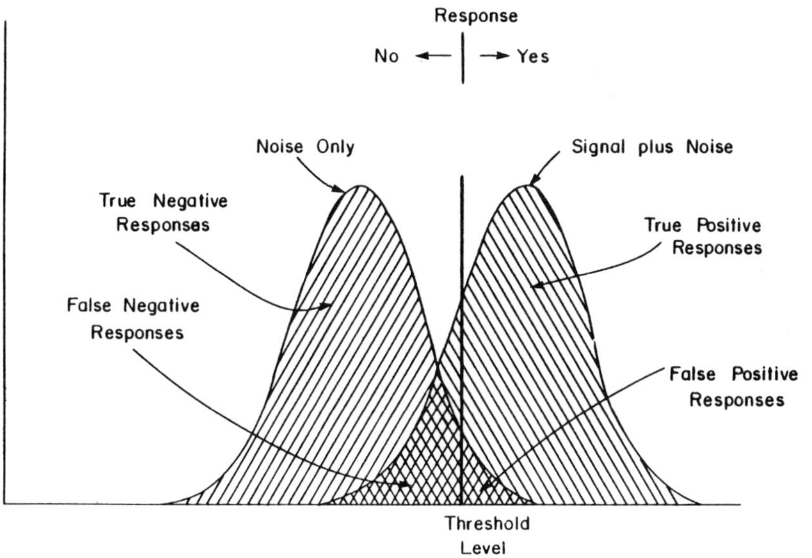

Figure 10.17. Observer noise and signal plus noise distributions with threshold or decision criterion level.

The observer decides whether or not a signal is present on the basis of whether the intensity is above or below a threshold or criterion level. The noise and the signal + noise distributions always overlap to some extent. This means that there will always be some false positive and false negative responses.

Perception theory says that each observer has an individual characteristic curve (the ROC curve) relating TPR and FPR which does not change. The observer can change the operating point on the curve but not the shape of the curve. Figure 10.18 illustrates the ROC curves for two observers. The dotted diagonal represents chance or random responses.

Observer A can change the operating point on the curve to increase the true positive rate, but only by accepting an increase in the false positive rate. Similarly, reducing the false positive rate will also decrease the true positive rate.

The area under the ROC curve is a measure of observer accuracy. Observer A is superior to observer B because the area under curve A is greater than under curve B.

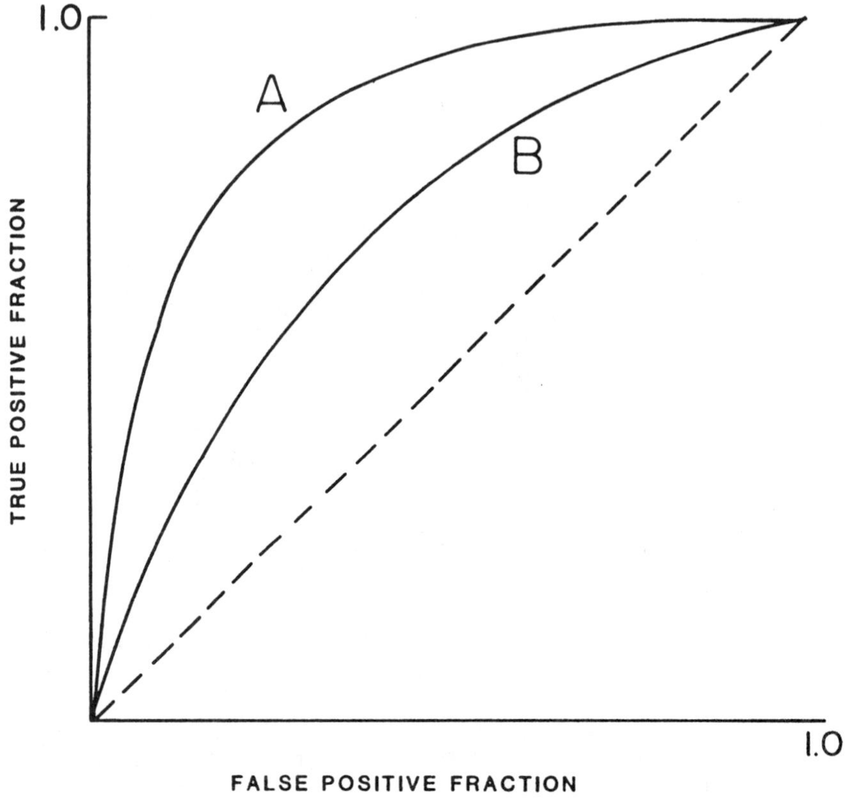

Figure 10.18. ROC curves for observers A and B.

CHAPTER 10 QUESTIONS

1. Which of the following techniques will produce the highest contrast?
   A. 100 kVp 100 MA 0.25 sec
   B. 70 kVp 200 MA 0.5 sec
   C. 85 kVp 100 MA 0.5 sec
   D. 85 kVp 200 MA 0.25 sec

A for True, B for False

2. The contrast will decrease if a three phase (6 pulse) generator is substituted for a single phase (2 pulse) generator.

3. The MTF values
   A. describes the system response as a function of input voltage rate.
   B. can be multiplied together to obtain the overall system repsonse.
   C. is used to obtain the true positive rate.
   D. describes the system response as a function of distance to the focal spot.

Questions 4 and 5

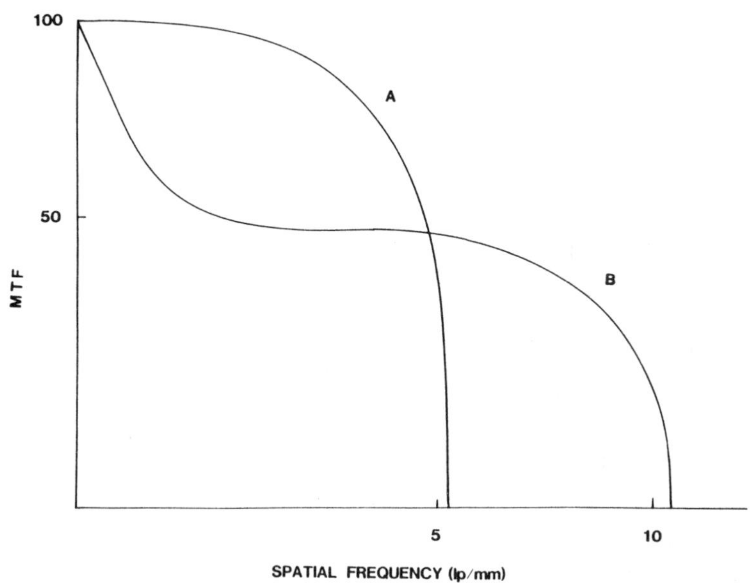

4. Which system would be better for imaging large low contrast objects?

5. Which system would be better for imaging small objects?

6.

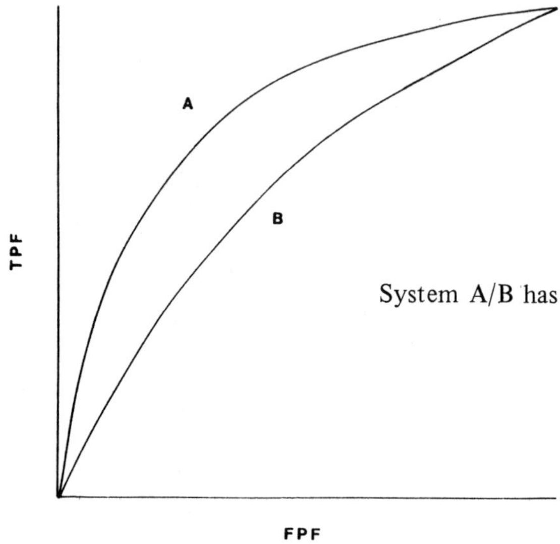

System A/B has superior performance.

7. Subject contrast is dependent on

1. kVp
2. MA
3. Beam Filtration
4. SID
5. Density

A. 1, 2, 3, 5
B. 1, 3, 4, 5
C. 1, 3, 4
D. 1, 3, 5

8-10, A for True, B for False

8. Increasing kVp will increase image latitude.

9. Changing from a 120 to a 70 kVp technique will result in a longer scale radiograph.

10. To detect an object with low subject contrast, short scale radiography should be chosen.

11. Image contrast

A. depends on patient thickness.
B. decreases with scatter.
C. depends on kVp.
D. All of the above.

12. Display contrast

A. is fixed by the kVp chosen.
B. is fixed by the film chosen.
C. is fixed by the CT scanner chosen.
D. is limited by the scan time of the digital system.

13. A display level control

A. sets the x-ray transmission level to be displayed as black.
B. sets the x-ray attenuation level to be displayed as black.
C. can be adjusted to obtain optimum subject contrast.
D. must be calibrated prior to every exam.

14. Display contrast

A. must be set before the CT scan.
B. can be changed after the CT scan.
C. requires a change in calibration factors for every change.
D. will not change the image appearance.

15. The window control

A. specifies how many transmission values are displayed as black.
B. specifies how long the CT scan will take.
C. specifies how many transmission values are required to change the display from black to white.
D. specifies which transmission level will be displayed as black.

16. A resolution of 2 line pairs per mm means that two objects _______ mm apart can be imaged as two objects.

A. 2 mm
B. 1mm
C. 0.5 mm
D. 0.25 mm

17. Two objects _________ mm apart can just be resolved with a 3 lp/mm imaging system.

A. .1
B. .17
C. .33
D. .67

18. Two objects __________ mm apart can just be resolved with a 10 lp/mm imaging system.

A. .1
B. .05
C. .5
D. .25

19. How large is the penumbra with a 2 mm focal spot used to image objects 14″ from a film with 40″ SID?

A. .7 mm
B. .9 mm
C. 1.1 mm
D. 1.3 mm

20. What is the penumbra with a 1.5 mm focal spot used to image objects 7″ from the film with 40″ SID?

A. .1 mm
B. .3 mm
C. .5 mm
D. .8 mm

21. Adjusting the decision threshold to reduce false positive responses will

A. decrease true positive responses.
B. increase false negative responses.
C. increase true negative responses.
D. All of the above.

22. Adjusting the decision threshold to increase true positive responses will

    A. increase true negative responses.
    B. decrease false negative responses.
    C. decrease false positive responses.
    D. All of the above.

CHAPTER 11

X-RAY FILM

X–rays produce a change in the film emulsion so that it will turn black when it is developed. More x–rays produce more blackening. X–ray film is made by coating an emulsion layer containing silver halide crystals on a blue tinted plastic base as illustrated in Figure 11.1. The plastic base is tinted to reduce eye strain while reading radiographs.

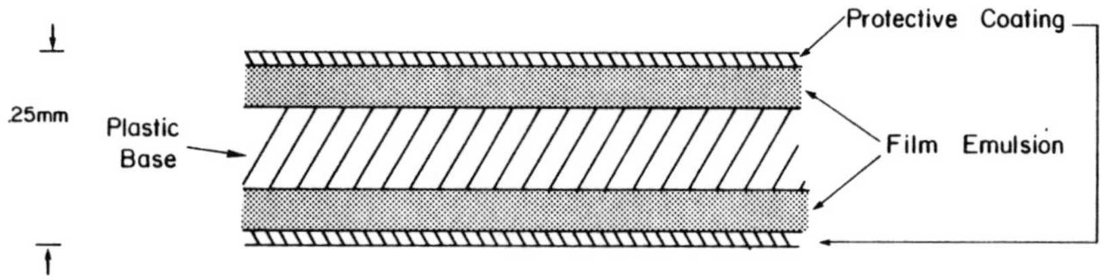

Figure 11.1. Film construction.

Most x–ray film has emulsion coated on both sides of the plastic base to double efficiency. The emulsion is a mixture of gelatine and silver bromide with a small amount of silver iodide added. The different film characteristics are determined by the number and size of the silver halide crystals in the emulsion.

For best resolution, **single coated** film with the emulsion coating on only one side of the plastic base is used. Single coated films are used in mammography and to image **Cathode Ray Tube (CRT)** displays in CT, digital imaging, ultrasound and nuclear medicine.

Optical Density

The optical density is defined as the logarithm of the ratio of the incident to transmitted light. Figure 11.2 illustrates schematically the transmission of light through a series of blackened films.

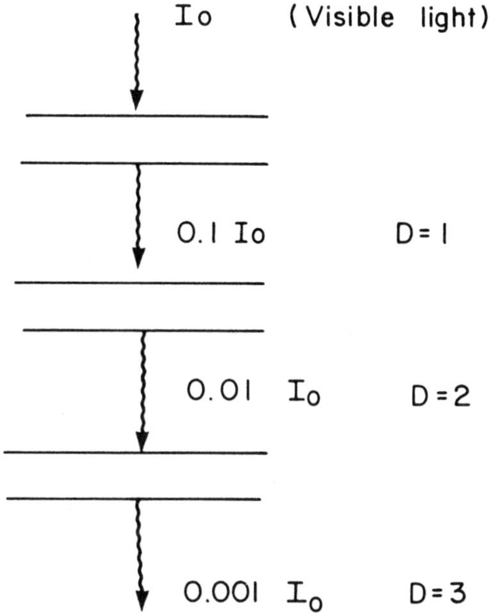

Figure 11.2. Transmission through films and the optical density.

The density of a film is defined as the logarithm of the ratio of incident to transmitted visible light intensities.

$$D = \log \frac{I_o}{I} \qquad 11.1$$

Where I_o is the incident intensity and I is the transmitted intensity.

Table 11.1 gives the transmission, the percent transmission, the ratio of incident to transmitted intensity, and the optical density of a series of films of increasing density.

The reason that topical densities are convenient is that **densities are additive.** If we have two films, each of density 1 (i.e., transmit 10% of the incident light), then their combination is the same as a single film of optical density 2 (i.e., the combination will transmit 1% of the light). X-ray films usually have optical densities in the range from 0.3 to 2.5 OD. It is just possible to read a newspaper through a film with OD = 1. A film of OD = 3 appears black.

TABLE 11.1
RELATION BETWEEN TRANSMISSION AND DENSITY

Transmission	*%T*	I_o/I	*Density*
1	100	1	0
.5	50	2	0.3
.1	10	10	1.0
.01	1	100	2.0
.001	.1	1,000	3.0
.0001	.01	10,000	4.0

The second reason that optical densities are convenient is that the optical density scale is logarithmic and the response of the eye is approximately logarithmic. Figure 11.3 illustrates the situation where four steps of brightness transmission through a film are examined.

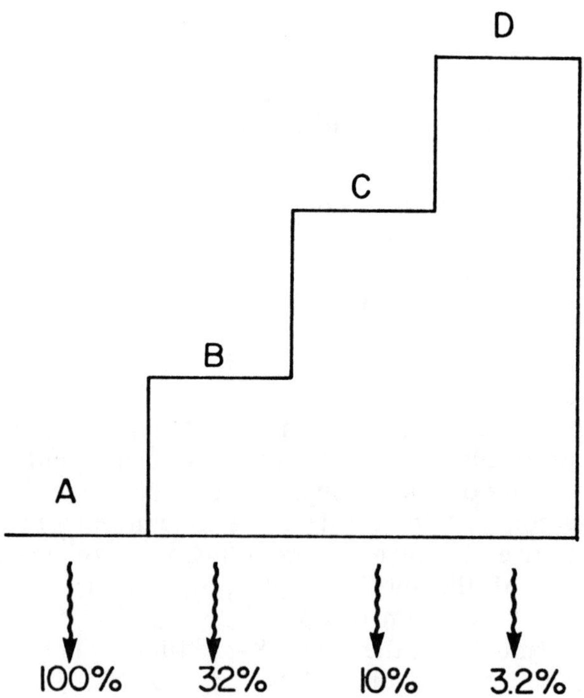

Figure 11.3. Transmission of x-rays through a step wedge.

Table 11.2 presents the x-ray transmissions through the wedge steps and the resulting OD values together with the changes in brightness.

TABLE 11.2
X-RAY TRANSMISSION THROUGH STEP WEDGE AND CORRESPONDING OPTICAL DENSITY VALUES

Region	*%T*	*O.D.*	*Change in OD*
A	100	0	
B	32	.5	.5
C	10	1.0	.5
D	3.2	1.5	.5

Notice that each step will appear to have a brightness change (change in OD) equal to the ones next to it. A radiograph of the step wedge shown in Figure 11.3 will appear to have equal brightness steps.

H and D Curves

The film response to a series of different exposures can be displayed as an H and D or characteristic curve where the optical density is plotted as a function of the logarithm of the relative exposures. This curve is named after Hurter and Driffield and is a characteristic of the film. Figure 11.4 illustrates an H and D curve for a typical x-ray film.

Base Fog and Toe Region

The base fog level is caused by background exposure and should be less than 0.2 OD. The toe region of the curve is present only with exposures produced with intensifying screens. Direct exposure to x-rays does not produce a toe region in the characteristic curve. One x-ray is sufficient to produce a latent image grain in the emulsion. However, it takes about four light photons from an intensifying screen to produce a latent image grain. Which grains get hit is a statistical process so the first part of an intensifying screen exposure doesn't produce enough hits on any one grain to produce a latent image grain.

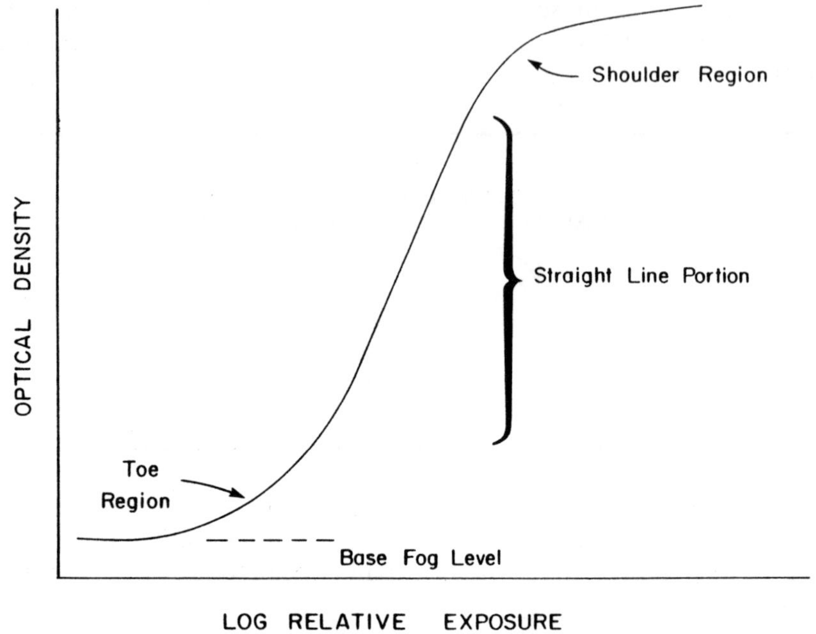

Figure 11.4. Typical characteristic curve plotting film optical density as a function of log relative exposure.

In the straight line portion of the curve, the density is proportional to the log of the exposure value.

In the straight line portion of the curve, the film gamma, Γ, is defined as

$$\Gamma = \frac{D_2 - D_1}{\log E_2 - \log E_1} \qquad 11.3$$

is the slope of the characteristic curve. Note that

$$\log E_2 - \log E_1 = \log E_2/E_1$$

so, we can rewrite Equation 11.3 as:

$$D_2 - D_1 = \Gamma \log E_2/E_1$$

Recall that E_2/E_1 is related to the subject contrast, i.e., the difference in exposures transmitted through two adjacent regions of the body. Thus, we see that the difference in optical density

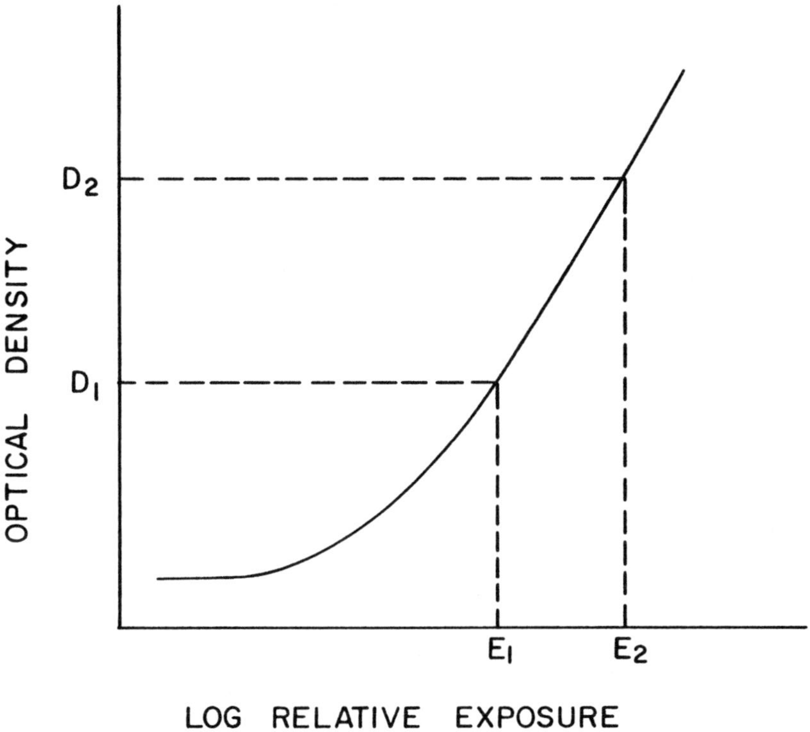

Figure 11.5. Relation between log relative exposures and change in optical density.

(the film contrast) is related to the subject contrast multiplied by the film gamma. Film gamma is usually greater than 1 and so the film contrast is greater than the subject contrast.

Example 11.1:
The Γ of a film is 2.3 and two portions of a film differ in exposure by a factor of two. If the thicker part of the subject produces a density of 1.1, what is the density of the thinner part?

$$D_2 - D_1 = \Gamma \log E_2/E_1$$

$$E_2/E_1 = 2$$

$$\log 2 = .3$$

$$D_2 - D_1 = 2.3 \times 0.3$$

$$= 0.69$$

$$D_1 = 1.1$$

$$D_2 = 1.1 + 0.69 = 1.79$$

In the shoulder region of the H & D curve, almost all the silver grains in the film have been exposed and so any increase in exposure will be wasted.

Film Speed

The film speed is defined as one over the exposure in Roentgens (1R = 260 μC/kg) required to produce an optical density of 1.0 above base fog.

Example 11.2:
A film screen combination required 5 mR to produce an optical density of 1 above base fog. What is the speed of this combination?

$$\text{Speed} = \frac{1}{.005\text{R}}$$

$$= 200$$

Figure 11.6 indicates two films. Film B is "faster" than Film A because it requires less exposure to produce OD = 1 above base fog.

Latitude

Film latitude refers to the range of exposures over which an acceptable radiograph can be obtained. This is usually taken to lie in the range of optical densities between 0.25 and 2.0. Film B has greater latitude. Notice that the film with the lower gamma has the wider latitude.

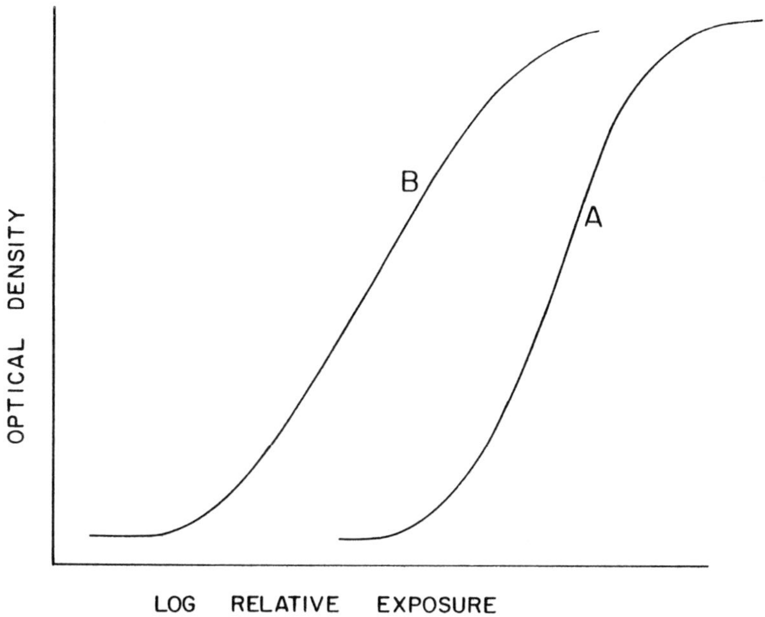

Figure 11.6. Two films of different speed and latitude.

Reciprocity Law Failure

The reciprocity law states that the same exposure will produce the same optical density regardless of the combination of current and time used to obtain the exposure. The reciprocity law holds for direct exposures to x–rays but not for visible light exposures from intensifying screens. Reciprocity law failure occurs with visible light from intensifying screens whenever the exposure factors vary by more than about a factor of 10. This means a 200 mAs exposure obtained at 50 MA four seconds would not give the same optical density as a 500 MA 0.4 second esposure.

Film Chemistry

Film consists of a suspension of silver bromide crystals in a gelatin emulsion. During the production of the film, the silver bromide crystals are combined with a small amount of iodine so that the crystals are actually silver iodobromide crystals. The presence of the iodine, which is a much larger atom, strains the crystal structure and allows the silver ions to move around. Small amounts of sulfur which are present form Ag_2 S molecules in the crystal. These areas are called **sensitivity specks** and have the ability to trap free electrons.

The presence of the free electrons produced by ionization either by visible light or radiation allows the silver ions to be reduced to silver atoms. The metallic silver atoms migrate to locations near the sensitivity speck and act as a catalyst when a weak reducing agent (the developer) is added. Those grains of silver bromide which have been altered by light contain 3 to 10 silver atoms and can be completely reduced to a pure silver grain by the developer.

Development

The **developer** must be a weak reducing agent so that it does not reduce the unexposed grains. After the x-ray exposure, the film contains a **latent** image. That is, some of the silver iodobromide grains have a few atoms of silver where x-rays passed; the unexposed grains remain unchanged. The term latent image refers to the distribution of the changed and unchanged grains. The fact that at least three silver atoms per crystal are required to permit the developing agent to operate is responsible for the toe region of the H and D curve. The first few mR of an exposure produce one or two silver atoms on each of many grains but do not produce very many grains capable of being developed. Any additional increase in exposure above the toe region will produce developable grains and changes in the optical density of the film.

Film development is a chemical process. As the developer temperature is increased, or as the developer is left in contact with the film longer, more of the unexposed film grains will be developed. This produces a uniform fogging effect. Increasing the development time or temperature will increase:

base fog
speed
contrast

Fixer

On completion of development, the exposed silver iodobromide grains are reduced to metallic silver. Most of the unexposed grains will be unaffected by the developer. In the next stage of development, the "fixer" is used to dissolve away the unexposed silver iodobromide grains while leaving the metallic silver grains unaffected. The grains of silver are so small that they appear black instead of the metallic silver color familiar on teapots and coins. Finally, any residual chemicals are washed away and the film is dried.

CHAPTER 11 QUESTIONS

1. A film emulsion
   A. turns dark when exposed to light or x-rays.
   B. is a mixture of silver oxide and gelatine.
   C. contains a latent image after exposure to light and x-rays.
   D. has a plastic base on both sides for easy processing.

2. Optical density is defined as
   A. the ratio of transmitted to incident light intensity.
   B. the ratio of incident to transmitted light intensity.
   C. the logarithm of the ratio of transmitted to incident light intensity.
   D. the logarithm of the ratio of incident to transmitted light intensity.

3. A film which transmits 1% of the incident light has an optical density of
   A. 1
   B. 1.5
   C. 2
   D. 2.5

4. A film which transmits 0.3% of the incident light has an optical density of
   A. 1
   B. 1.5
   C. 2
   D. 2.5

5. A film of optical density 1.5 is placed in front of a film of optical density 1.2. The combination has an optical density of
   A. 1.2
   B. 1.5
   C. 1.8
   D. 2.7

6. Equal changes in optical density
   A. are caused by equal changes in transmission.
   B. appear to have equal brightness changes.
   C. are caused by logarithmic changes in optical density.
   D. All of the above.

7. An H & D curve
   A. plots log linear density against relative exposure.
   B. relates the optical density of the film to the light intensity from the screen.
   C. plots optical density against log relative exposure.
   D. relates subject contrast to kVp and beam filtration.

8. A film exposed to x-rays without an intensifying screen:
   A. has no toe region of the HD curve.
   B. has no base fog region of the HD curve.
   C. has no shoulder region of the HD curve.
   D. All of the above.

9. The toe region of the HD curve represents
   A. the region where x-ray photons have produced a latent image.
   B. the region where light photons have not yet formed a latent image.
   C. the region where almost all the silver halide grains have been exposed.
   D. the region where the Γ of the film is a straight line.

10. The gamma of a film
   - A. relates optical density to patient thickness.
   - B. relates optical density to patient transmission.
   - C. relates the shoulder region of the HD curve to the toe region.
   - D. is measured at OD = 1 above base fog.

11. If two portions of a film whose Γ is 1.8 differ in exposure by a factor of 10, what is the density difference between them?
   - A. 0.18
   - B. 1.0
   - C. 1.8
   - D. 18

12. Two portions of a film whose Γ is 2.1 differ in exposure by a factor of 5. If the lighter portion has a density of 0.8, what is the density of the darker portion?
   - A. 1.5
   - B. 2.3
   - C. 2.6
   - D. 5.8

13. A film with wide latitude cannot have
   - A. high contrast.
   - B. high speed.
   - C. low sensitivity.
   - D. low base fog.

14. Film speed
   - A. is measured at the point where $\Gamma = 1$.
   - B. is measured at the point where OD = 1 above base fog.
   - C. is equal to the exposure in R required to produce OD = 1.
   - D. is independent of silver halide content of the film.

15. A film screen combination requires 10 mR to produce an optical density of 1 above base fog. The speed of this combination is
   A. 10
   B. 100
   C. 200
   D. 250

16. Increasing the development temperature increases
   A. base fog.
   B. film speed.
   C. contrast.
   D. All of the above.

17–20

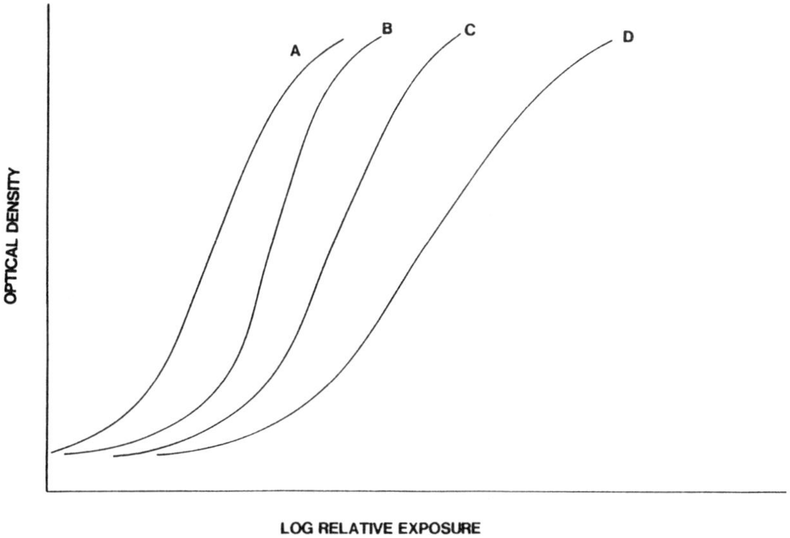

17. Which film has the widest latitude?
18. Which film has the highest gamma?
19. Which film is fastest?
20. Which film is the slowest?

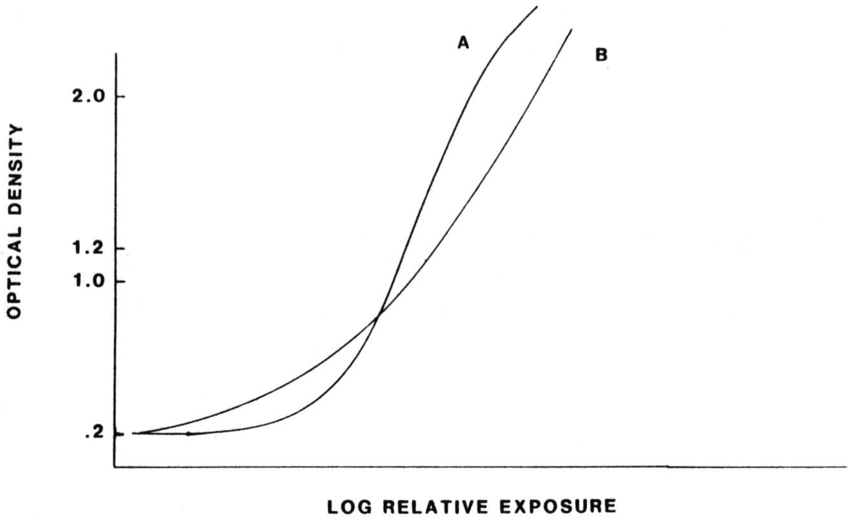

21. Which film is faster?

CHAPTER 12

INTENSIFYING SCREENS

Direct x-ray exposure produces only about 2% of the film blackening with modern film systems. The other 98% is produced by intensifying screens located on either side of the films. Figure 12.1 illustrates the arrangements of the screens in a typical film screen cassette.

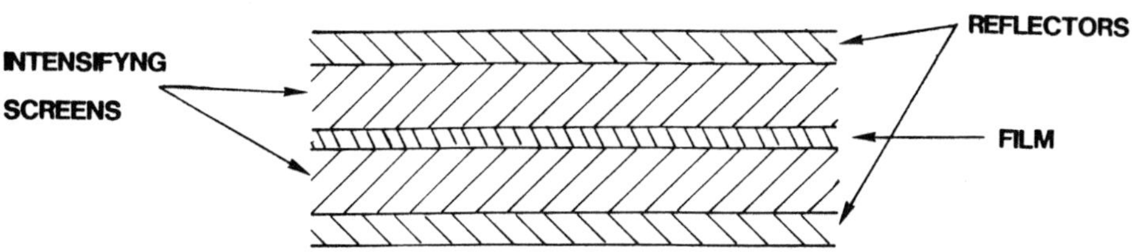

Figure 12.1. Construction and arrangement of intensifying screens.

The crystals of fluorescent materials are uniformly mixed in a plastic binder laid on top of a reflective layer and coated with a protective layer. The plastic binder is tinted to absorb some of the light emitted laterally. Reduction of lateral diffusion of the screen light improves resolution.

The intensifying screens act as amplifiers to convert more of the x-ray energy into visible images. The **intensification factor** measures how much improvement is provided by the intensifying screens and is given by:

$$\text{Intensification factor} = \frac{\text{Exposure without Screens}}{\text{Exposure with Screens}} \qquad 12.1$$

Intensifying screens can produce either **fluorescence** or **phosphorescence.**

Fluorescence = Light emitted within 10^{-8} s after x-ray interaction.

Phosphorescence = Light emitted as afterglow at times longer than 10^{-8} s after x–ray interaction.

In the early 1900's, Thomas Edison discovered that calcium tungstate ($CaWO_4$) produced fluorescent light when struck by x–rays. Calcium Tungstate screens were the accepted standard screens in all Radiology Departments from then until the early 1970's.

Intensifying Screen Speed

The speed of the screen relates to the number of x–rays required to produce an optical density of one on a film (the film must be specified). Most screen speeds are relative and fall in one of three categories:

Slow or Detail
Par or Regular
Fast or High

Higher speed screens can produce the same optical density with smaller x–ray exposures.

The speed of the intensifyiing screen depends on

A) Thickness
B) Crystal Size
C) Material

Thickness

Thicker screens have higher speed but poorer resolution because the screen light can diffuse laterally. Thinner screens trade improved resolution for slower speeds.

Crystal Size

Larger crystals have higher efficiency but poorer resolution than smaller crystals. Lateral diffusion of light in the screen produces a loss of resolution. Just as tiny fog droplets produce more scattering and attenuation than raindrops, so the smaller screen crystals reduce lateral light diffusion more than larger crystals.

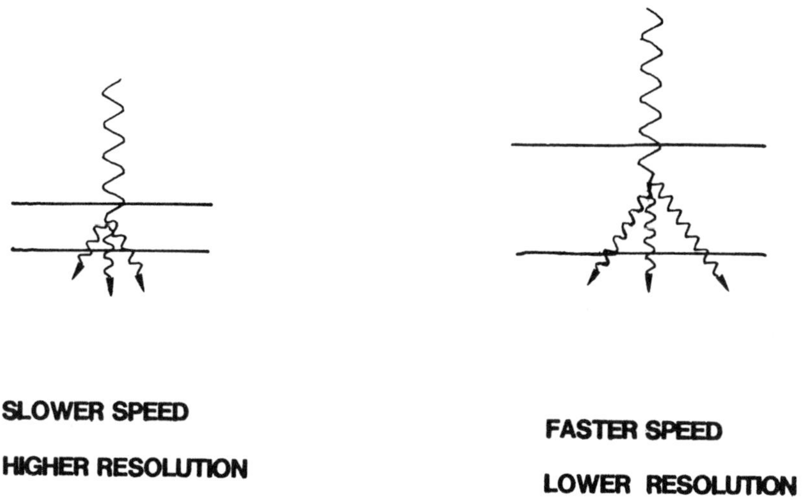

Figure 12.2. Trade-offs between screen thickness and resolution.

Materials

In order to improve the performance of intensifying screens over that of $CaWO_4$, new materials had to be developed. Two approaches were possible:

A. Develop compounds with more efficient x–ray absorption, i.e., they have higher **absorption efficiency**.

B. Develop compounds which emit more visible light per absorbed x–ray photon. These compounds are more efficient at converting x–ray energy to light energy, i.e., they have higher **conversion efficiency**.

In the early 1970's, a group of Rare Earth Screens were introduced which used different materials and had higher absorption and conversion efficiencies. Table 12.1 gives the atomic number and K absorption edge energy for some of the most common screen materials.

If the K absorption edge is close to the x–ray photon energy, the probability of interaction is greatly increased. This is reflected in the increase in μ_m the mass absorption coefficient. Figure 12.3 illustrates the variation of absorption with x–ray energy in the diagnostic range.

TABLE 12.1
ELEMENTS USED IN INTENSIFYING SCREENS

Element	*Z*	*K Absorption Edge Energy (KeV)*
Yittrium	39	17
Barium	56	37
Lanthanium	57	39
Gadolinium	64	50
Tungsten	74	70

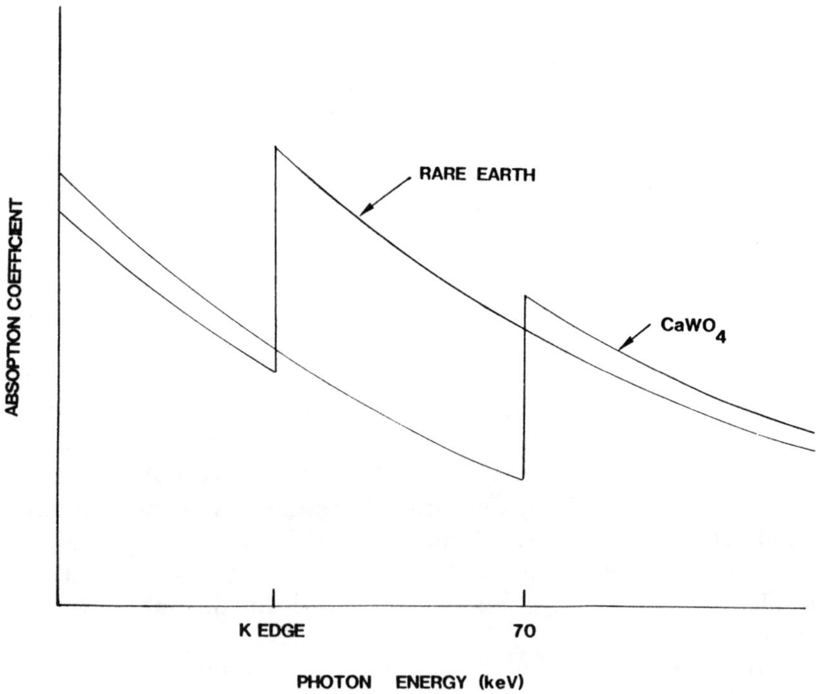

Figure 12.3. Absorption of calcium tungstate and rare earth screens as a function of energy.

Note that Gadolinium and Lanthanium have significantly higher absorption coefficients than $CaWO_4$ in the diagnostic energy range. Yittrium has an absorption coefficient equal to $CaWO_4$ but its conversion efficiency is almost four times greater. Table 12.2 details some of the characteristics of the rare earth compounds used in screens.

TABLE 12.2
CHARACTERISTICS OF INTENSIFYING SCREEN COMPOUNDS

	Formula	*Light Emitted*
Calcium Tungstate	$Ca\,WO_4$	Blue
Gadolinium Oxysulfide	$Gd_2\,O_2\,S$	Green
Lanthanium Oxysulfide	$La_2\,O_2\,S$	Green
Barium Lead Sulfate	$Ba\,Pb\,SO_4$	Blue
Yittrium Oxysulfide	$Y_2\,O_2\,S$	Blue
Barium Fluorochloride	BaFCl	Blue
Lanthanium Oxybromide	LaOBr	Blue

Barium Lead Sulfate screens have essentially the same characteristics as $CaWO_4$ screens. Both Gadolinium Oxysulfide and Lanthanium Oxysulfide screens emit green light which is not energetic enough to activate conventional **panchromatic** x–ray film to produce a latent image. Special **orthochromatic** film with increased sensitivity in the lower energy (green) region of the spectrum must be used with these screens. Figure 12.4 illustrates the sensitivity of regular and orthochromatic film as a function of wavelength. Figure 12.5 presents the light emitted from $CaWO_4$ and rare earth screens together with the sensitivity of panchromatic (regular) and orthochromatic films.

Note that the rare earth screens will not expose regular blue sensitive panchromatic film.

Advantages of Rare Earth Screens

Rare earth screens are two to ten times faster than conventional $CaWO_4$ screens. This means that tube loading and patient dose can be reduced for the same resolution as with the conventional screens. It is also possible to obtain better resolution with

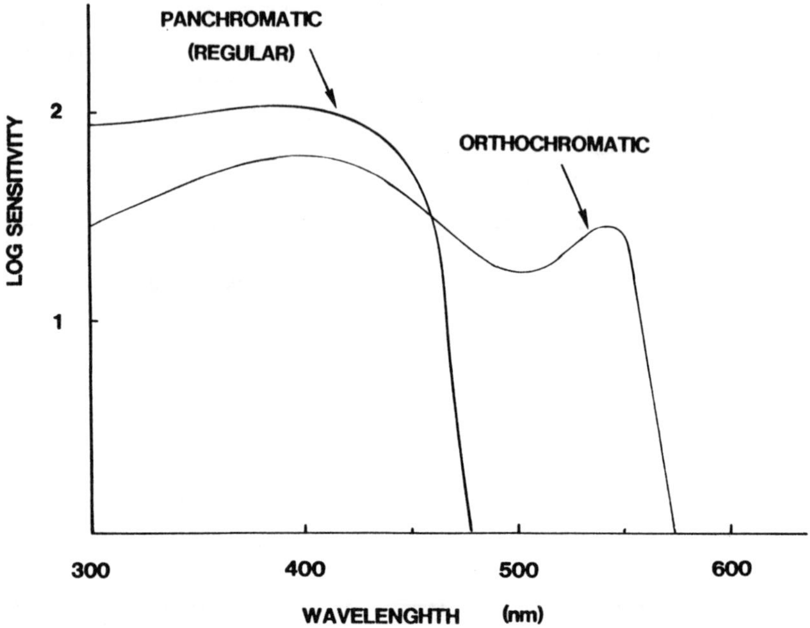

Figure 12.4. Response of pan- and orthochromatic film as a function of wavelength.

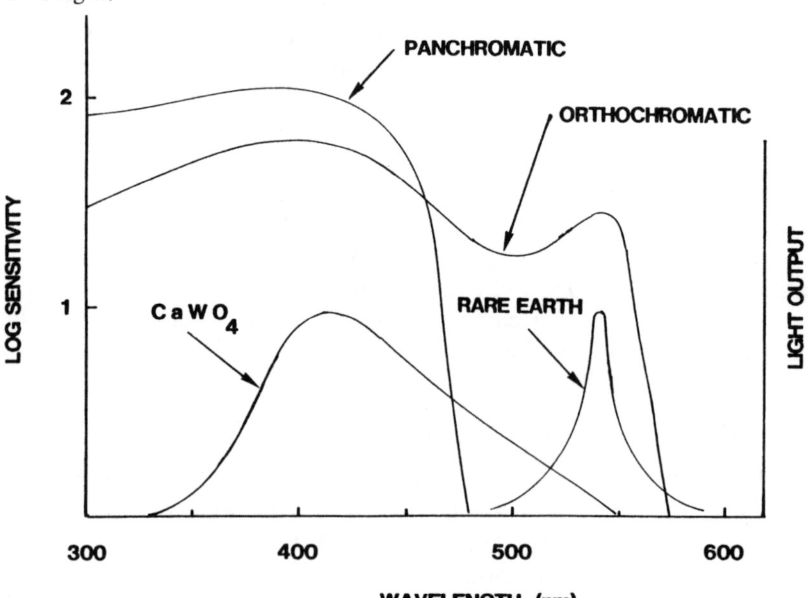

Figure 12.5. Light emission characteristics of Ca WO_4, and rare earth screens.

the rare earth screens at the same speed rating as $CaWO_4$ screens, i.e., trade some speed improvement for an improvement in resolution. This is done by using a thinner (better resolution) rare earth screen with the same speed as a thicker $CaWO_4$ screen.

Disadvantages of Rare Earth Screens

Disadvantages of the rare earth systems include:

a) a different kVp response than $CaWO_4$ screens,
b) increased quantum mottle,
c) some phototimers which cannot respond rapidly enough.

KVP Response

Figure 12.6 illustrates the relative response of rare earth screens compared to $CaWO_4$ screens as a function of kVp.

The green sensitive films have a slight increase in sensitivity relative to blue sensitive films at higher energies so the only significant difference in response is at low energies. The rare earth screens are less sensitive at low energies so they respond less to scattered radiation than $CaWO_4$ screens. This property slightly improves contrast.

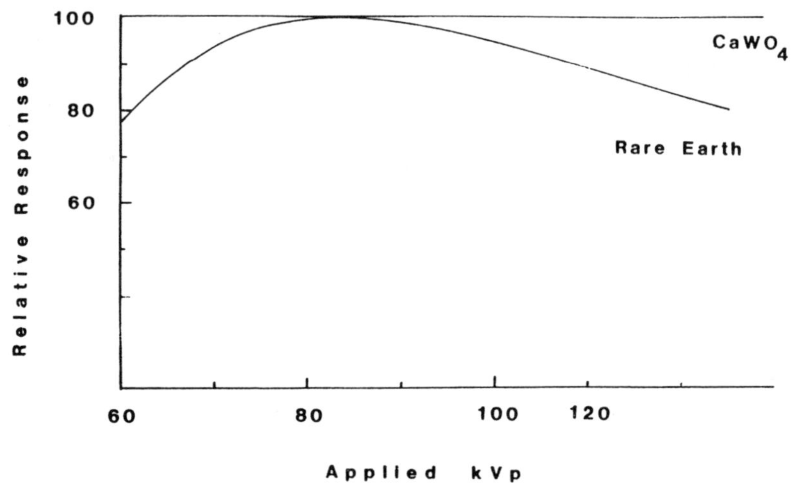

Figure 12.6. Energy response of Ca WO_4 and rare earth screens.

Increased Quantum Mottle

The amount of **quantum mottle** is determined by the number of photons present at the **quantum sink**. The quantum sink is that step in the imaging process which has the fewest photons. For film screen systems the quantum sink occurs at the input to the intensifying screen. Quantum mottle is determined by the number of x–ray photons interacting in the intensifying screen. Rare earth screens which are more efficient at converting x–ray energy into visible light will require fewer x–ray photons to form an image. Such screens will exhibit increased quantum mottle.

Limited Response of Phototimers

Some automatic exposure circuits designed to terminate the exposure when enough x–rays have reached the film require about 30 ms to sense the x–ray exposure and turn off the x–ray beam. With rare earth screens, some views (i.e., chest) need only a 3–5 ms exposure. Either a new circuit must be installed or a lower MA station used to extend the exposure time so the phototimer can react properly.

Fast vs. Detail Screens

Changing the absorption efficiency of a screen does not change the quantum mottle of the final image. Figure 12.7 illustrates schematically the substitution of a fast for a detail screen of the same material.

The same optical density is obtained in both cases. Fewer photons are incident on the patient with the faster screen but **the same number of photons interact** in the screen in both cases. Thus, the Quantum Noise is the same.

For the same screen material, changes in thickness do not produce changes in noise level. Instead, spatial resolution is traded for speed.

Replacement of a $CaWO_4$ screen with a rare earth screen whose improved intensification factor is due solely to increased absorption efficiency will not change the quantum mottle. Fewer x–ray photons will strike the patient but the same number will be absorbed by the screen. Thus the number of photons at the quantum sink will be the same.

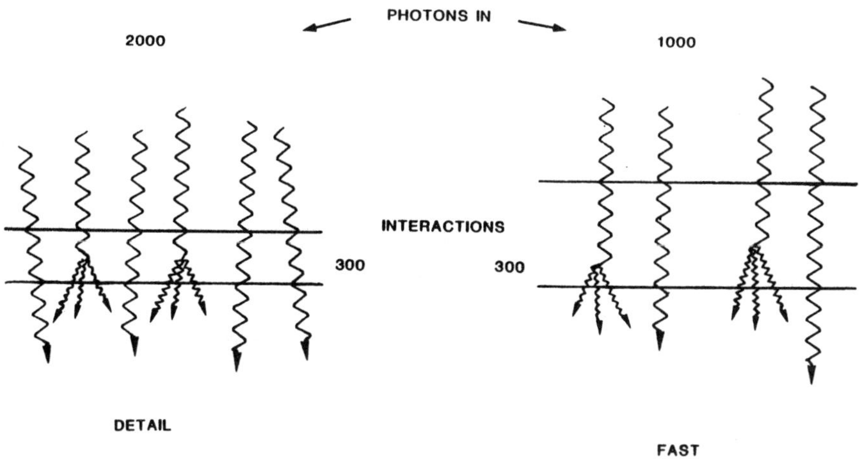

Figure 12.7. Substitution of a fast for a detail screen of the same material reduces the patient dose but does not change the quantum mottle.

If the increased speed of the replacement screen is produced by higher conversion efficiency, then fewer x-rays will be needed to produce the same optical density and the Quantum Noise will be increased. This is the same effect as using a faster film.

Safe Lights

The orthochromatic film used with the green emitting rare earth screens is sensitive to the brown light of most safelight filters. A special reddish brown filter must be used in dark rooms where orthochromatic film is used.

CHAPTER 12 QUESTIONS

1. Fluorescence is light emitted __________ seconds after an x-ray interaction
   A. within 10^{-8}
   B. longer than 10^{-8}
   C. within 10^{-6}
   D. longer than 10^{-6}

2. The intensification factor
   A. is the ratio of exposure with to exposure without screens.
   B. is the ratio of exposure without to exposure with screens.
   C. measures the efficiency of converting light to x-ray energies.
   D. measures the efficiency of x-ray absorption conversion.

3. Phosphorescence is light emitted __________ seconds after an x-ray interaction.
   A. within 10^{-8}
   B. longer than 10^{-8}
   C. within 10^{-6}
   D. longer than 10^{-6}

4. Afterglow is another name for fluorescence/phosphorescence.

5. Higher speed screens require more/less exposure.

6. High speed screens have ________ than par speed screens.
   A. greater thickness
   B. larger crystals
   C. poorer resolution
   D. All of the above.

7. Lateral light diffusion is greater/less with larger crystals.

8. With $CaWO_4$ screens __________ can be traded for __________.

A. speed - resolution
B. conversion efficiency - speed
C. speed - latitude
D. latitude - contrast

9. A screen with smaller crystals will have improved

A. resolution
B. speed
C. latitude
D. phosphorescence

10. An improvement in __________ results in more of the incident photons being absorbed.

A. conversion efficiency
B. absorption efficiency
C. contrast efficiency
D. resolution.

11. Matching the K edge of the screen material to the incident x-rays results in improved

A. conversion efficiency.
B. absorption efficiency.
C. contrast efficiency.
D. resolution.

12. Increasing the screen thickness will increase

A. absorption.
B. resolution.
C. contrast.
D. All of the above.

13. Blue/Green light is more energetic.

14. Advantages of rare earth screens include

A. thicker screens.
B. improved speed.
C. greater tube loading.
D. increased patient dose.

15. A rare earth screen with the same absorption efficiency and twice the conversion efficiency is substituted for a $CaWO_4$ screen. The quantum mottle will

A. increase.
B. decrease.
C. stay the same.

16. A rare earth screen with the same conversion efficiency and twice the absorption efficiency is substituted for a $CaWO_4$ screen. The patient dose will

A. increase.
B. decrease.
C. stay the same.

17. A rare earth screen with the same conversion efficiency and twice the absorption efficiency is substituted for a $CaWO_4$ screen. The quantum mottle will

A. increase.
B. decrease.
C. stay the same.

18. When a high speed $CaWO_4$ screen is substituted for a par speed, $CaWO_4$ screen the exposure factors must be reduced by 200 MAS. The quantum mottle will

A. increase.
B. decrease.
C. stay the same.

19-23, Rare earth screens having both increased absorption and conversion efficiencies are substituted for $CaWO_4$ screens. Both the new and the old screens have the same speed. What happens to: (Answer A for increase; B for decrease; C for remains the same)

19. Quantum Mottle
20. Resolution
21. Patient Dose
22. Geometric Unsharpness
23. Motion Unsharpness

CHAPTER 13

SCATTER AND SCATTER REDUCTION

An x–ray beam which has passed through a patient contains both **primary** and **scattered** radiation. An x–ray beam incident on a patient consists of **primary radiation.** Inside the patient the x–rays can:

a. pass through the patient without interacting.
b. undergo a photoelectric interaction.
c. undergo Compton scattering.

Photons that undergo photoelectric interactions are completely absorbed in the patient. Characteristic x–rays from tissue materials have such low energies that they do not get out of the patient.

Photons emerging from the patient are either primary photons or Compton scattered photons. The secondary or Compton scattered photons have changed direction and lost energy.

At diagnostic x–ray energies Compton scattered photons are **isotropic**, that is, they are scattered equally in all directions, and they have almost the same energy as the primary photons. As an example, a 30 keV photon loses only 2 keV in scattering through 90°.

Secondary photons carry no diagnostic information because of their changes in direction. The effect of scatter on loss of contrast was discussed in Chapter 10. Scatter also results in a loss of resolution. Figure 13.1 presents two radiographs of a bar phantom under no scatter and full scatter conditions.

The loss of resolution due to scatter is obvious. To improve image contrast and resolution, techniques have been developed to reduce scatter.

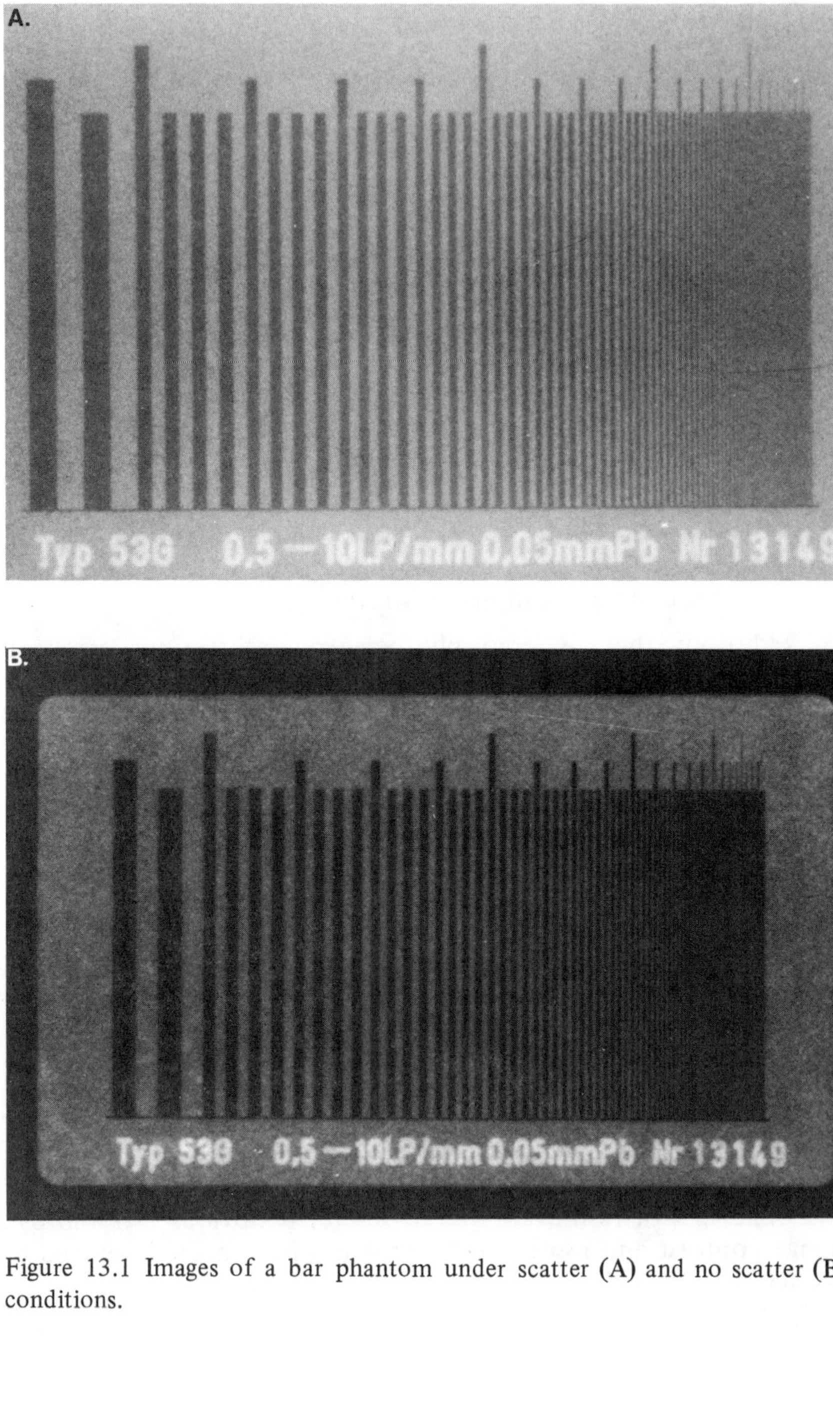

Figure 13.1 Images of a bar phantom under scatter (A) and no scatter (B) conditions.

Scatter reduction techniques currently in use are:

- Field Size Reduction
- Grids
- Air Gap
- Moving Slit

Field Size

The amount of scatter is directly proportional to the field size. Dramatic reduction in scatter can be obtained by reducing the field size.

Example 13.1:
How much is scatter reduced when the field size is reduced from 10 x 10 in. to 7 x 7 in.?

$$\text{Area of } 10 \times 10 \text{ field} = 100 \text{ in}^2$$

$$\text{Area of } 7 \times 7 \text{ field} = 49 \text{ in}^2$$

Scatter is reduced by the ratio of the areas, i.e., more than a factor of 2.

Grids

Grids are thin flat sheets made of alternate lead and aluminum or plastic layers. Grids are placed between the patient and the detector. The lead strips are designed to attenuate the scattered radiation and the plastic or aluminum interspaces to allow the passage of the primary radiation. Figure 13.2 illustrates the action of a grid in eliminating scattered radiation.

Grid Ratio

The penetration and attenuation characteristics of the grid are described by the **grid ratio.**

The grid ratio is given by:

$$\text{Grid Ratio} = \frac{h}{D} \qquad 13.1$$

where h is the height of the lead strips and D is the distance between the lead strips.

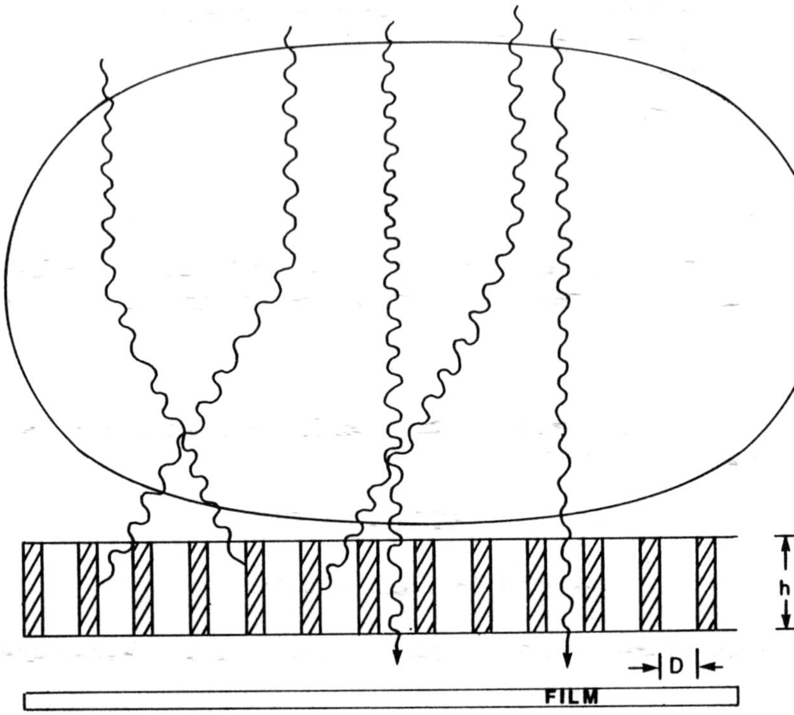

Figure 13.2. Scatter reduction through the use of a grid.

Notice that the lead thickness and the interseptal spacing are not equal. Typical grid ratios range from 8:1 to 16:1. Grid ratios of 8:1 or less are generally used for energies less than 90 kVp while grid ratios of 12:1 or greater are used at higher energies.

The number of lines per inch determines how fine the grid lines will appear on the image. The modern grids contain between 80 and 120 lines per inch. The higher the grid ratio the smaller the acceptance angle and the less transmitted scatter. Figure 13.3 illustrates the change in scatter acceptance angle with changes in grid ratio.

Increasing the grid ratio increases the:

Bucky Factor
Patient Dose
Film Contrast
Contrast Improvement Factor

and decreases the transmission of the primary beam.

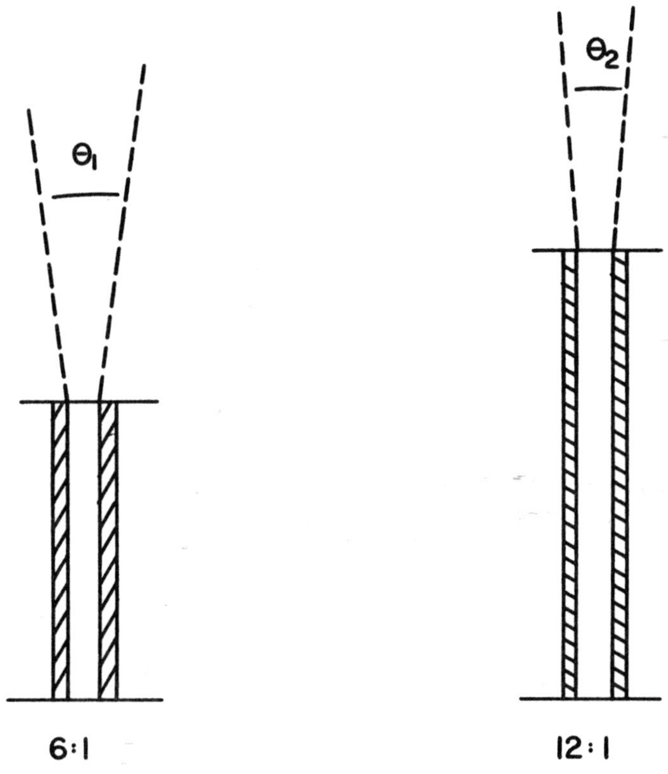

Figure 13.3 Decrease in acceptance angle with increasing grid ratio.

Grid Cut-off

Linear grids made up of parallel strips suffer from **grid cut-off** at large field sizes perpendicular to the grid lines. Grid cut-off is evidenced by a decrease in exposure and display density near the edges of the detector. Figure 13.4 illustrates how grid cut-off occurs.

The half width, w, at which total grid cut-off occurs is given by:

$$w = \frac{SID}{GR} \qquad 13.2$$

where SID is the source image distance and GR is the grid ratio.

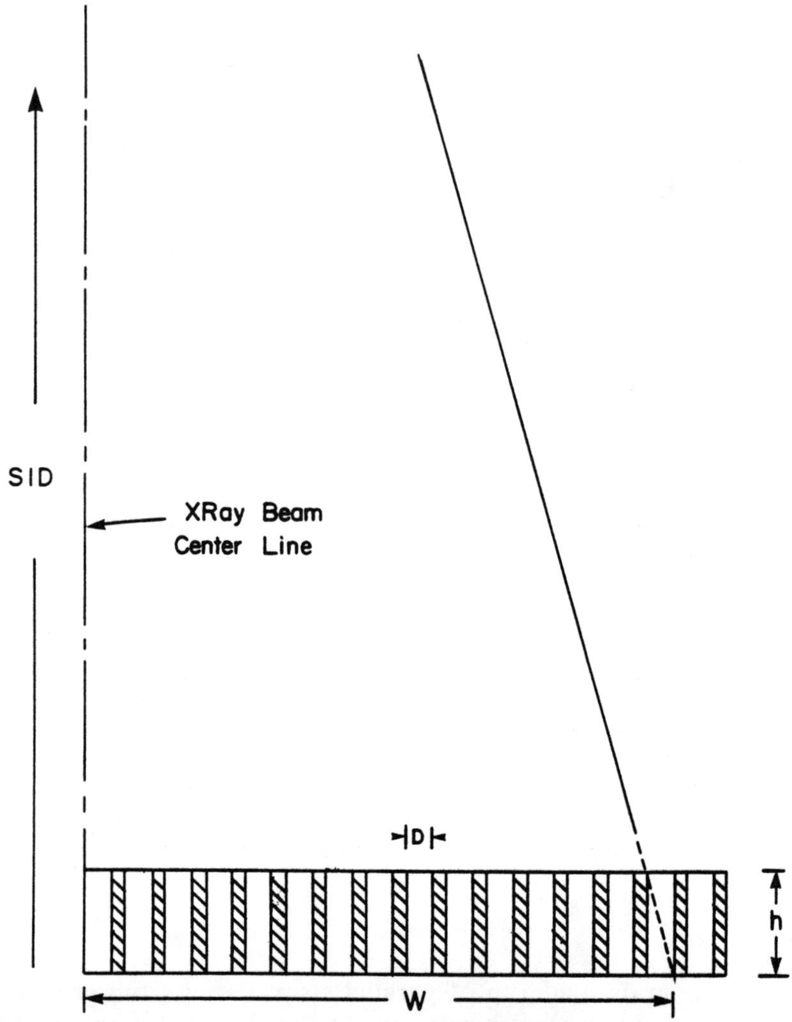

Figure 13.4. Grid cut-off at a distance W from the x-ray beam center line.

Example 13.2:
At what half width will total grid cut-off occur with an 8:1 linear grid if the SID is 40"?

$$w = \frac{40}{8/1}$$

$$w = 5''$$

Focused Grids

To eliminate the problem of grid cut–off with wide fields **focused grids** are designed with their lead strips pointing toward a convergent point. Figure 13.5 presents a schematic view of a focused grid.

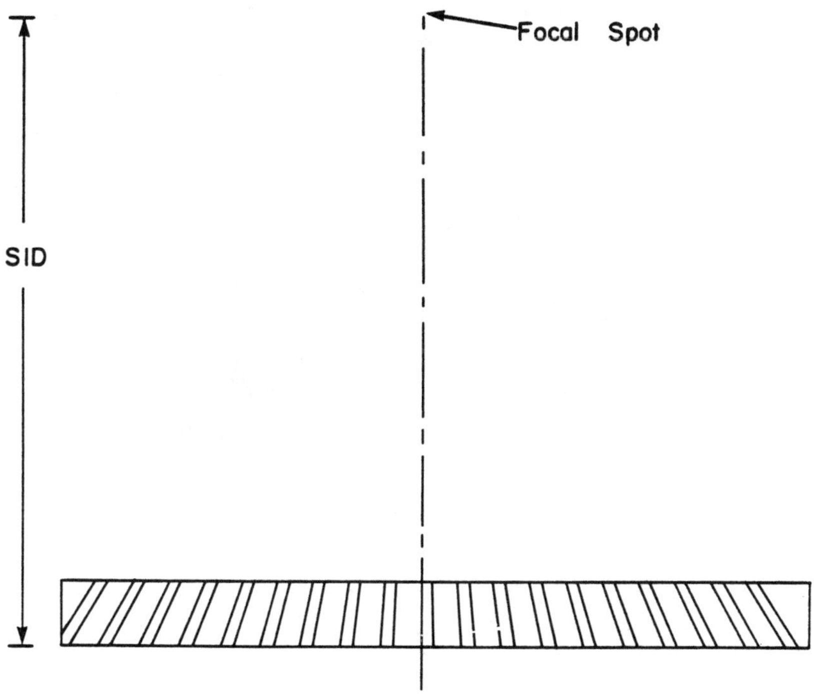

Figure 13.5. Focused grid at a source image.

Focused grids can only be used in the designed distance range and must not be used off center or upside down. Use of a focused grid upside down will produce "grid cut–off" resulting in a strip with correct exposure down the middle with underexposed regions on either side of the center. Figure 13.6 presents an example of grid cut–off produced by an upside down grid.

A focused grid shifted off center will exhibit lateral grid cut–off on only one side of the image even if it is facing the tube correctly and at the correct distance to the source. Grids with grid ratios of 12:1 or higher are especially susceptible to **lateral decentering cut–off.**

Figure 13.6. Grid cut-off due to upside down focused grid.

About 70% of the primary beam penetrates a typical grid. Penetration of the grid by scattered radiation is usually one-tenth or less for grid ratios of 8:1 or greater.

Moving Grids

Moving or **Bucky** grids are designed to move during the exposure and blur out the grid lines. Most radiologists do not notice the grid lines when 80 (or more) lines per inch stationary grids are used so Bucky grids are not as widely used as they once were. Moving grids require about 15% higher MAS than an identical stationary grid.

Measures of Grid Effectiveness

There are several methods of describing how well grids remove scattered radiation. The **contrast improvement factor**, K, is defined as:

$$K = \frac{\text{Contrast with grid}}{\text{Contrast without the grid}} \qquad 13.2$$

The contrast improvement factor describes the improvement in contrast obtained by the use of the grid. It depends not only on the grid effectiveness but also on the patient size, field size, kVp and beam filtration. The contrast improvement factor increases with increasing grid ratio. Figure 13.7 A and B illustrate the effectiveness of a grid in improving image quality.

The **Bucky Factor** is defined as:

$$B = \frac{\text{Exposure at the film without Grid}}{\text{Exposure at the film with Grid}} \qquad 13.4$$

The Bucky Factor is related to the required increase in MAS when a grid is added to a non-grid technique. A rule of thumb is that the exposure factor (MAS) has to be **increased by a factor of 4** when a grid is added. This is to make up for the portion of the primary beam intercepted by the lead and the scatter which has been removed from the beam.

Example 13.3:
An exposure taken at 85 kVp, 200 MA 1/4 s demonstrates acceptable density but too much scatter. What technical factors will be required if a 10:1 grid with a Bucky factor of 4 is added?

Need to increase exposure by a factor of 4.

These would be possible choices

85 kVp	800 MA	1/4 s
85 kVp	200 MA	1 s
100 kVp	200 MA	1/2 s

The latter choice results from the rule that a 15% increase in kVp is equivalent to a factor of two increase in MAS.

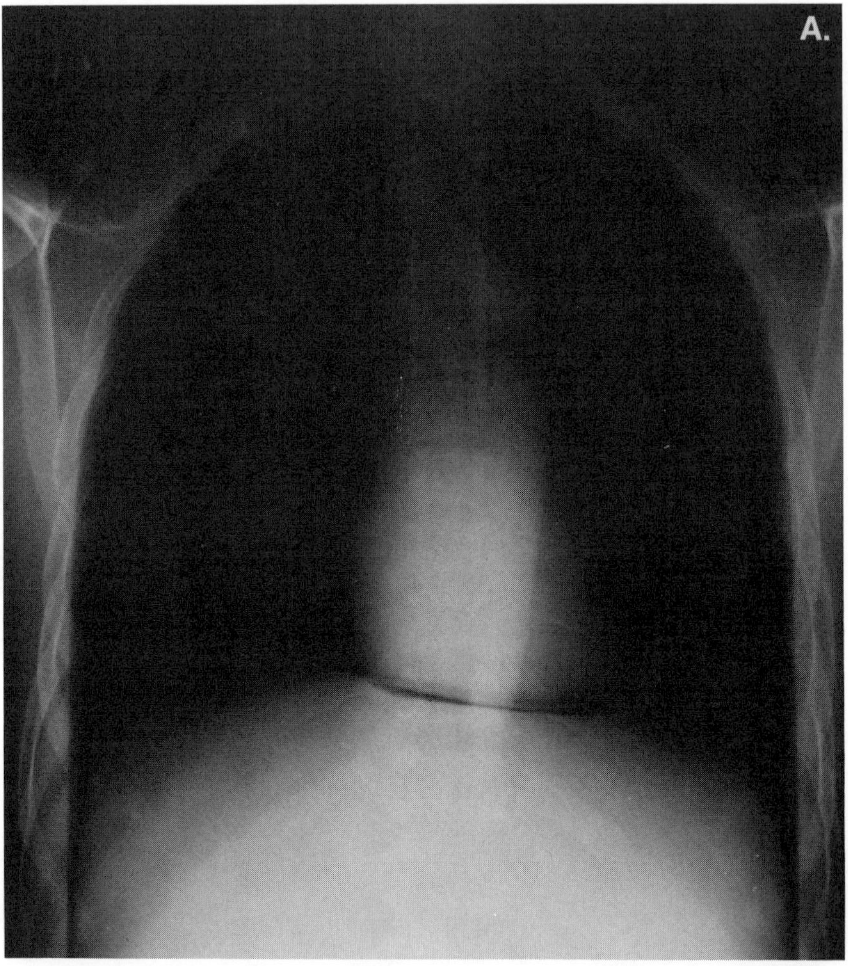

Figure 13.7 (A). Chest radiograph taken at 120 kVp with a grid.

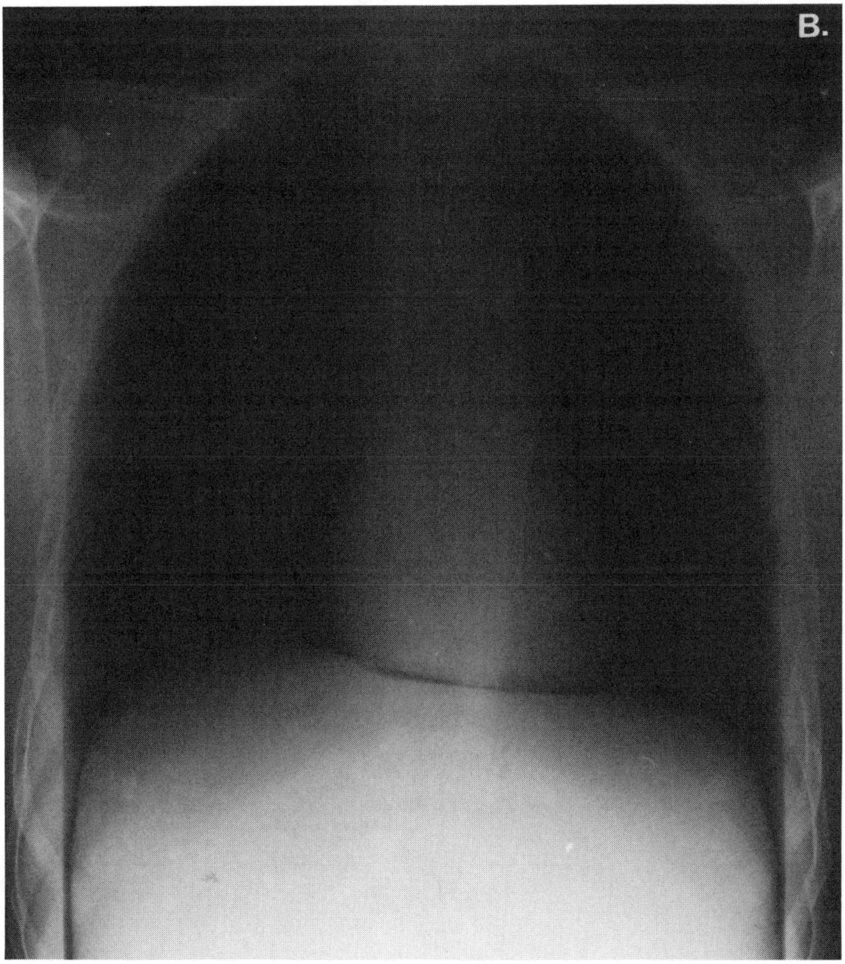

Figure 13.7 (B). Chest radiograph taken as 120 kVp without a grid.

Air Gap Scatter Reduction Technique

Air gap technique involves interposing an air gap between the patient and the radiation detector. Since much of the scattered radiation is wide angle scattering, the greater distance to the detector means that some of the scattered radiation will miss the detector. This is the source of the scatter reduction and **not** attenuation by the air gap. Because the increased patient–film distance would change the magnification if the source–detector distance remained the same, the source to patient distance is increased, usually from 72 to 120", to keep the magnification the same as obtained with a conventional 72" radiograph. A 6 to 8 inch air gap can provide as much scatter reduction as an 8:1 grid. Patient dose with the air gap technique is about one fourth the exposure with a grid technique. Figure 13.8 illustrates the air gap technique.

By changing from 72" to 120" SID, the tube loading would increase by about a factor of three but the patient dose would remain the same because the patient is farther from the source. By eliminating the grid, the MAS can be reduced by about a factor of 4 resulting in a net decrease in tube loading and patient dose.

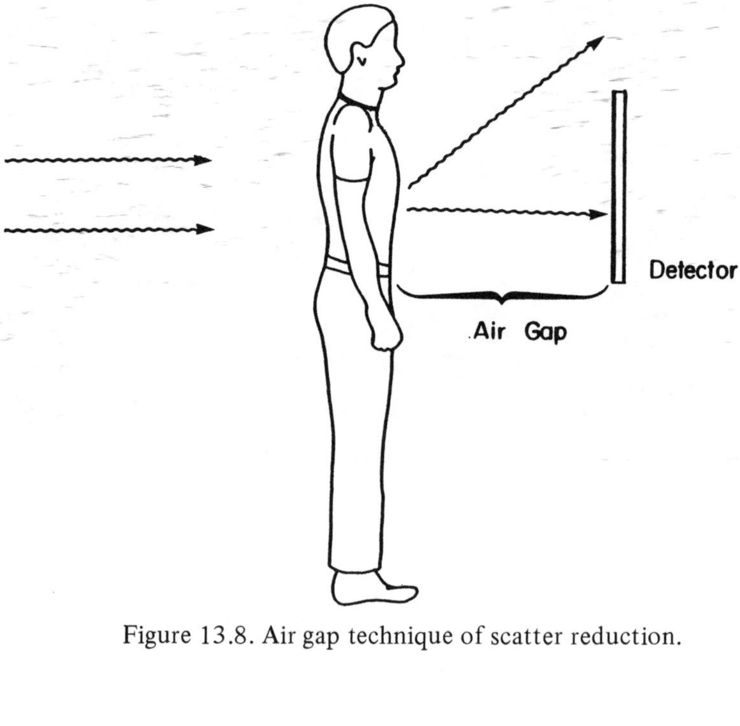

Figure 13.8. Air gap technique of scatter reduction.

Moving Slit Techniques

Almost perfect scatter elimination can be achieved using a moving slit technique as shown in Figure 13.9.

A slit between the x-ray tube and the patient allows only a small strip of radiation to strike the patient. A second slit between the patient and the detector allows only the primary beam to reach the detector. The efficacy of this technique has been clearly demonstrated. It is not in widespread clinical use because of the excessively high loading of the x-ray tube and consequent long time required for an exposure. The patient dose is not increased because only a narrow slit of radiation strikes any portion of the patient.

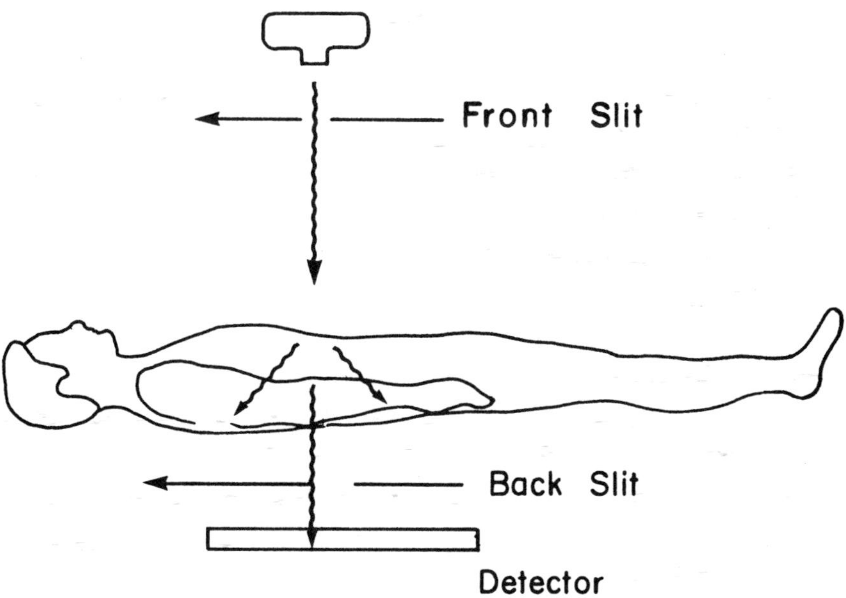

Figure 13.9. Moving slit technique for scatter elimination.

CHAPTER 13 QUESTIONS

1-2, A for True, B for False

1. Primary radiation is radiation that has not passed through the patient.

2. Secondary radiation consists of radiation that has undergone photo-electric of Compton interactions.

3. If a radiation field is reduced from 10 x 10 to 5 x 5 the new scatter is __________ of the old scatter value.
   A. 10%
   B. 25%
   C. 50%
   D. 75%

4-7, Increasing the grid ratio __________ (A for increases, B for decreases, C for stays the same) the __________

4. Scattered Beam Transmission
5. Bucky Factor
6. Contrast Improvement Factor
7. Subject Contrast

8-10, A for True, B for False

8. A grid with a higher grid ratio will allow more scattered radiation to reach the film than one with a lower grid ratio.

9. A grid with a higher grid ratio will have a higher Bucky Factor.

10. A grid with a higher grid ratio will have a lower Contrast Improvement Factor.

11. Grid cut-off
   A. can result from lateral decentering.
   B. can result from a focused grid used at the wrong distance.
   C. can be eliminated by using small fields with a parallel grid.
   D. All of the above.

12. Grid cut-off will occur at a field width of ________ with a 10:1 grid at a 48" SID.

    A. 2.4"
    B. 3.6"
    C. 4.8"
    D. None of the above.

A for True, B for False

13. A focused grid at the correct field size will not exhibit grid cut-off at the widest field sizes.

14. About ______ of the scattered radiation is intercepted by a 10:1 grid.

    A. 10%
    B. 50%
    C. 90%
    D. 99%

15. Moving grids are designed to

    A. blur out the grid lines.
    B. blur out the patient motion.
    C. blur out the grid MTF.
    D. None of the above.

16. The contrast improvement factor

    A. increases the grid ratio.
    B. increases with increasing field sizes.
    C. increases with patient thickness.
    D. All of the above

17. An 85 kVp 100 MA 1/2 sec exposure produces an acceptable density with too much scatter. Which technique would produce an acceptable exposure with a 12:1 grid in place?

    A. 100 kVp 200 MA 1/2 sec
    B. 85 kVp 400 MA 1 sec
    C. 100 kVp 100 MA 1/2 sec
    D. 115 kVp 200 MA 1 sec

18. The Air Gap Technique

A. increases the grid to patient distance to reduce scatter.
B. increases the film to patient distance to reduce scatter.
C. increases the SID to decrease contrast resolution.
D. None of the above.

19. The Moving Slit Technique reduces scatter

A. by allowing only primary radiation to strike the patient.
B. and tube loading by detecting only primary radiation.
C. by allowing only primary radiation to strike the detector.
D. by eliminating all secondary radiation in the patient.

CHAPTER 14

RADIATION DETECTORS

Radiation detectors can be divided into three categories:

1. Gas filled or solid ionization detectors
2. Scintillation detectors
3. Thermoluminescent Dosimeters

All detectors respond to ionization produced by the radiation.

Gas Filled Detectors

The simplest gas filled detector is shown schematically in Figure 14.1. It consists of a metal tube surrounding a central wire connected to a battery. When radiation passes through the detector tube, some of the gas molecules are ionized. The positive ions are pulled to the outer walls and the negative electrons are attracted to the positive center wire. The charge collected on the center wire is measured by the meter.

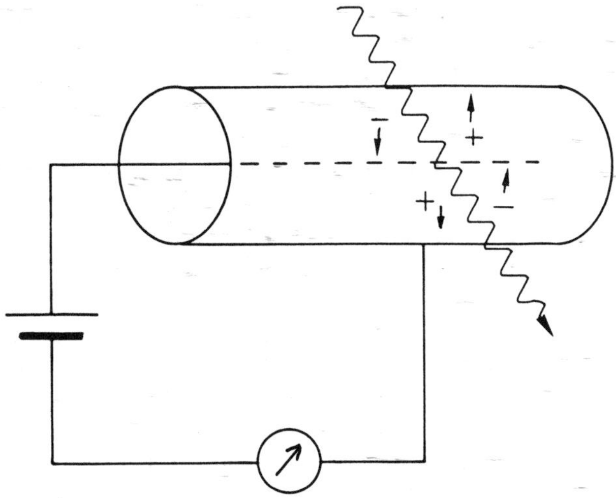

Figure 14.1. Gas filled ionization detector.

The gas in the tube can be air or some other gas. The charge collected as a function of voltage applied to the center wire is shown in Figure 14.2.

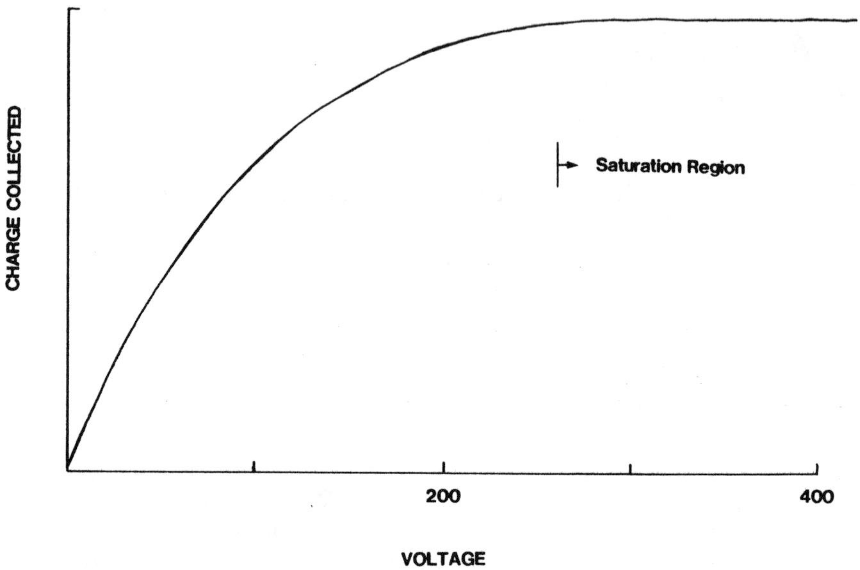

Figure 14.2. Charge collected in an ionization chamber as a function of voltage.

At low voltages, some of the electrons are collected at the center wire but most recombine with positive ions before they reach the center wire. If the applied voltage is increased, the electrons move faster, there is less time for recombination to take place and more electrons are collected at the center wire.

If more than a few hundred volts is applied to the center wire, almost all the ionization electrons are collected at the center wire and the output is said to be **saturated.** The flat region of the curve above an applied voltage of a few hundred volts is known as the saturation region.

Ionization detectors have a small response to radiation; they have **low sensitivity**. Ionization detectors require high amplification to respond to small amounts of radiation. One advantage of ionization detectors is that they have a wide intensity response range, that is they can respond to high and low intensity signals equally well.

The energy response of an ionization detector depends on the detector gas. Air has almost the same atomic number as tissue so an air filled ionization detector has the same energy response as tissue.

Gas filled ionization detectors are used as dose calibrators in nuclear medicine; to calibrate the output of x-ray machines and as detectors in some CT scanners.

Proportional Counters

If the voltage applied to the center wire is increased above the saturation region, the ionization electrons gain enough energy to cause **secondary ionizations** in the gas before reaching the center wire. These secondary ionizations result in a **gas amplification** producing a larger signal than obtained with an ionization detector. In this voltage region, the output signal is **proportional** to the ionization in the detector. Proportional counters are not used in diagnostic Radiology.

Geiger Mueller Counters

If an even higher voltage is applied to the center wire, the detector can be operated in the Geiger Mueller (GM) region. Under these conditions, there is so much amplification that a single ionizing event produces complete ionization of the gas in the tube. This is called the avalanche effect. Figure 14.3 illustrates the response of a gas filled detector as a function of applied voltage. The voltages presented in Figure 14.3 are typical although the actual voltage values depend on the size of the tube and the type of gas.

GM counters usually have a thin window on the sleeve protecting the tube. The thin window allows low energy radiation to enter the tube so it can be detected.

The sensitivity of a GM counter depends strongly on the ability of the radiation to penetrate into the tube. For this reason, GM counters are not used as calibration instruments.

Geiger Mueller counters are extremely sensitive (they can detect a single ionizing event) and are used primarily as survey instruments to detect spilled isotopes or lost radioactive sources. They do not require large amplification and can be made small and rugged for portable use.

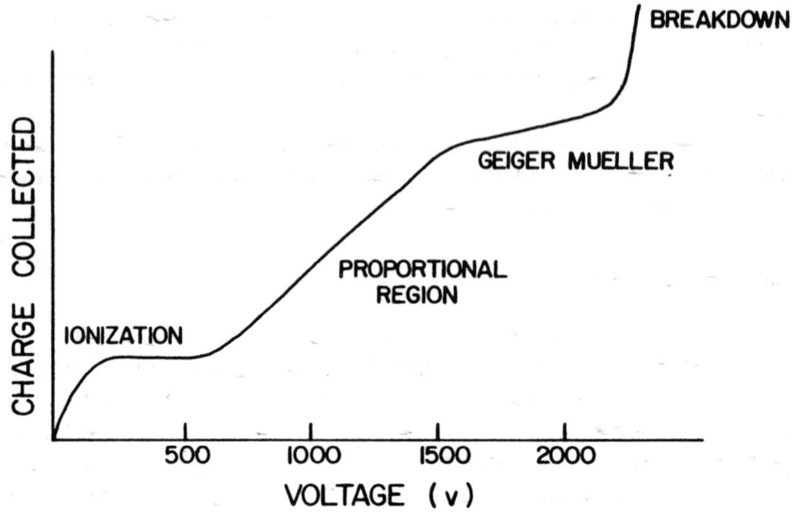

Figure 14.3. Charge collected as a function of applied voltage on a gas filled detector.

Dead Time

With a GM tube and certain other detectors, there must be an interval of at least τ seconds (called the dead time) between events for an event to be recorded. For a GM tube, the dead time may be as high as 100 milliseconds. Any radiation events occurring during the dead time will not be detected. If a counter with dead time τ records an observed Count Rate R_o, the true Count Rate is:

$$R_t = \frac{R_o}{1 - R_o\tau} \qquad 14.1$$

Example 14.1:
A GM tube with a dead time of 40 ms has a recorded count rate of 300 counts/min. What is the true count rate?

$$R_t = \frac{R_o}{1 - R_o\tau}$$

$$R_o = 300 \text{ cpm}$$

$$= \frac{300}{60} \text{ cps}$$

$$= 5 \text{ cps}$$

$$= \frac{5}{1 - 5 \times .040}$$

$$= \frac{5}{1 - .2}$$

$$= \frac{5}{.8}$$

$$= 6.25 \text{ cps}$$

Solid State Detectors

A solid state detector operates in the same way as a gas filled detector except the ionization occurs in a solid instead of a gas. The solid is a **semiconductor.** One simple example of a solid state detector is an n-p junction operated under reverse or back-bias conditions. Under forward-bias conditions, a negative voltage is applied to the n side of the junction and positive voltage applied to the p side and a current flows in the circuit. Figure 14.4 illustrates the schematic operation of a solid state detector.

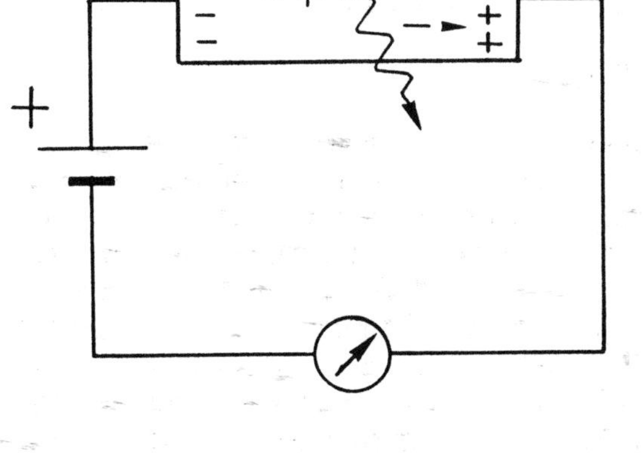

Figure 14.4. Solid state detector

Under back-bias conditions, all free charges are swept out of the depletion layer and there is an electric field in the depletion layer. There is no current in the circuit until an x-ray passes through the detector. Then the charges produced by the ionization are swept out of the region by the electric field and recorded as a current or charge collected. A solid state detector can be operated as an ionization detector but not as a proportional detector of a GM detector. Solid state detectors are small and more sensitive than gas filled detectors because the solid has greater density. They can collect all the energy deposited by the x-ray photons and can determine the energy of the detected photons.

Thermoluminescent Dosimeters (TLD)

TLD detectors give off light when heated, the amount of light depends on the radiation exposure of the TLD. TLD detectors are manufactured out of selected materials with small amounts of added impurities. The impurities alter the crystal structure so that some of the electrons formed by radiation ionization are captured in crystal traps. These electrons are held in the traps until the crystal is heated to release the trapped energy as visible light. The amount of light released depends on the radiation dose accumulated since the last heating. TLD detectors are **integrating detectors**, that is they add up the radiation dose and give off light proportional to the accumulated dose when heated. Their response to radiation is very similar to tissue so they are used widely as personnel dosimeters. TLD detectors must be heated to over 200°C during readout so they cannot be accidently heated to readout temperatures.

Scintillation Detectors

Scintillators are materials which give off light when struck by gamma or x-ray photons. Sodium Iodide, NaI (Tl) is the most commonly used scintillator. A photomultiplier tube converts light into an electrical signal. A scintillation crystal connected to the photomultiplier tube produces an electrical signal output proportional to the amount of light released by the scintillator. The Tl in the NaI (Tl) is used as a wavelength shifter to match the light output from the sodium iodide crystal to the photocathode sensitivity. Figure 14.5 illustrates the operation of a scintillation crystal and photomultiplier.

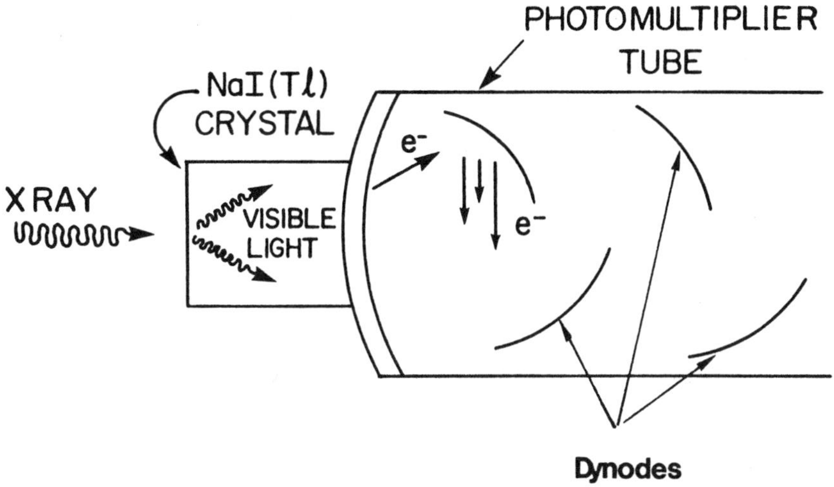

Figure 14.5. Schematic view of a photomultiplier tube.

The photocathode emits electrons when activated by visible light from the NaI crystal. The electrons from the photocathode are accelerated to the first dynode. Figure 14.6 shows an x-ray of a photomultiplier tube. Each dynode in the photomultiplier tube emits four or five electrons for every incident electron.

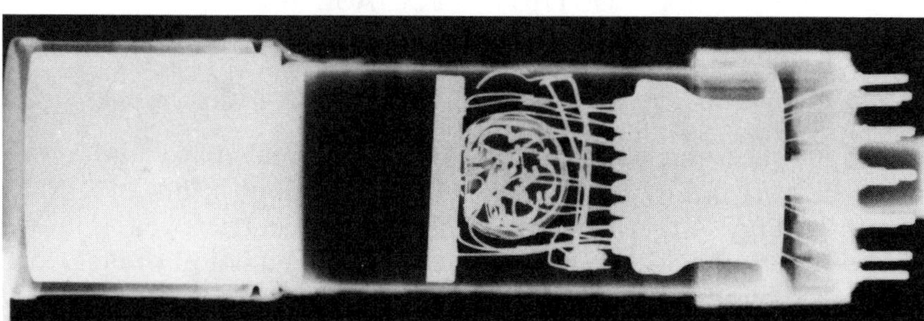

Figure 14.6. X-ray of photomultiplier tube.

Output of Scintillation Detectors

Gamma or x-rays striking a sodium iodide crystal can interact via either a Compton or photoelectric interaction. A photoelectric interaction absorbs all the photon energy in the crystal. A Compton interaction results in a sharing of the energy between the recoil electron and the scattered photon which may escape from the crystal. Larger crystals increase the chance of a photoelectric interaction following an initial Compton scattering. Complete absorption of the photon energy results from such a two step process. Figure 14.7 illustrates a spectra obtained from a scintillation detector. The pulses from the photoelectric and Compton interactions are indicated.

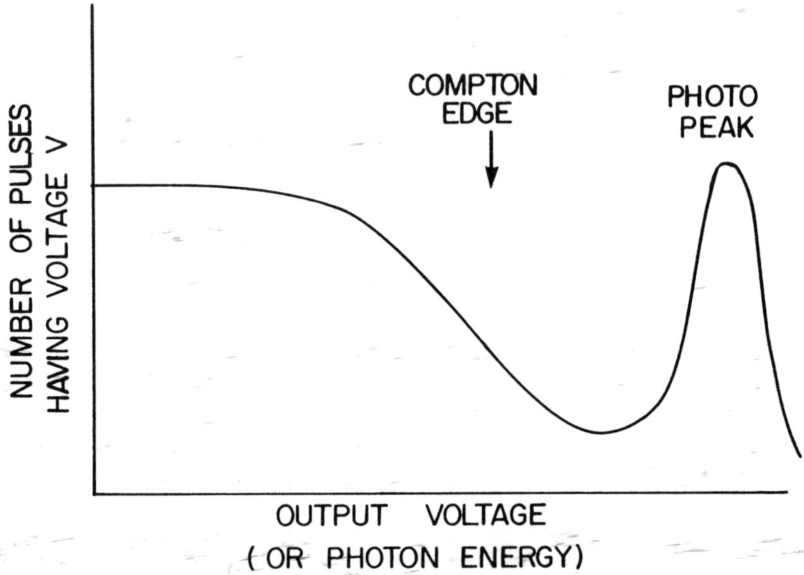

Figure 14.7. Pulse height spectrum from scintillation crystal.

The photo peak represents photons which have undergone photoelectric interactions resulting in the deposition of all the photon energy into the crystal. The photoelectric peak is not a narrow line but has some width because the emission of electrons from the photocathode and from the dynodes is a statistical process. Some events result in more electrons being collected than others.

The Compton edge represents the maximum energy a scattered electron can obtain from a photon from the Compton interaction. Figure 14.8 illustrates an idealized gamma ray spectrum observed when Cs–137 (E_γ = .66 MeV) gamma rays strike a sodium iodide detector.

The voltage output of the photomultiplier tube is proportional to the energy deposited in the crystal.

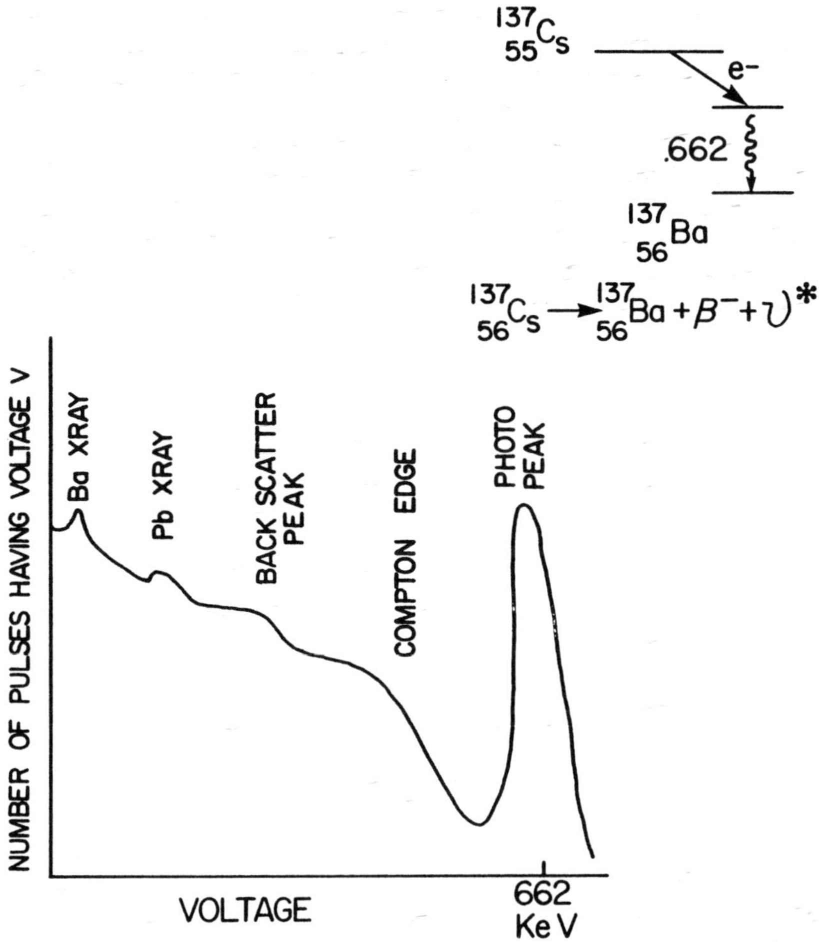

Figure 14.8. Pulse height spectrum from Cs-137 gamma rays.

The **photoelectric peak** is produced by photons which are completely absorbed in the sodium iodide crystal. The **Compton edge** is produced because there is a maximum energy which Compton scattered photons can deposit into the crystal. This maximum energy for Compton scattered photons is always less than the photo peak energy.

The **backscatter peak** is produced by photons which are scattered backwards from the surrounding shielding (usually lead) and which usually have energies between 200 and 250 KeV.

The **lead x–ray peak** is caused by characteristic 88 KeV lead x–rays from the surrounding lead shielding. The barium x–ray peak results from characteristic x–rays from the daughter nucleus Ba - 56.

One other peak which may appear in a scintillation spectrum is the **escape peak.** It is produced by interactions in which the K x–ray of iodine escapes from the crystal. Thus, the escape peak is 30 KeV below the photo peak. Figure 14.9 illustrates the example of an escape peak which could be observed from the decay of Mercury 197 ($E_\gamma = 77$ KeV).

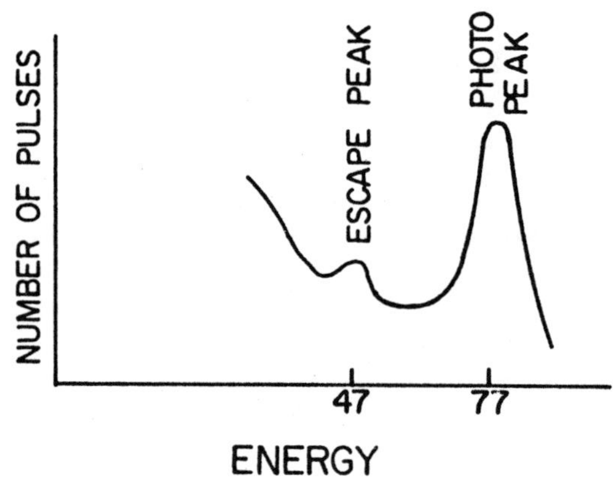

Figure 14.9. Photopeak from Mercury 197 decay together with the escape peak resulting from 30 KeV iodine K x–ray escaping from the scintillation crystal.

The escape peak is recorded at about 47 KeV. Escape peaks are noticeable only with low energy gamma rays. The photo peak produced by high energy gamma rays is so wide it completely obscures the escape peak.

Energy Resolution

Resolution of a detector is measured as the full width at half maximum of the photopeak signal. Figure 14.10 illustrates the measurement of the resolution from a photo peak.

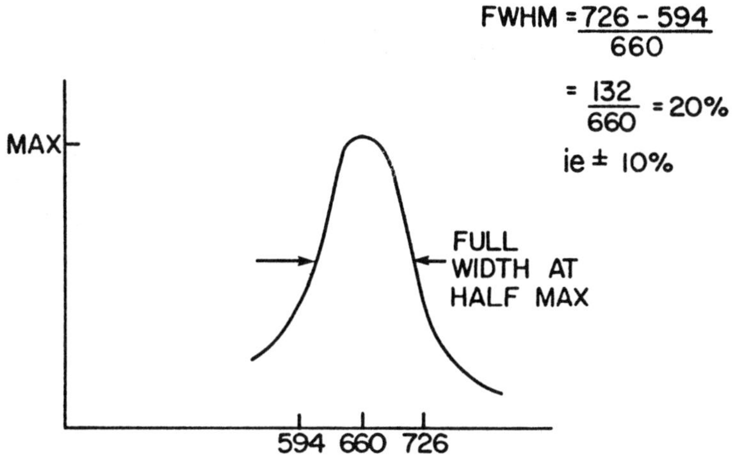

Figure 14.10. Example of detector resolution.

It is possible to electronically reject pulses which are above or below a specified level. This is called setting a detector window width. Usually, the detector **window width** is set at 10%, i.e., plus or minus 10% of the photo peak energy.

The advantage of selecting only pulses that lie in the photo peak is that most scattered radiation can be rejected with such a window setting. Pulses in the photo peak guarantee thay were produced by x–ray photons which have not been scattered prior to reaching the detector. Using a wider window, increases detection efficiency but decreases scatter rejection.

Xenon Gas Detectors

Xenon gas detectors are used in some CT scanners because the density of Xenon (3.52 gm/cc) is comparable to that of NaI (Tl) – (3.67 gm/cc) and a shorter duration signal is obtained. This means higher count rates can be tolerated with a Xenon detector than with a NaI (Tl) detector.

Other Scintillators

Sodium iodide detectors have high efficiency (about 20%) but some of the light from the sodium iodide crystal comes off for about one quarter of the microsecond (250 ns). If another radiation event occurs during this decay time, the energy measurement of the second event will be erroneous. Figure 14.11 illustrates this "pileup effect."

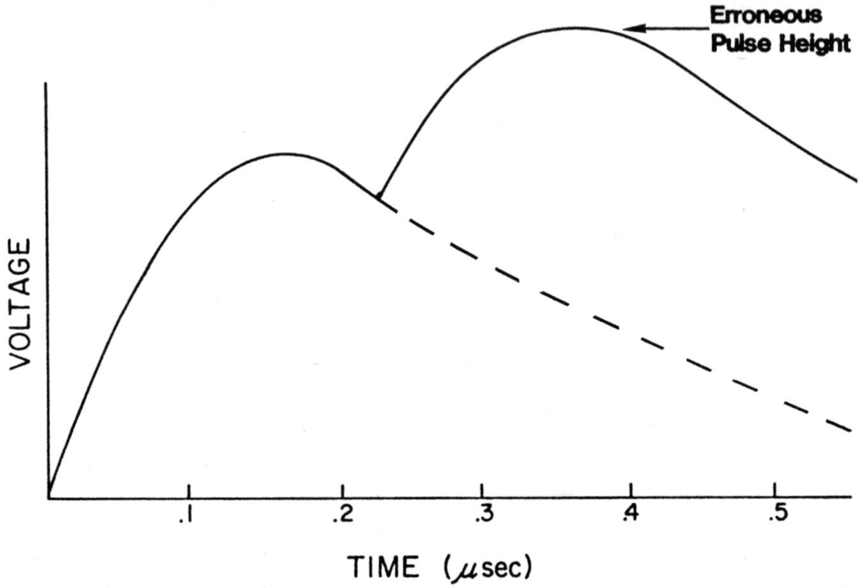

Figure 14.11. Example of pulse pileup.

Two solutions are possible, one is to limit the number of events which occur per second, the other is to employ a detector with a shorter decay time. Bismuth germinate (BGO) and Cesium iodide (CsI) are also being used as scintillation detectors because their decay times are shorter than NaI (Tl).

CHAPTER 14 QUESTIONS

1. A gas filled detector
   - A. collects the gas molecules to measure the ionization density.
   - B. collects the charged ions to detect the presence of radiation.
   - C. produces a light output when struck by radiation.
   - D. produces light output when heated after exposure to radiation.

2-8, Match the uses and characteristics of these radiation detectors. The answers can be used more than once.

- A. Ionization Chamber
- B. G.M. Counter
- C. NaI Scintillator
- D. TLD Detector

2. Used for personnel dosimeters
3. Used to search for lost source
4. Used to calibrate radiation output
5. Gives off light while irradiated
6. Gives off light when heated after irradiation
7. Has a long (200 ms) dead time
8. Has a long (200 ns) decay time

9. In the saturation region of an ion chamber
   - A. essentially all the ions are collected.
   - B. an increase in voltage will collect more ions.
   - C. the charge collected depends on the relative humidity.
   - D. more negative than positive ions are collected.

10. An air filled ionization detector

A. can detect single ionizing events.
B. has a long dead time.
C. has an energy response equal to tissue.
D. must be heated after irradiation.

11. A scintillation detector

A. converts visible photons into x-ray photons.
B. can detect the amount but not the energy of the x-ray photons.
C. can detect the amount and energy of the x-ray photons.
D. uses Tl to convert visible to x-ray wavelengths.

12-16, A ___________ detector can be used to determine the energy of the radiation. (A for True, B for False)

12. Ionization Chamber
13. GM Counter
14. Scintillation Crystal
15. TLD Detector
16. Solid State Detector

17. A larger scintillation crystal is more efficient because

A. there will be more Compton interactions
B. there will be more coherent interactions.
C. there is an increased chance of a photoelectric interaction followed by one or more Compton interactions.
D. there is an increased chance of one or more Compton interactions followed by a photoelectric interaction.

18. The Compton edge in a pulse height spectrum
A. is always half the photopeak value.
B. is a peak of photons 30 KeV less than the photopeak.
C. represents the maximum energy of a Compton scattered photon.
D. represents a photon that has been Compton scattered from the lead shielding.

19. The backscatter peak
A. represents photons backscattered into the crystal from the surrounding shielding.
B. represents photons backscattered into the surrounding shielding from the crystal.
C. represents characteristic x-rays backscattered into the crystal.
D. represents Iodine x-rays which are backscattered into the crystal.

20-23, Match

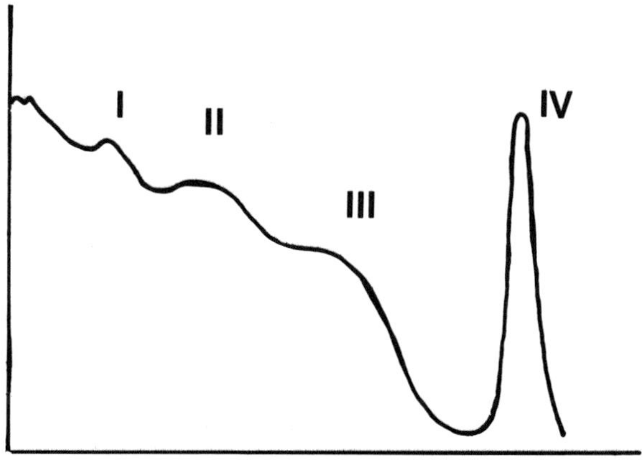

20. I
21. II
22. III
23. IV

A. Photo Peak
B. Lead X-ray
C. Backscatter Peak
D. Compton Edge

24. The full width at half maximum of a 200 KeV photo peak is 40 KeV. The resolution of this crystal is

A. ±20%
B. ±10%
C. ±40%
D. ±5%

25. Pulse pile up

A. is caused by low energy photons.
B. is caused by long pulse rise times.
C. produces erroneous resolution values.
D. produces erroneous energy values.

CHAPTER 15

FLUOROSCOPIC IMAGING

Dynamic imaging allows the radiologist to view the internal structures of the patient in action. Dynamic imaging is usually performed using image intensified fluoroscopic systems. Early direct fluoroscopy (not image intensified) systems consisted of lead glass coated with a fluorescent material. The radiologist viewed the patient's internal organs while protected from the x-rays by the lead glass.

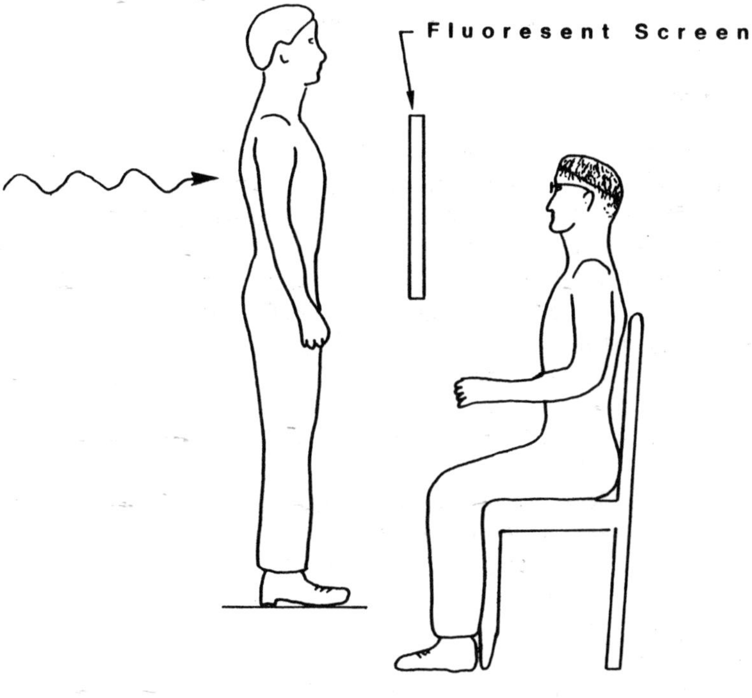

Figure 15.1. Direct fluoroscopy.

Unfortunately, the direct fluoroscopic image was dim and it was impossible to see small objects.

Radiation doses to the patient under direct fluoroscopy varied from .07–.25Sv/min. (7–25 rad/min).

Direct fluoroscopy resolution is limited by the resolution of the eye rather than the resolution of the screen.

Visual Properties

The eye collects photons for about 200 ms and no longer. This means the image quality of a dim fluoroscope image cannot be improved by watching for a longer time.

There are two types of vision:

Scotopic Vision at low light levels
Photopic at high light levels

When we move from regions of high light intensity to low light intensity (a movie theater for example) our vision gradually shifts from photopic to scotopic vision over about a 20 minute period. This is known as **dark adaptation.**

Scotopic Vision

Low light levels require scotopic vision (rod vision) which has **high sensitivity but poor visual acuity**. Scotopic vision has a resolving power of about 1 mm, and poor contrast perceptability. Contrast differences of 15–20% are just noticeable with scotopic vision. Dark adapted vision is not destroyed by red light so radiologists used to wear red goggles before fluoroscopy to protect their dark adaptation.

The fovea of the eye has no rods. This means that with scotopic vision:

a. The viewer must look slightly to the side to see things with rod vision.
b. Rod vision is improved by motion. Visual acuity with rod (scotopic) vision is about 10 times worse than with cone vision (photopic vision).

Photopic Vision

Photopic vision (cone vision) has **low sensitivity but high visual acuity** (.03 mm resolution) and good contrast perception.

Under photopic vision it is easy to detect a 1–2% difference in contrast.

Image Intensifiers

The purpose of an image intensifier tube is to add enough energy to the fluoroscopic system so that brightness levels permit photopic vision (cones) instead of scotopic vision (rods).

Dark adaptation is not necessary to view image intensifier images.

Figure 15.2 illustrates the basic operation of an image intensifier.

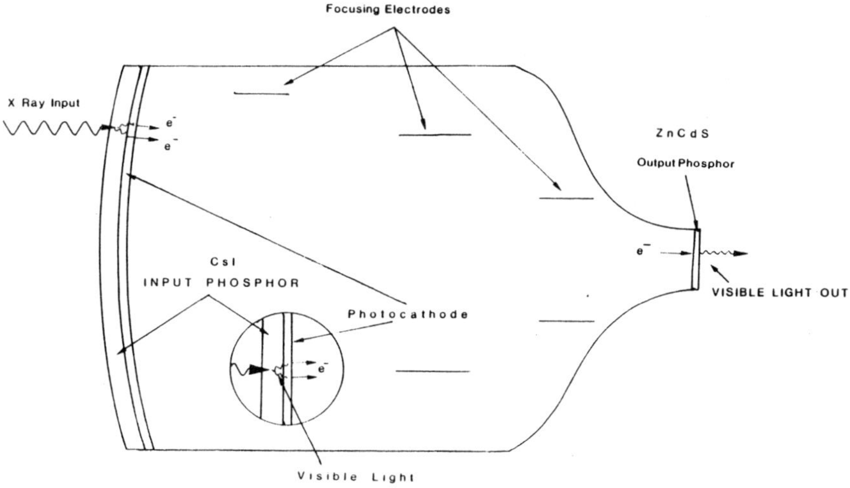

Figure 15.2. Operation of an image intensifier.

The steps in image formation with an image intensifier are:

A. Convert incoming x–rays to visible light in the CsI input phosphor layer.
B. Convert the visible light into photoelectrons at the photocathode.
C. Accelerate the photo electrons to the output phosphor.
D. Convert electrons to visible light at the (ZnCd)S output phosphor.

Input Phosphor

The original input phosphors were (ZnCd)S, the newer image intensifier tubes have CsI input phosphors. CsI has K edges closer to the x–ray beam average energy and can be vacuum deposited to provide more dense packing and a needle–like crystal shape that channels the light more efficiently onto the photocathode. Modern input phosphors absorb about 50% of the incident x–rays.

Output Phosphor

The output phosphor is made of (ZnCd)S because it is more efficient at converting electron energy into visible light and has excellent resolution in thin layers.

Brightness Gain

Brightness gain is made up of two components:

1. Minification gain the same light energy is concentrated in a smaller area.
2. Voltage or flux gain from the acceleration of the electrons. Acceleration voltages of 25–50 KV are used.

Minification Gain

Minification gain, Gm, is given by:

$$G_m = \frac{(\text{Input diameter})^2}{(\text{Output diameter})^2}$$

The usual output diameter is 25 millimeters. The input phosphor diameter varies from 13 to 30 centimeters. Table 15.1 gives typical input phosphor diameters, minification gain and relative exposures for the same light output.

TABLE 15.1

Input Diameter	*Minification Gain*	*Relative X-ray Exposure*
13 cm (5")	25	1.0
23 cm (9")	81	0.3
30 cm (12")	144	0.19

Flux Gain

Typical flux or voltage gains range between 30 and 50. The total brightness gain is the product of the voltage or flux gain and the minification gain.

Example 15.1:
A 15 cm diameter (input) image intensifier tube with an output diameter of 2.54 cm has a flux gain of 42. What is the brightness gain of this tube?

First calculate the minification gain:

$$\text{Minification Gain} = \frac{(\text{Input Diameter})^2}{(\text{Output Diameter})^2}$$

$$= (15)^2/(2.54)^2$$

$$= 225/6.45$$

$$= 34.9$$

$$\text{Total brightness gain} = \text{Flux gain} \times \text{Minification gain}$$

$$= 42 \times 34.9$$

$$= 1466$$

Dual Mode Image Intensifiers

Many image intensifiers have the provision for two input diameters. Such tubes are known as **dual mode** image intensifiers. Figure 15.3 illustrates a dual mode 9 inch and 6 inch image intensifier.

To change the field of view from 9" Dia to 6" Dia, the image intensifier tube accelerating and focus voltages are changed so that only the central 6" diameter circular area is focused on the output phosphor.

In the 6 inch mode, the central six inches of the input phosphor covers the **same** output phosphor diameter resulting in a **magnified image**. There is less minification gain so the exposure rate must be boosted to maintain the same output image brightness. For a change from 9" to 6" mode, the increase in exposure

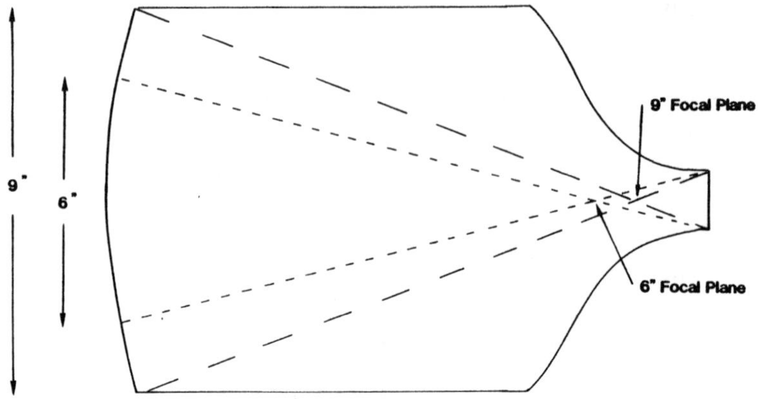

Figure 15.3. Dual mode image intensifier.

(2.25 greater) is the ratio of the areas, i.e., 81 divided by 36. The spatial resolution of the image intensifier is increased in the magnified mode.

Example 15.2:
What is the new patient exposure rate if the image intensifier mode is changed from 6" to 9"? The entrance exposure rate in the 6" mode is 1860 C/kg – min (7.2 R/min).

Changing from 6" to 9" mode increases the brightness gain by the ratio:

$$\frac{9^2}{6^2} = \frac{81}{36}$$

$$= 2.25$$

The entrance exposure rate can be decreased by this same factor

$$\text{New Exposure Rate} = \frac{1860}{2.25}$$

$$= 830 \text{ C/kg} - \text{min}$$

$$= 3.2 \text{ R/min.}$$

The exposures are smaller for the larger input image intensifiers because light is collected from a larger area.

Conversion Factor

The **conversion factor** is the ratio of the light output in Candela/m^2 to the x-ray input. Typical values are 190–380 Cd/m^2 per μC/kg–s (50–100 Cd/m^2 per mR/s).

Optical Systems

Figure 15.4 indicates a typical optical system containing the collimator lens, a beam splitter, an aperture, and an imaging lens for a cine camera.

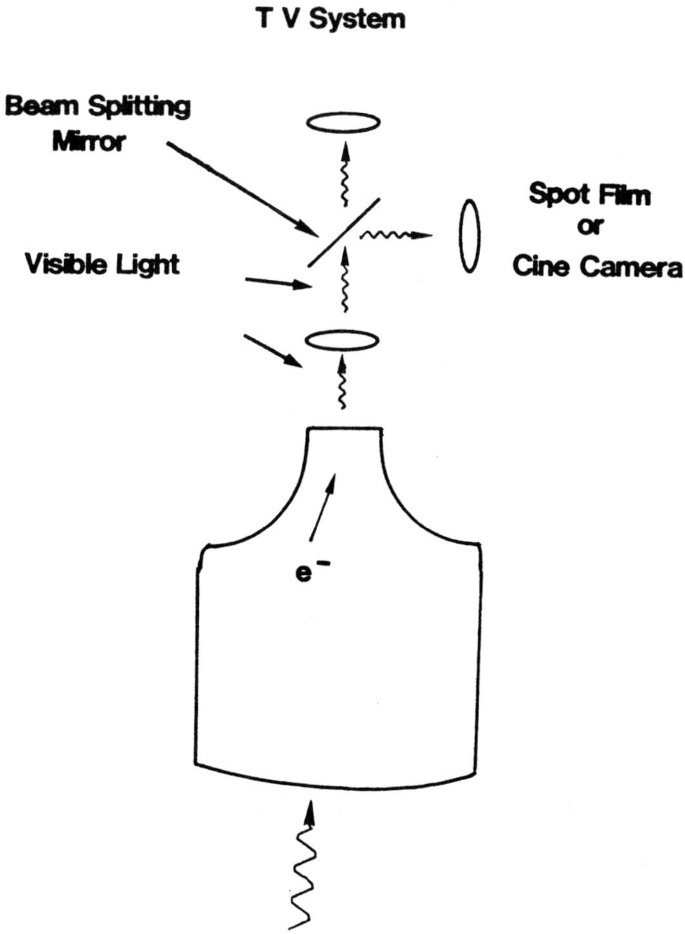

Figure 15.4. Image intensifier optical system.

The collimator lens collects the light from the image intensifier screen and the beam splitter sends light to both a viewing and a recording system. A mirror viewing system has better resolution than a TV or cine camera system.

Magnification

The magnification of the image intensifier optical system is given by:

$$M = \frac{\text{focal length of camera lens}}{\text{focal length of collimator lens}}$$

Optical System Efficiency

The f–number is given by the following equation:

$$f = \frac{\text{focal length of lens}}{\text{diameter of lens}}$$

The f–number is changed by adjusting the aperture. There are a series of standard f–stop numbers which are given in Table 15.2. f–stop numbers are written as f/4. f/8, f/16.

TABLE 15.2

f-Stop	*Relative Area or Efficiency*
16	1
11	2
8	4
5.6	8
4	16
2.8	32
2.0	64
1.4	128
1	256

Notice that changing the aperture by one f–stop changes the light collection efficiency by a factor of 2. Smaller f–stop numbers have larger apertures.

Veiling Glare

Veiling glare is a general brightness over the entire output phosphor. Veiling glare is the image intensifier equivalent of background fog. It is caused by retrograde light from the output phosphor striking the photocathode. The higher the veiling glare the smaller the contrast resolution of the image intensifier tube.

Vignetting

Vignetting is a light cutoff near the edges of an image so that the image appears with full brightness only in the central portion. The diameter of the image is set by the diameter of the output phosphor of the image intensifier tube. If there is too large an aperture, i.e., too small an f–stop, in the intermediate stages of the lens system the final image will show a dim area of decreased intensity around the edges. If the camera lens is located at position I as shown in Figure 15.5, there will be no vignetting; if it is placed in location II there will be vignetting. To eliminate vignetting, the camera lens should be placed close to the collimating lens or have a smaller diameter than the collimating lens, or both.

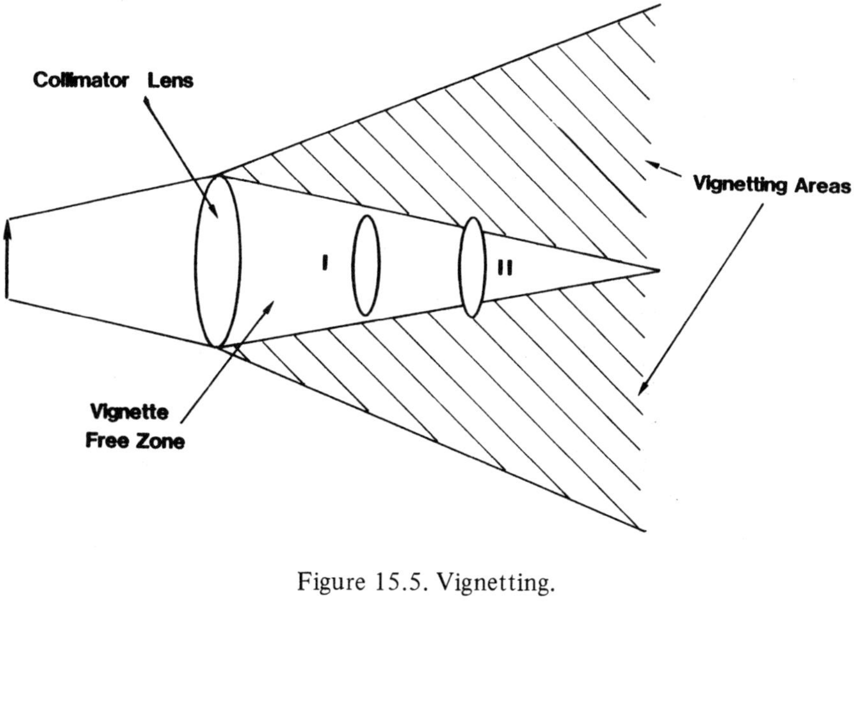

Figure 15.5. Vignetting.

Statistical Noise of Image Intensified Images

The statistical quality of the image intensified image is determined by the number of photons at the point where the fewest photons are present. This location is called the **quantum sink.** The **quantum noise** or **quantum mottle** of the final image is determined by the number of photons present at the **quantum sink.** In an image intensifier system the quantum sink is at the **input phosphor.** Increasing the brightness gain of the system will make the output image brighter but will **not** decrease the quantum mottle.

Figure 15.6 illustrates how the noise level is set by the photon flux at the input to the image intensifier tube.

Quantum mottle can be reduced **only** by increasing the x-ray flux at the image intensifier input.

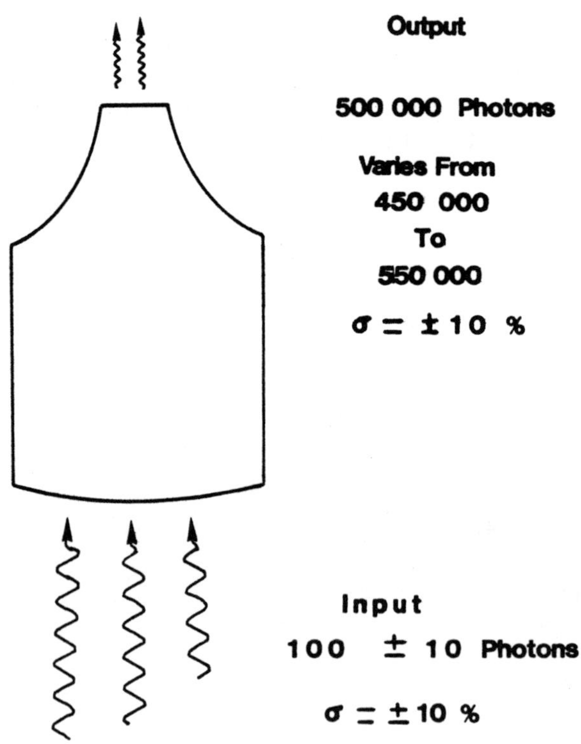

Figure 15.6. The noise level of the output depends on the number of photons at the input.

If an image is too noisy, the kVp and/or MA must be increased to increase the photon flux. To avoid overexposing/overloading TV circuits, the increase in x–ray flux can be balanced by a reduction in the size of the aperture in the lens system (i.e., increasing the f–stop number). Figure 15.7 illustrates how changes in flux and aperture size are balanced to maintain the same output brightness under changes in input x–ray intensity.

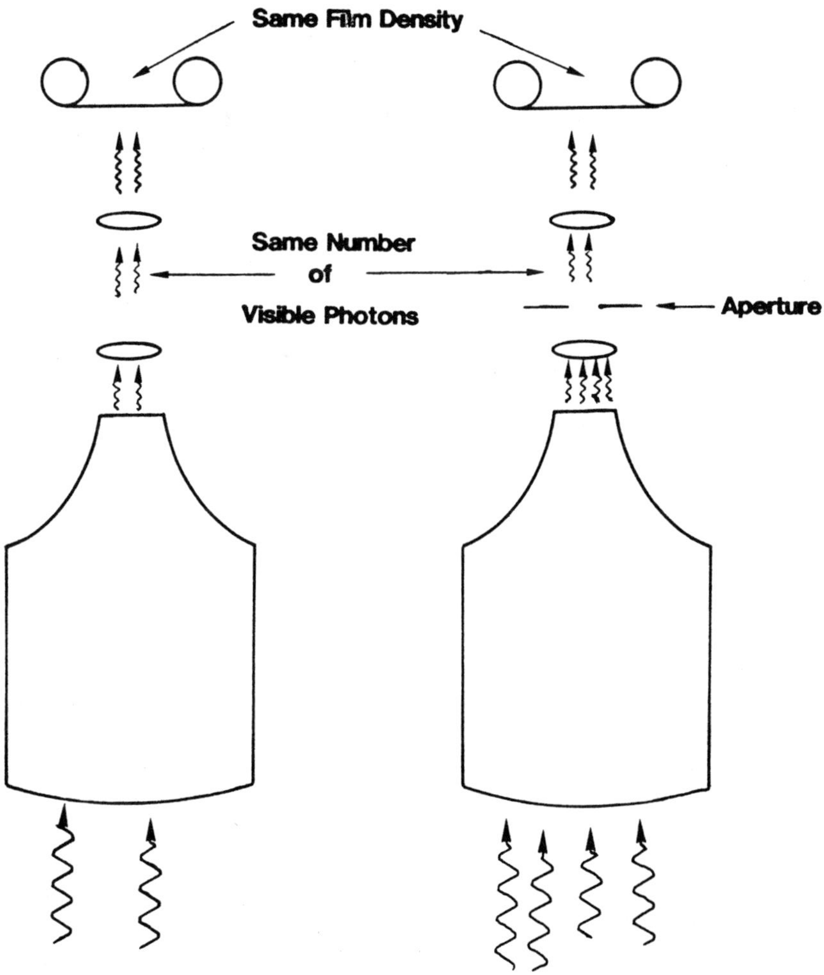

Figure 15.7. Decreasing the quantum mottle is accomplished by decreasing the aperture and increasing the input x–ray intensity.

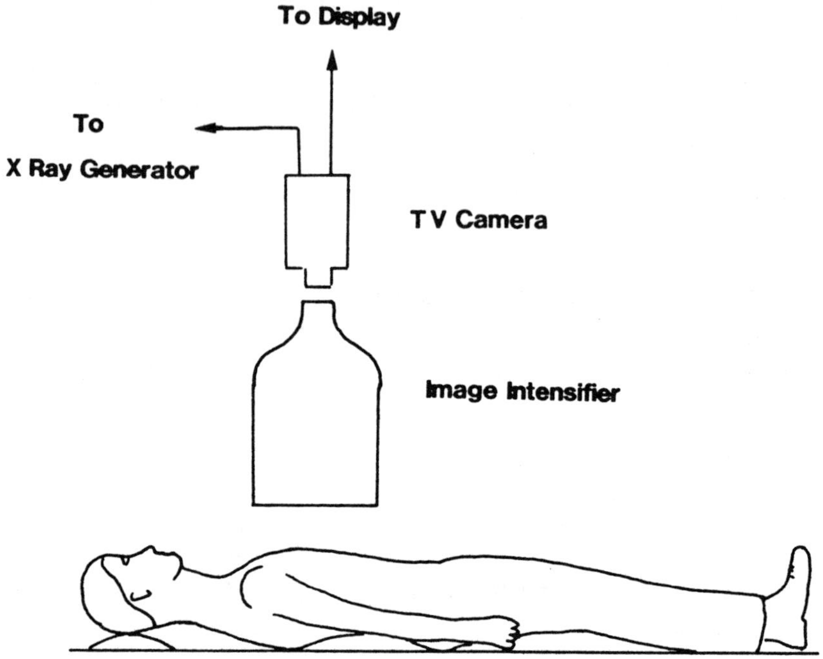

Figure 15.8. Automatic brightness control of fluoroscopy.

Automatic Brightness Control

Under Automatic Brightness Control a sensor samples the output of the image intensifier system to control the light output. When the fluoroscopic system is moved from the chest to the abdomen the x–ray intensity must be increased to compensate for the increased absorption. The x–ray tube output is altered by changing either the MA or the kVp to maintain constant light output from the image intensifier tube.

For many years the preferred method of changing the brightness was by changing the kVp. The kVp could be changed more radiply than the MA which was changed by changes in the filament temperature MA changes have a relatively slow response time. Changes in kVp affect the contrast as well as the x–ray intensity. Recently, grid pulsed tubes have been used in fluoroscopy to change the MA. Grid pulsed tubes can change the MA by changing the amount of time the grid allows the tube current to flow. This allows the output brightness to be changed rapidly without changing the contrast.

Recording Fluoroscopic Images

Most fluoroscopic images are recorded either on film or video tape.

Cineradiographs recorded on film provide better spatial resolution but require a higher patient dose than video tape recordings. Cine film must be processed for viewing whereas video tape images can be reviewed immediately to verify the study was successful and complete. The contrast and brightness of video recorded images can be adjusted during viewing but cine images cannot. Cine film provides superior slow motion and stop frame images.

Cine–fluoroscopy records the image intensifier images on cineradiographic film. A cine–camera is a movie camera which photographs the image intensifier tube output phosphor.

Figure 15.9 illustrates the operation of a cine camera.

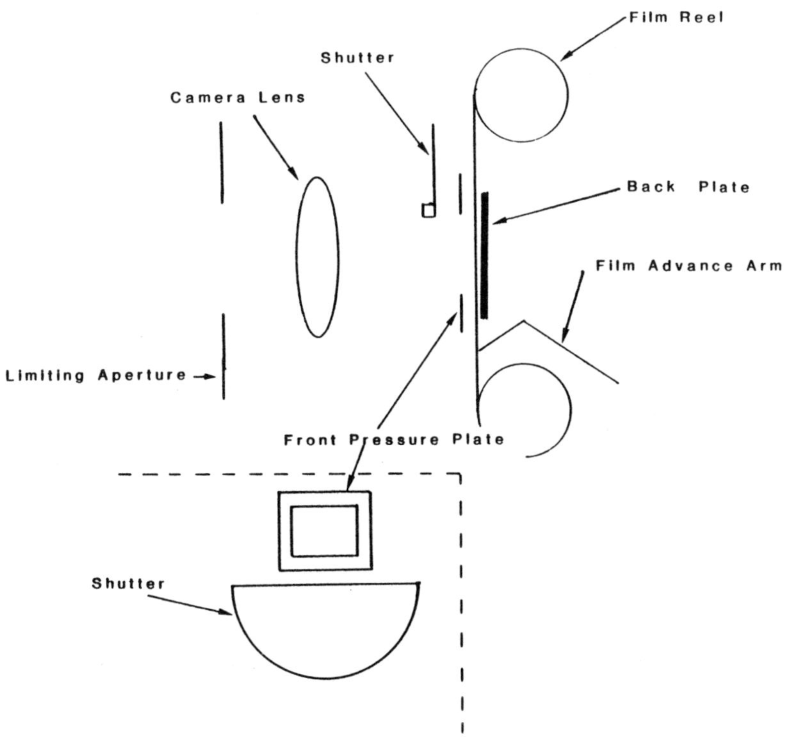

Figure 15.9. Cine camera shutter and film transport operation.

Film Transport

During the transport of the film for the preparation of the next exposure, the shutter rotates in front of the aperture and the advance or pull–down arm moves the film one frame forward. A pressure plate moves forward to hold the film against the back plate. By this time the shutter has rotated around to allow light to strike the film.

For ease in timing the frame speed is a multiple of 60 cycles, i.e., 15, 30, 60 or 120 frames/sec. The shutter mechanism sends a signal to the x–ray generator to indicate when the film is in place and ready to be exposed. The x–ray pulses are synchronized with the shutter open time to reduce patient exposure and tube loading.

Image Framing

A 35 mm film has an image area of 18 mm high by 24 mm wide. There is no way to put the output phosphor's circular image exactly on the film. The two extreme choices are:

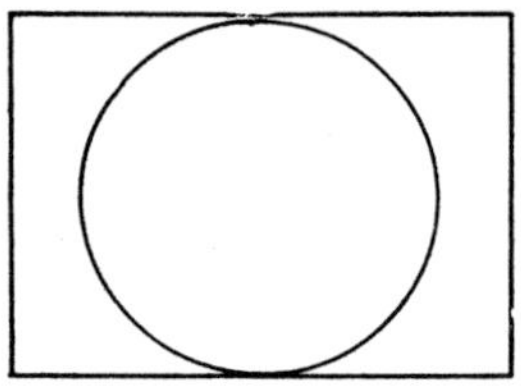

EXACT FRAMING
100% of image is recorded on 60% of film area, 40% of film is unused.

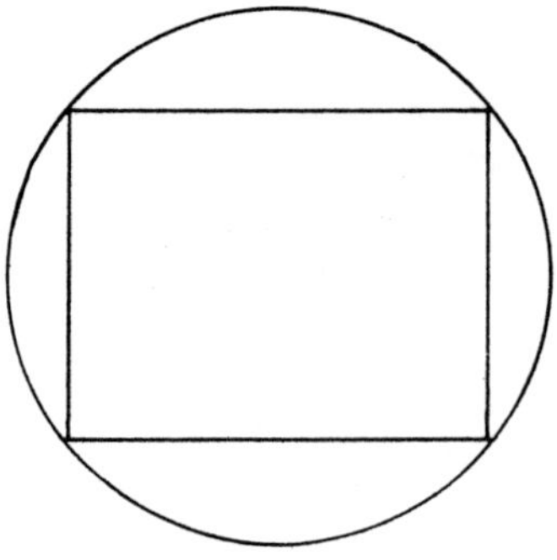

OVERFRAMING
100% of film area is used to record 60% of the image - 40% of image area is unused.

Figure 15.10. Exact and overframing of Cine Images.

Overframing results in a magnified image and unused exposure to the patient. Overframing requires higher patient exposure because only a fraction of the output is used to expose the film.

Exposure Rates for Cine Fluorography

Typical exposure values at the face of the image intensifier range between 5–26 nC/kg (20–100 μR) per frame. Entrance skin exposures to the patient are about 100 times as large, i.e., typical exposure rates are .5–2.5 μC/kg (2–10 mR) per frame. This results in an entrance skin exposure rate between 2–9 mC/kg (7–35R) per minute at a frame rate of 60 frames per second. If the frame rate is reduced, the exposure is reduced by the same factor.

Example 15.3:
What is the exposure rate to the patient in R/min at a frame rate of 15 f/s if the entrance exposure is 4mR/frame?

$$\text{Entrance exposure rate in mR/sec} = 4\ \text{mR/frame} \times 15\ \text{frames/s}$$

$$= 60\ \text{mR/s}$$

$$\text{Entrance exposure rate in R/min} = 3.6\ \text{R/min}$$

Exposure From 16 and 35 mm Films

The question of whether to use 16 mm or 35 mm film to record a fluoroscopic exam rests on the amount of quantum mottle that is acceptable. The 35 mm film area is about four times greater than 16 mm film area. If everything else is the same (film optical density, image intensifier tube, film type, frame rate, etc.), 35 mm film requires about **four times** the number of photons, and hence four times the x-ray flux as a 16 mm film. Because the quantum sink is the input to the image intensifier tube, the quantum mottle is about halved with the 35 mm film. Many departments use 16 mm film for lower abdominal studies because they are willing to accept the greater image mottle in return for lowered patient and scattered radiation doses.

Spot Film Cameras

The exposure for a 105 millimeter abdominal spot film is about 100 mR. This can be compared with the exposure for a

14 by 14 spot film of about 300 mR. The difference in exposure is because the 105 spot film is recording an image off the image intensifier tube output whereas the 14 x 14 spot film uses a film screen detector. These are exposures at the detector, entrance skin exposure are about 100 times greater. The difference in exposure is due to the added brightness amplification of the image intensifier.

TV Viewing and Recording

A basic TV system operation is shown in Figure 15.11.

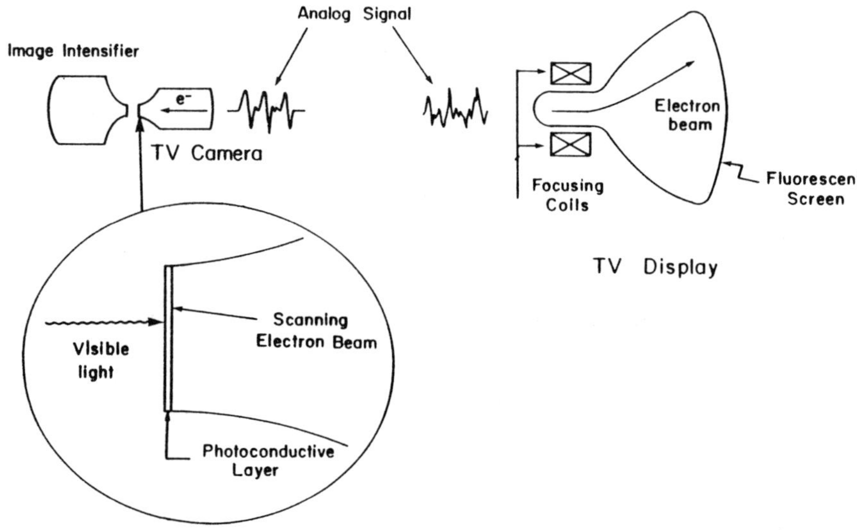

Figure 15.11. TV recording and display system.

TV Camera Operation

The image is focused on a photosensitive layer (antimony trisulfide) plated on the front face of the TV camera. An electron beam is swept across this photo sensitive layer and the electron current which passes through the target plate is collected as the video signal. The resistance of the layer varies with the amount of light striking the plate. If the conductivity of the photosensitive layer is large because a lot of light is striking that area of the target then most of the electron beam will pass through the target plate and will appear as a large video signal. When the scanning electron beam reaches a dark area of the picture the conductivity will be low and little of the electron beam will appear as the video signal. The video signal consists of voltage changes representing light and dark areas of the photosensitive layer. The layer is scanned with 525 scan lines every 1/30 second.

Vidicon tubes suffer from image lag when the light levels change rapidly as when the fluoroscopy system is moved from the abdomen to the chest. The light sensitive layer does not respond instantly but lags behind increases or decreases in light level. The **plumbicon** tube uses a lead monoxide photosensitive layer. It has much less lag than a vidicon tube.

TV Display System

The display or picture tube has an electron beam which is scanned in synchrony with the camera electron beam. The intensity of the electron beam allowed to strike the picture tube phosphor is modulated so that it reproduces the light and dark areas as picked up by the camera.

By convention, in the United States a television picture is made up of 525 line frames. One frame is displayed every 1/30th of a second. A frame is made up of two fields, each containing half (262–1/2) the total lines and presented in 1/60th of a second. The two fields are interlaced so that the even numbered lines are presented during the first field and the odd numbered lines are presented in the second field. The interlacing of two fields eliminates flicker of the final image. Figure 15.12 illustrates how the two fields are interlaced to form one frame.

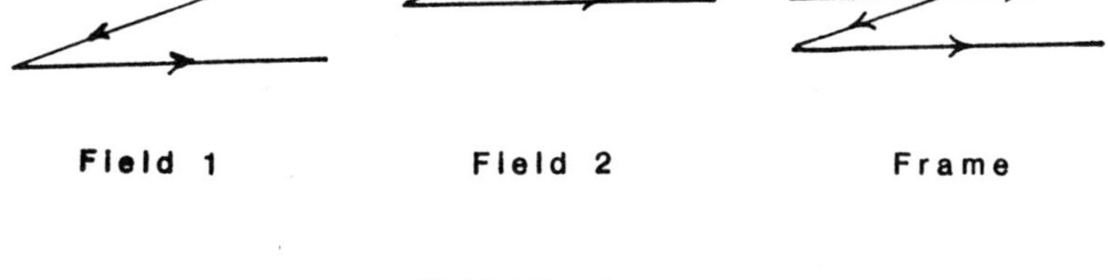

Figure 15.12. Display interlace of two fields to make one TV frame.

Band Pass Requirements

Band pass or **band width** refers to the range of frequencies which will be passed by an electrical system. Better resolution requires higher frequencies. We can ask **what frequency is required to produce a particular resolution** in a video system. We are interested in how many cycles can be displayed in a scan line. As an example, consider Figure 15.13 in which we would like to ask what frequency is required to display five cycles per scan line.

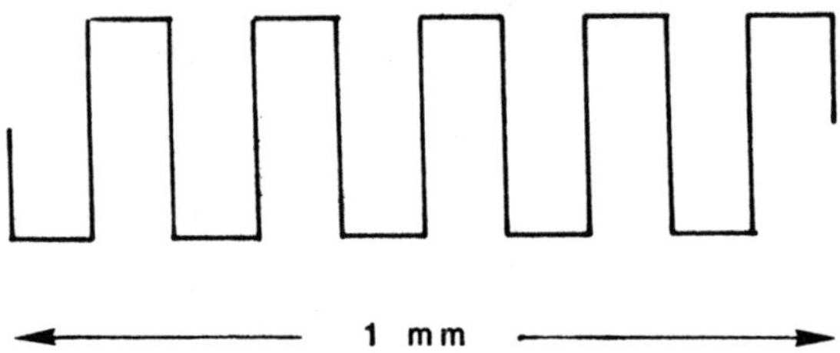

Figure 15.13. Five cycles/scan line display. One cycle consists of one bright and one dark line.

Notice that one cycle presents on line pair, i.e., one dark and one light line.

Example 15.4:
What band width is needed to display five line pairs per scan line.

$$5\frac{\text{cycles}}{\text{line}} \times 525\ \frac{\text{scan lines}}{\text{frame}} \times 30\ \text{frames/sec} \qquad 15.1$$

$$= 78750\ \text{cycles/sec}$$

$$= 79\ \text{kHz}$$

The required band width can be calculated for a typical medical TV system by asking what is the lowest and highest frequency necessary to display the required information. The lowest frequency would be 1 cycle per scan line (i.e., half the screen is black and half the screen is white) but there is some question as to what should be the highest frequency. A conventional compromise is a system which has **equal horizontal and vertical resolution.** The vertical resolution in a 525 line system is limited by the number of horizontal lines, i.e., 525. In this case, there would be 262–1/2 line pairs, i.e., every other scan line would be black or white and the minimum and maximum frequencies would be:

Minimum Frequency:

$$1\ \frac{\text{cycle}}{\text{line}}\ \text{x}\ 525\ \frac{\text{scan lines}}{\text{frame}}\ \text{x}\ 30\ \text{f/s} = 15750\ \text{c/s} \qquad 15.2$$

$$= 16\ \text{kHz}$$

Maximum Frequency:

$$262.5\ \frac{\text{cycles}}{\text{line}}\ \text{x}\ 525\ \frac{\text{scan lines}}{\text{frame}}\ \text{x}\ 30\ \text{f/s}$$

$$= 4.134\ \text{x}\ 10^6\ \text{c/s}$$

$$= 4.1\ \text{MHz}$$

Recall that 1 Hertz = 1 cycle/s

Actually, about 10% of the scan time is used for image retracing and synchronization, so it is not available for actual image display. Thus, the required band pass for a 525 line system is about 4.5 MHz.

Stop Action Resolution

When a TV display is in the Stop Action mode, only one field is displayed. If the vertical and horizontal resolutions are equal during dynamic display, the vertical resolution is half the horizontal resolution with a stop action display from a video tape recorder. Stop action images displayed from a video disk recorder do not suffer from this loss of resolution during playback.

CHAPTER 15 QUESTIONS

1-4, A for True, B for False

1. Scotopic vision has better detail resolution than photopic vision.
2. Photopic vision has superior contrast resolution.
3. Scotopic vision has superior sensitivity.
4. Dark adapted vision is sensitive to red light.

5. Dark adaptation requires about ________ min.
   A. 5
   B. 10
   C. 20
   D. 45

6. Image intensifier tubes
   A. raise the light levels into the scotopic vision range.
   B. raise the light levels into the photopic vision range.
   C. raise the light levels so that red goggles are necessary.
   D. raise the light levels through magnification gain.

7. The entrance exposure rate of an image intensifier in the 9″ mode is 3 R/min. What is the entrance exposure rate in the 6″ (magnification) mode?
   A. 4.5
   B. 6.75
   C. 7.5
   D. 9

8-15, A dual mode image intensifier is switched from 6″ to 9″ mode. For the same output brightness how will the following change?

Answer
A. Increase
B. Decrease
C. Remain the same.

8. Field of View
9. Spatial Resolution

10. Quantum Mottle

11. Scattered Radiation

12. Magnification

13. Minification Gain

14. Flux Gain

15. Entrance Exposure

16. The photocathode in an image intensifier

    A. converts visible light to x-rays.
    B. converts x-rays to visible light.
    C. converts electrons to visible light.
    D. converts visible light to electrons.

17. An image intensifier input phosphor is made of __________ and the output phosphor is made of _________

    A. Cs I – Cs I
    B. Zn Cd S – Cs I
    C. Cs I – Zn Cd S
    D. Cs I – NaI

18. A 12″ image intensifier has a 1″ output phosphor. The minification gain is:

    A. 12
    B. 48
    C. 144
    D. 256

19. A 6″ image intensifier with a 1″ output phosphor has a flux gain of 45. What is the brightness gain of this tube?

    A. 36
    B. 45
    C. 81
    D. 1620

20. The brightness gain of a 9″ image intensifier with a 1″ output phosphor is 2270. What is its flux gain?

    A. 81
    B. 22.7
    C. 28
    D. 36

21. The conversion factor of an image intensifier is 80 Cd/m^2 per mR/sec. If the light output of this image intensifier tube is 40 Cd/m^2 what is the input exposure rate?
    A. 0.5 mR/sec
    B. 1.0 mR/sec
    C. 20 mR/sec
    D. 40 mR/sec

A for True, B for False

22. Doubling the f-stop number will increase the light reaching the film.

23. Veiling glare
    A. is caused by scattered photons reaching the input phosphor.
    B. always reduces output contrast.
    C. is dependent on input subject contrast.
    D. is reduced by voltage minification.

24. Vignetting
    A. produces a dim region in the center of a bright image.
    B. produces a dim image due to scattering of electrons in the image intensifier.
    C. produces a dim image area surrounding a bright central image.
    D. can be eliminated by using lenses of larger diameter than required by the output phosphor.

25. The noise level of an image intensified image
    A. depends on the number of photons striking the input phosphor.
    B. depends on the number of electrons striking the output phosphor.
    C. increases with increasing x-ray flux.
    D. decreases with increased flux gain.

26. A noisy image intensified image
    A. has too much quantum mottle.
    B. has too few input photons.
    C. can be improved by increasing the aperture f-stop number.
    D. is statistically unstable.

27-32, A cineradiograph recording system is substituted for a video recording system. How will the following be affected? (A for increase, B for decrease, C for remains the same)

27. Spatial Resolution
28. Contrast Adjustability
29. Scattered Radiation
30. Patient Exposure
31. Slow Motion Display Resolution

33-37, A 35 mm camera is substituted for a 16 mm camera. For the same film density, how will the following be affected? (A for increase, B or decrease, C for remains the same)

33. Spatial Resolution
34. Subject Contrast
35. Processing Time
36. Quantum Mottle
37. Patient Dose

38-41, A for True, B for False

38. Exact framing utilizes the entire intensifier image.
39. Exact framing provides a magnified image.
40. Exact framing requires smaller patient exposure than overframing.
41. Overframing provides superior spatial resolution.

42. Two fields are combined to form one frame
    A. every 1/60 sec.
    B. to reduce motion artifacts.
    C. to reduce quantum mottle.
    D. to reduce flicker.

43. What band width is needed to display 150 cycles/scan line?
    A. 79 kHz
    B. 2.4 MHz
    C. 3.6 MHz
    D. 4.1 MHz

CHAPTER 16

DIGITAL IMAGING

Digital imaging involves detection and recording of both the number and position of x-ray photons which pass through the patient. More than a dozen methods of producing digital images have been suggested. The most widely used method utilizes conventional image intensifier output which is converted into digital values. The digital values (i.e., numbers) are stored in a regular array of rows and columns, a **matrix**.

Conversion of images into a matrix of digital values allows the images to be added or subtracted, to apply contrast enhancement, filtering, edge enhancement and other forms of manipulation to the image prior to display.

Figure 16.1 illustrates the steps in the formation of a digital image. The video signal from the image intensifier is digitized by the Analog-to-Digital Converter (ADC) and sent to the computer. After processing in the computer's central processing unit (CPU), the signal is either stored (on tape or on a disk) or is sent to the Digital-to-Analog Converter (DAC) for conversion back into an analog signal and then to the display terminal.

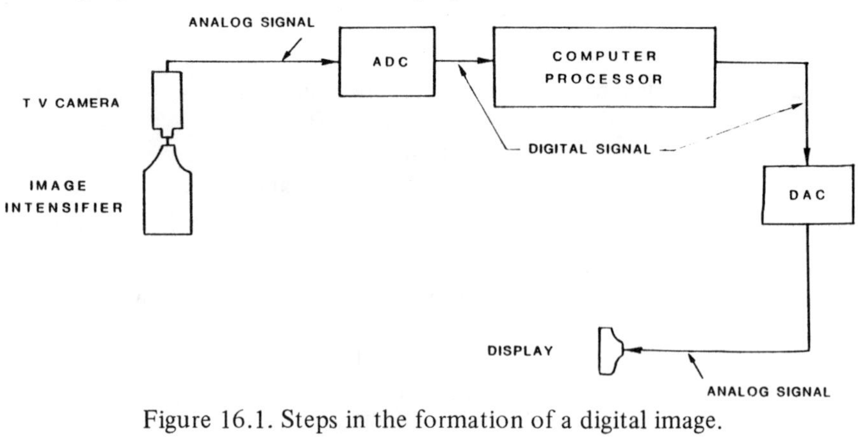

Figure 16.1. Steps in the formation of a digital image.

Analog-to-Digital Converters

Analog–to–Digital Converters (ADC) convert a time varying voltage (analog) signal to a digital signal by sampling the voltage at regular times called the sampling interval. The signal is assigned a digital value for each of the sampling intervals. Figure 16.2 illustrates the operation of an ADC.

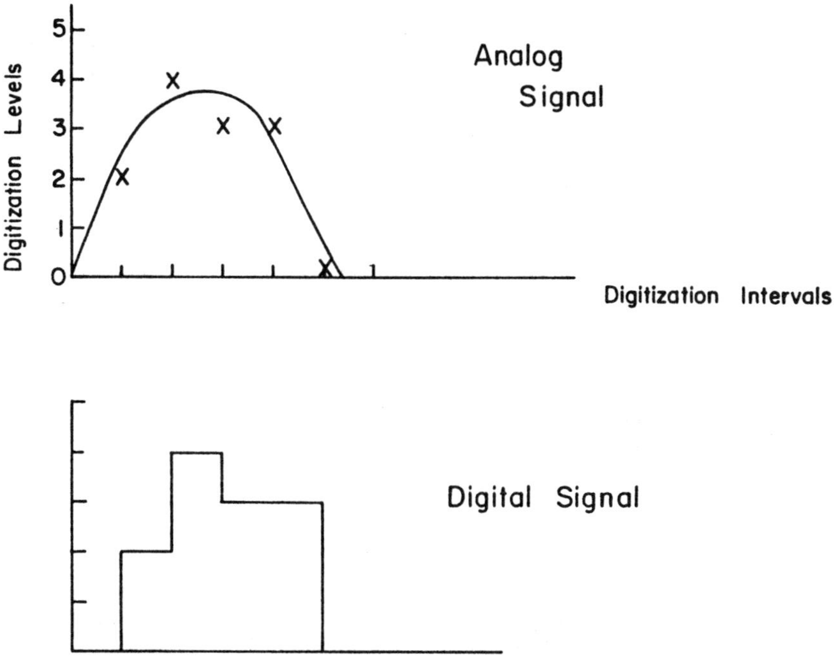

Figure 16.2. Analog signal and resulting digitized signal.

Note that higher sampling frequencies are required to digitize higher signal frequencies. The sampling frequency should be at least twice as great as the highest frequency in the signal.

Computers

Computers are made up of hardware and software systems. The hardware system consists of the Central Processing Unit (CPU) and peripheral devices such as the keyboard, console, disk drives, and display terminals. Software systems are the instructions and programs (algorithms) that tell the computer what to do. A good rule of thumb is "If you can touch it, it's hardware." The CPU has two types of memory chips, Read Only Memory (ROM) which permanently stores instructions and programs, and Random Access Memory (RAM) which can be revised by the user.

Binary Numbers

All computers deal with binary (on–off, yes–no) numbers instead of the more familiar decimal numbers. Any decimal number can be expressed in terms of its equivalent binary number by calculating how it is made up of powers of two.

For example, the number 7 can be considered as made up of 4 (2^2) plus 2 (2^1) plus 1 (2^0). Table 16.1 presents examples of decimal numbers and their corresponding binary numbers.

TABLE 16.1
DECIMAL AND BINARY NUMBERS

Decimal	*Binary*				
	2^4	2^3	2^2	2^1	2^0
1	0	0	0	0	1
2	0	0	0	1	0
3	0	0	0	1	1
5	0	0	1	0	1
21	1	0	1	0	1

Each on–off condition or power of two is called a **bit**. Eight bits are combined to form a **byte**. The maximum number of bits that a computer can use at one time is called a **word**. Computers with eight, sixteen or thirty–two bit words are common.

Spatial Resolution

Spatial resolution describes how close together two objects can be and still be recognized as separate objects. Spatial resolution is measured in pixel size (in mm) or in line pairs per mm (lp/mm). A line pair consists of one bright and one dark line.

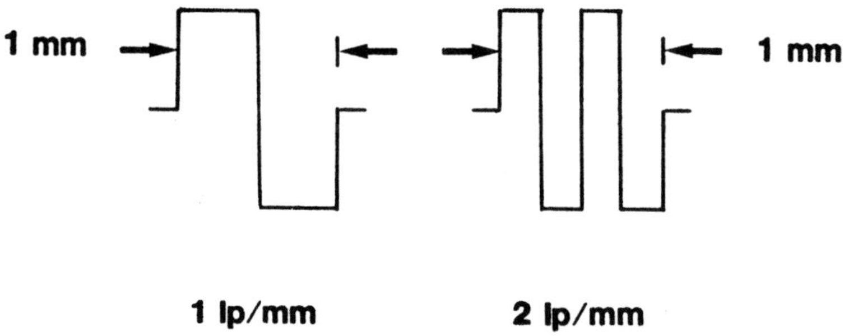

Figure 16.3. Resolution expressed in line pairs per mm.

Pixel size is calculated by dividing largest side of an image by number of pixels along 1 side of matrix.

$$\text{pixel size} = \frac{\text{image size in mm}}{\text{number of pixels}} \qquad 16.1$$

LP Resolution is calculated by:

$$1/2 \times \frac{1}{\text{pixel size}}$$

At least two pixels are required to display one line pair.

Example 16.1:
What is the pixel size in mm and the resolution in lp/mm if a 256 x 256 matrix used to image a 23 cm diameter image intensifier?

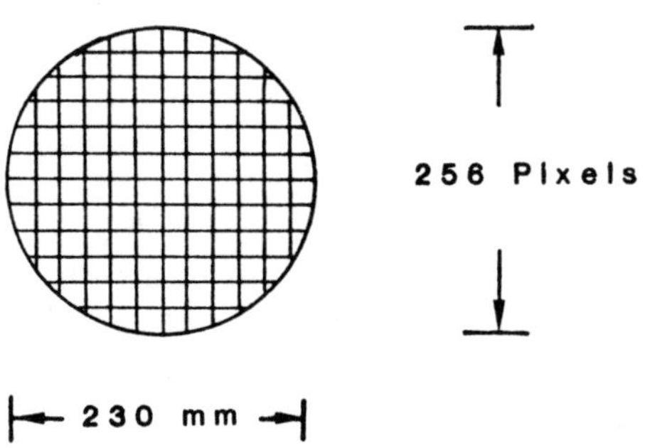

$$256 \text{ pixels} = 230 \text{ mm}$$

$$\frac{230 \text{ mm}}{256 \text{ pixels}} = 0.9 \text{ mm/pixel}$$

There are 2 pixels/line pair

$$\frac{1 \text{ lp}}{2 \text{ pixels}} \times \frac{1 \text{ pixel}}{.9 \text{ mm}} = \frac{1 \text{ lp}}{1.8 \text{ mm}}$$

$$= 0.55 \text{ lp/mm}$$

Example 16.2:
If the matrix size of Example 16.1 is increased to 512 x 512, what is the new pixel size in mm and the resolution in lp/mm?

The pixel size in mm:

$$230 \text{ mm}/512 \text{ pixels} = .45 \text{ mm/pixel}$$

Resolution in lp/mm:

$$.45 \text{ mm/pixel} \times 2 \text{ pixels/lp} = .9 \text{ mm/lp}$$

or

$$1/.9 = 1.1 \text{ lp/mm}$$

Typical image intensifiers have resolutions of 3–5 lp/mm.

Digital System Noise

Noise degrades contrast resolution. The principle sources of noise are quantum noise caused by x-ray input fluctuations, electronic noise in the TV camera chain and quantitization noise from the analog-to-digital converters. The total noise is a combination of the individual sources of noise.

$$\sigma_n = \sqrt{\sigma_q^2 + \sigma_e^2 + \sigma_d^2} \qquad 16.2$$

where σ_n is the total noise of the system, σ_q is the quantum or statistical noise, σ_e is the electronic noise in the TV system and σ_d is the digitization noise.

In radiology we would like to have image noise dominated by quantum noise, i.e., the image is limited by dose, otherwise we are wasting dose because something else is limiting the image quality.

Signal to Noise Ratio

The ratio of the object contrast to the background noise is known as the signal to noise ratio (SNR). For an input signal of one the SNR is:

$$\text{SNR} = \frac{1}{\sqrt{\sigma_q^2 + \sigma_e^2 + \sigma_d^2}} \qquad 16.3$$

Contrast Resolution

Contrast resolution describes how large a contrast difference is required for two areas to be reliably perceived as separate. The number of gray scale steps or levels and the overall system noise determine the contrast resolution.

Minimal Detectable Contrast

In the absence of noise the minimal detectable contrast level is one gray scale step. This is sometimes called a **Just Noticeable Difference** (JND). The contrast represented by 1 step depends on the number of steps. This depends on the number of bits used to represent the contrast. Table 16.2 presents the minimum detectable contrast difference for different number of bits and gray levels available. The step size or gray level size refers to the percent contrast change represented by one gray level.

TABLE 16.2
MINIMUM DETECTABLE CONTRAST AS A FUNCTION OF NUMBER OF BITS AND GRAY LEVELS AVAILABLE

Bits	*Gray Levels*	*Minimum Detectable Contrast*
2	4	25%
3	8	12.5%
4	16	6.25%
5	32	3.1%
6	64	1.6%
7	128	0.8%
8	256	0.4%

Example 16.3:
What memory size (in bits) is needed to store a 128 x 128 matrix with 64 shades of gray?

Memory size for 128 x 128 matrix = 16384

For 64 shades of gray each pixel requires 6 bits

Total memory size required:

16384 x 6 = 98304 bits

Quantum Noise

The quantum noise is given by:

$$\sigma_q = \sqrt{n}$$

where n is the average number of photons per pixel at the entrance to the image intensifier, **the quantum sink.**

Digital Subtraction Angiography

The most widespread use of digital imaging is in digital subtraction angiography (DSA) which is illustrated in Figure 16.4.

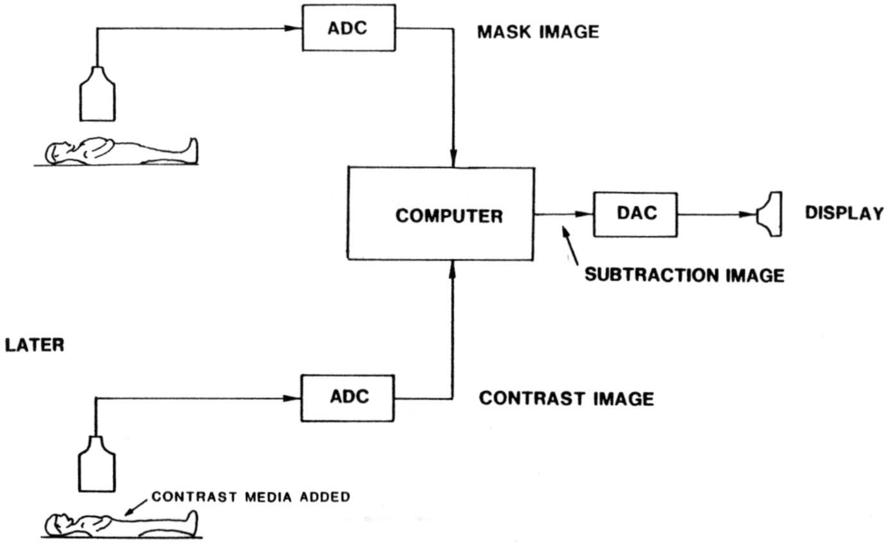

Figure 16.4. Schematic view of digital subtraction angiography.

In DSA, a mask image is made and stored prior to injection of a contrast agent. After the contrast medium is injected, a second image is obtained and stored and the mask image is subtracted from the contrast image to form the subtracted image. Although the subtracted image is always noisier than either the mask or the contrast image, the removal of distracting overlying structures more than makes up for the increased noise.

Example 16.4:
Calculate the signal and statistical noise in a DSA image if the mask image has an average of 1300 photons per pixel per exposure and 1150 photons per pixel in the contrast image.

Noise in the Mask image:

$$\sigma_m = \sqrt{1300}$$

$$\sigma_m = 36$$

$$\%\sigma_m = \frac{36}{1300}$$

$$\%\sigma_m = 2.8\%$$

Noise in the Contrast image:

$$\sigma_c = \sqrt{1150}$$

$$\sigma_c = 34$$

$$\%\sigma_c = 2.9\%$$

Subtraction signal:

$$s = 1300 - 1150$$

$$s = 150$$

Uncertainty in Subtraction signal:

$$\sigma_s = \sqrt{1300 + 1150}$$

$$\sigma_s = 49$$

$$\%\sigma_s = \frac{49}{150}$$

$$\%\sigma_s = 33\%$$

Uncertainty in Gray Levels

The uncertainty or quantum noise in terms of the number of photons in a pixel is given by $\sqrt{n}$. It is more convenient to express this in terms of uncertainty in gray levels. The uncertainty in terms of gray levels is given by:

$$\sigma_g = \sqrt{g \times \frac{N}{G}} \qquad 16.4$$

where g is the gray level of the pixel, G is the total number of gray levels and N is the number of photons per pixel required to give the brightest (highest) gray level. The value N/G is the number of counts per pixel per gray level. The relative uncertainty is given by:

$$\%\sigma_g = \frac{\sigma g}{N/G} \times 100 \qquad 16.5$$

As the total number of gray levels (G) increases, the relative noise also increases because the same number of photons is divided among a larger number of gray scale steps.

Example 16.4:
What is the relative uncertainty in the fourth gray level (midrange) in a system that has 8 shades of gray (8 gray levels) if the brightest level requires 5000 counts per pixel?

$$N/G = \frac{5000}{8}$$

$$= 625 \text{ counts/pixel per level}$$

The fourth level has:

$$625 \times 4 = 2500 \text{ counts}$$

$$\sigma_g(4) = \sqrt{g\,N/G}$$

$$= \sqrt{2500}$$

$$\sigma_g(4) = 50$$

Relative Uncertainty

$$\%\sigma_g = \frac{50}{625} \times 100$$

$$\%\sigma_g = 8\% \text{ of a level}$$

Example 16.5:
What is the relative uncertainty in the eighth gray level (midrange) of the system in Example 16.4 if the number of levels is increased to 16?

$$N/G = 312 \text{ counts/pixel/level}$$

The eighth level has:

$$g \times N/G \text{ counts/pixel}$$

$$= 2500 \text{ counts/pixel}$$

i.e., the midrange gray level counts per pixel remains the same.

The uncertainty in the eighth level is:

$$\sigma_g = \sqrt{g\, N/G}$$

$$= \sqrt{8 \times 312}$$

$$= \sqrt{2500}$$

$$= 50$$

The relative uncertainty is:

$$\%\sigma_g = \frac{\sigma g}{N/G}$$

$$\%\sigma_g = \frac{50}{312} \times 100$$

$$\%\sigma_g = 16\%$$

The SNR decreases with an increase in the number of gray levels unless the number of photons increases too. This means that the contrast sensitivity can be increased by increasing the number of gray levels but the dose to the patient must also increase to maintain the same signal to noise ratio.

The quantum noise depends on the gray level. This means that pixels with few counts (dark pixels) have very little quantum noise. The relative noise may be large but the absolute value of the noise is small.

Digitization Errors

Digitization errors arise because a signal will be assigned to one of two adjacent gray levels by the analog to digital converter. The digitizer does not round off the analog value but assigns it to one of the two adjacent gray levels essentially at random. These digitization errors give rise to a signal to noise ratio which depends on the number of gray levels employed. Table 16.3 presents the digitization SNR for some representative gray levels.

TABLE 16.3
DIGITATION ERRORS

Bits	*Number of Gray Levels*	*Digitization SNR*
7	128	440
8	256	890
9	512	1770
10	1024	3550

Electronic Noise

The electronic noise can be obtained from the dark field signal and is expressed in terms of signal to noise ratios. Typical TV cameras have SNR values of 500:1 or 1000:1. This means that the noise is 1/500 or 1/1000 the signal.

Example 16.6:
What is the overall SNR in a digital system with a 500:1 TV camera and 8 bit digitization?

$$\text{Noise} = \sqrt{g\left(\frac{N}{G}\right) + \left(\frac{1}{500}\right)^2 + \left(\frac{1}{890}\right)^2}$$

and the signal to noise ratio is:

$$\text{SNR} = \frac{1}{\sqrt{g\left(\frac{N}{G}\right) + \left(\frac{1}{500}\right)^2 + \left(\frac{1}{890}\right)^2}}$$

At **low light levels,** quantum noise is very small and the signal is limited by the electronic noise. In the lighter parts of the image, the signal is quantum noise limited.

If a low noise 1000: 1 SNR Camera is substituted in the system then the SNR becomes:

$$\text{SNR} = \frac{1}{\sqrt{g\left(\frac{N}{G}\right) + \left(\frac{1}{1000}\right)^2 + \left(\frac{1}{890}\right)^2}}$$

In this case, the signal is quantum limited at high light levels and digitization limited at low levels. The system would require at least a 9 bit digitization to avoid digitization limits.

As the number of gray scale steps (i.e., contrast resolution) increases, the signal to noise ratio **decreases** unless there is a corresponding increase in N and the total photon flux.

Dose Requirements in Digital Radiology

About 1 mGy (100 mrad)/image are required to produce an image with 16 shades of gray but over 30 mGy (3000 mrad) are required for 128 shades of gray. To reduce the dose requirements, either the spatial resolution (pixel size) or contrast resolution (number of gray scale steps) or both can be relaxed. Clinical experience indicates that more than 16 shades of gray are rarely required.

Temporal Averaging

Another way to reduce the noise without increasing the patient dose is to combine several signals through signal averaging. The noise will decrease by the square root of the number of frames averaged. Such temporal averaging suffers from patient motion which introduces still another source of image noise. Averaging over several frames results in the loss of spatial resolution and produces decreased contrast resolution if patient motion takes place during the averaging process.

Figure 16.5 from Erickson, *et al.* Radiographics *1* 1981 illustrates the effect of changes in digitization level and matrix size on the appearance of the image. Note that changes in number of gray scale levels (digitization bits) is almost imperceptible after at least 4 levels are present.

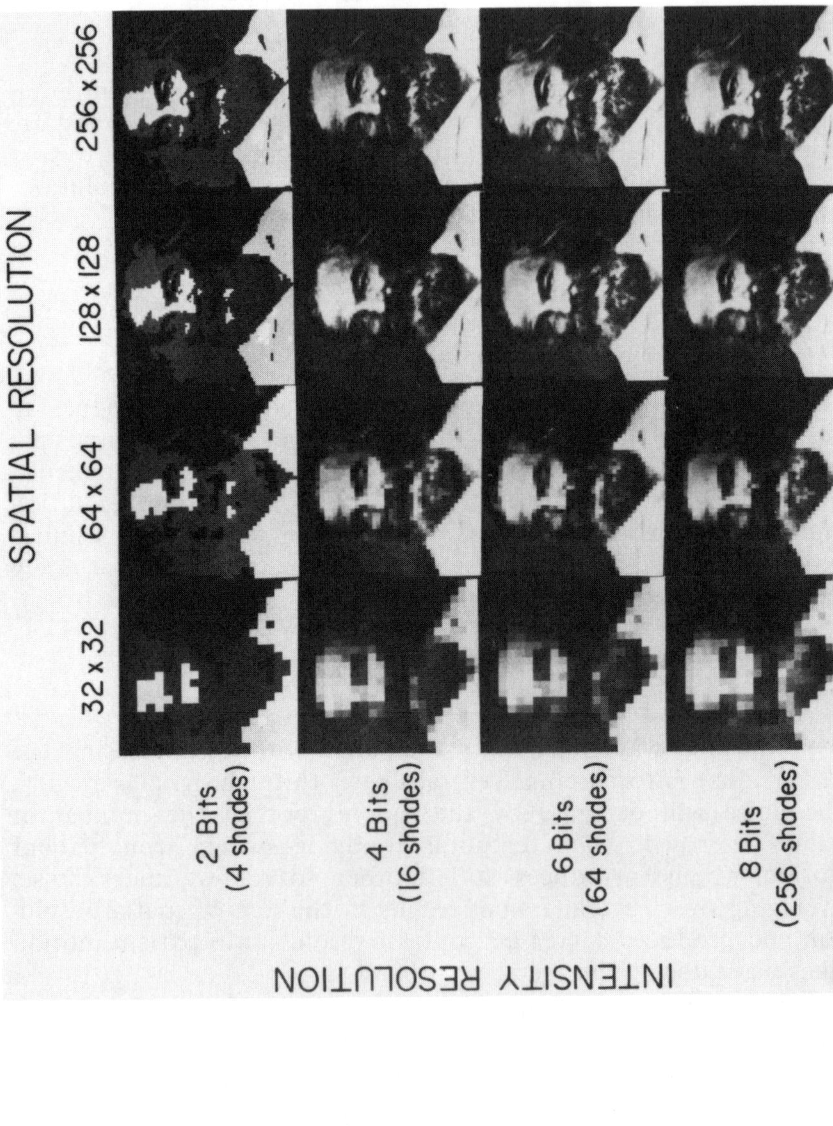

Figure 16.5. Effect of changing the resolution matrix and number of gray scale levels.

CHAPTER 16 QUESTIONS

1. Digital images
   - A. require a pixel of matrix values.
   - B. can be processed prior to acquisition.
   - C. must pass through a DAC prior to display.
   - D. always contain more information than the corresponding signal.

A for True, B for False

2. An analog signal is made up of discrete values.

3. The CPU of a computer system
   - A. is a peripheral device.
   - B. is part of the computer hardware.
   - C. is part of the computer software.
   - D. converts analog to digital signals.

4. A RAM chip
   - A. stores instructions which can be revised by the user.
   - B. stores instructions which cannot be revised by the user.
   - C. is a peripheral device.
   - D. is part of software package.

5. A keyboard
   - A. stores instructions which can be revised by the user.
   - B. stores instructions which cannot be revised by the user.
   - C. is a peripheral device.
   - D. is part of a software package.

6. A statistical analysis program
   - A. stores instructions which can be revised by the user.
   - B. stores instructions which cannot be revised by the user.
   - C. is a peripheral device.
   - D. is part of a software package.

7. An ROM chip

A. stores instructions which can be revised by the user.
B. stores instructions which cannot be revised by the user.
C. is a peripheral device.
D. is a part of a software package.

8. An ADC unit

A. converts a voltage signal to a digital signal.
B. converts a digital signal to a voltage signal.
C. modifies the pixel size to fit the matrix size.
D. must be used with an antiscatter grid.

9. What is the percent noise in a system where 1800 counts/pixel are collected?

A. 42.4%
B. 4.2%
C. 2.4%
D. 0.24%

10-14, A 1000 line TV system is substituted for a 525 line system without changing the band width for the electronics. (A for True, B for False)

10. The vertical resolution is improved.

11. The horizontal resolution is improved.

12. The dose to the patient is increased.

13. The subject contrast is increased.

14. The number of gray levels remains the same.

15. In DSA

A. the mask image is displayed before the contrast image.
B. the mask image is displayed after the contrast image.
C. the sum of the mask and contrast images are displayed.
D. the difference between the mask and contrast images are displayed.

16. The binary number 10011 corresponds to
    A. 11
    B. 17
    C. 19
    D. 23

17. A 152 mm diameter image is stored in a 256 x 256 matrix. The pixel size is
    A. .3 mm
    B. .6 mm
    C. .9 mm
    D. 1.2 mm

18. A 23 cm diameter image is stored in a 512 x 512 matrix. The pixel size is
    A. .45 mm
    B. .6 mm
    C. .9 mm
    D. 1.2mm

19. The minimal detectable contrast in a digitized image
    A. depends on the ADC.
    B. depends on the MAS.
    C. depends on the SID.
    D. is one gray scale step.

20. What memory size in bits is required to store a 256 x 256 image with 128 shades of gray?
    A. 8,400,000
    B. 87,000
    C. 2,620,000
    D. 460,000

21. Temporal averaging of digital imaging
    A. averages outpatient motion.
    B. improves spatial contrast.
    C. increases patient dose.
    D. reduces statistical noise.

CHAPTER 17

COMPUTERIZED TOMOGRAPHY

CT scanning obtains cross-sectional images through the body and eliminates distracting overlying images. An x-ray beam about 10 millimeters thick is passed through the patient as shown schematically in Figure 17.1 and the number of transmitted photons is measured and stored in a computer memory. These transmission data are related to the sum of all the attenuation coefficients in the x-ray beam path.

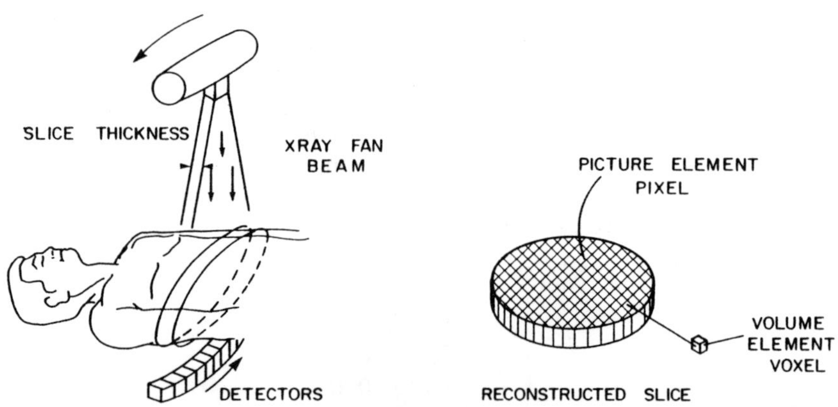

Figure 17.1 CT scanning geometry.

The average transmission for each beam path is measured and stored in the computer. The patient cross section is divided into a matrix of **voxels** (volume elements). By collecting data at many angles and paths, enough information is obtained to calculate the attenuation coefficient of each voxel. The attenuation coefficients are calculated using computer instructions called **algorithms** and converted to a CT number measured in **Hounsfield Units** given by:

$$HU = 1000 \frac{(\mu object - \mu water)}{\mu water} \qquad 17.1$$

The CT numbers are displayed as picture elements (pixels). An image is formed by assigning gray scale values to different CT numbers. Each pixel has a gray scale value corresponding to its CT number and the final image is formed by combining the individual pixels. Representative values of CT numbers are given in Table 17.1.

TABLE 17.1
REPRESENTATIVE CT NUMBERS OF SOME BODY MATERIALS

Material	*CT Number in Hounsfield Units*
Bone	+100 to 1000 HU
Liver	40 to 60
Muscle	10 to 40
Kidney	30
Water	0
Fat	-50
Air	-1000

It is only necessary to collect data through 180° rotation, but the data are usually collected over a larger angle to **overdetermine** the matrix and achieve a more accurate reconstruction.

Equipment

The first CT unit used a single pencil beam of x-rays with the detector and x-ray source moving on parallel tracks in a translate rotate motion. After each linear scan was completed, the support frame holding the x-ray tube and detector rotated through 1° and another linear scan was completed. This data collection continued until a complete 180° rotation had been accomplished. The geometries of second, third and fourth generation scanners are shown in Figure 17.2.

Second generation scanners use a **fan beam** about 10° wide and more (30) detectors. Data can be collected much faster with

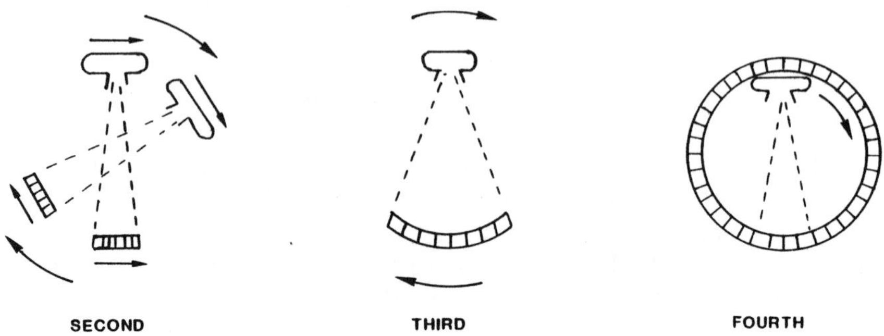

Figure 17.2. Second, third and fourth generation scanner geometries.

this combination of multiple detectors and a fan beam. The rotation angle between scans is increased to about 10° so that only 18 or 20 sets of measurements are needed to collect data for a complete image.

Third generation scanners utilize a 30° fan beam with rotational motion of both the x-ray tube and group of detectors. There are some problems with detector calibration with this geometry. The third generation scanners are especially susceptible to **ring artifacts** produced by slight differences in detector gains.

Fourth generation CT scanners employ a stationary ring of detectors with the x-ray tube rotating inside the ring. Only the x-ray source rotates. Table 17.2 summarizes the characteristics of the CT scanners.

TABLE 17.2
CHARACTERISTICS OF CT SCANNERS

Generation	*Motion*	*X-ray Beam*	*Rotation Angle*	*Detectors*	*Scan Time*
First	Translate-Rotate	Pencil	180	one	5 min
Second	Translate-Rotate	Fan	180	20	20 sec
Third	Rotate-Rotate	Fan	360	60	2 sec
Fourth	Rotate-Stationary	Fan	360	600	2 sec

In all systems, collimators are located near the source and the detectors to prevent scatter from reaching the detectors.

Detectors

Early CT scanners used NaI (Tl) crystals attached to photomultiplier tubes. The thickness of the detectors was chosen to have at least 90% detection efficiency. Sodium iodide crystals are efficient but they have a long afterglow component in the light output. The afterglow limits dose rates and prevents shorter scan times.

To collect enough data for acceptable images requires long scan times with an NaI crystal. Present CT units use Bismuth Germanate (BGO), Cesium Iodide (CsI) scintillation crystals or solid state detectors. The scintillator's efficiency is less than NaI (Tl) but the absence of afterglow means that much higher dose rates and shorter scan times are possible with BGO or CsI scintillators or with solid state detectors.

Packaging and mounting requirements prevent crystal detectors from being placed immediately adjacent to each other. Some x–rays pass through the interspaces between the crystals resulting in an overall detector efficiency of about 50%.

Gas–filled Ionization Detectors

High pressure ionization chambers filled with xenon gas are also used for CT detector systems. Xenon is a high Z (54) gas. At relatively high pressures (25 atm), the detection efficiency is about 50%. The interspaces in a gas filled detector are so thin that the overall efficiency is about the same as a scintillation detector system.

X–ray Tube Requirements

Although the heat load from a typical CT exposure of 120 kVp, 100 MA 3 sec for one slice is not greater than many other diagnostic examinations, it is common to obtain 10 to 20 slices in a few minutes. The total heat load from a complete CT examination can range from one half to one million HU. Anode heat capacity is usually the primary limitation on CT scanning sequences. X–ray tube failure is the primary cause of CT downtime. Anode heat capacities of 500,000 to 1 million HU are commonly found in CT tubes. The focal spot size is not as important in CT scanning as in conventional radiography because the beam size is limited by source collimation.

Image Display

CT images are displayed as a matrix of picture elements (pixels). The matrix size chosen for a CT scanner is a compromise between high spatial resolution (larger matrix, small pixels) and computer storage and image processing time (smaller matrix). Usual compromises are matrix sizes of 128 x 128; 256 x 256; 320 x 320 or 512 x 512.

SPATIAL RESOLUTION

Spatial resolution refers to how close together two objects can be located and still be distinguished as two separate objects. Spatial resolution depends on:

pixel size
matrix size
detector size
detector spacing
scan field size

Matrix and Pixel Size

Matrix size and pixel size are inversely related. Larger matrices result in smaller pixel sizes and vice versa. A larger scan field results in larger pixel sizes.

Example 17.1:
What is the pixel size with a 256 x 256 matrix and a 20 cm diameter scan field?

$$\frac{200 \text{ mm}}{256 \text{ pixel}} = 0.78 \text{ mm/pixel}$$

Example 17.2:
What is the pixel size with a 256 x 256 matrix and a 36 cm diameter scan field?

$$\frac{360 \text{ mm}}{256 \text{ pixel}} = 1.4 \text{ mm/pixel}$$

Example 17.3:
What is the pixel size with a 512 x 512 matrix and a 36 cm diameter scan field?

$$\frac{360 \text{ mm}}{512 \text{ pixel}} = 0.70 \text{ mm/pixel}$$

Detector Size and Spacing

Resolution improves as the detector size is reduced and the detector spacing is reduced.

Scan Field Size

If the scan field is reduced, the resolution increases because the same number of pixels is displaying a smaller field size.

Example 17.4:
The scan field is reduced from 40 cm diameter to 20 cm diameter. What are the initial and final pixel sizes if a 256 x 256 matrix is used?

Initial pixel size:

$$\frac{400 \text{ mm}}{256 \text{ pixel}} = 1.6 \text{ mm/pixel}$$

Final pixel size:

$$\frac{200 \text{ mm}}{256 \text{ pixel}} = 0.8 \text{ mm/pixel}$$

Contrast or Density Resolution

Contrast resolution refers to how different in contrast two objects must be to be perceived as objects with different densities. Contrast is defined as:

$$C = \left| \frac{N_O - N_S}{N_S} \right| \times 100 \qquad 17.2$$

where N_O is the number of counts per pixel in the object and N_S is the number of counts per pixel in the surrounding areas. (The difference in counts per pixel must be greater than the statistical noise for reliable perception.) Density or contrast resolution depends on:

scan time
radiation dose
pixel size
voxel size

Scan Time and Radiation Dose

As scan time and/or radiation dose increases, the number of photons collected in each pixel increases. The statistical noise decreases and the contrast resolution increases.

Pixel and Voxel Size

Increasing either the pixel size (smaller matrix) or the voxel size (larger slice thickness) increases the counts collected per pixel and decreases the statistical noise. The contrast resolution increases.

Perception of Objects in Noise

Human perception studies have established that the signal to noise ratio (SNR) must be about 5 before observers can reliably detect the presence of a signal in a noise field. That is, **the signal must be five times greater than the noise** for reliable detection.

Using this criterion, we can calculate whether an object can be seen and how many counts must be collected for perception.

Example 17.5:
What is the SNR of an object with 2240 counts per pixel surrounded by pixels with 2000 counts?

$$\begin{array}{rl} 2240 & \text{object} \\ \underline{2000} & \text{counts in surround} \\ 240 & \end{array}$$

$$\text{Contrast } \frac{240}{2000} = 12\%$$

$$\text{Signal} = 12\%$$

$$\text{Noise } \frac{2000}{2000} = 2.2\%$$

$$\text{SNR} = \frac{12}{2.2} = 5.5$$

This object **can** be seen.

Example 17.6:
Can an object with 8% contrast be perceived in a scan with 1000 counts/pixel?

This is the same as asking:
Is the SNR of this system greater than 5?

The signal is 8%

$$\text{The noise is } \frac{\sqrt{1000}}{1000} = 3.2\%$$

$$\text{SNR} = 8/3.2$$

$$= 2.5$$

No; this object with 8% contrast **cannot** be perceived in this scan.

Example 17.7:
How many counts must be collected in order to reliably see an object with 8% contrast?

$$\text{SNR} > 5$$

$$\frac{8\%}{\%\sigma} = 5$$

$$\%\sigma = .08/5$$

$$= .016$$

$$\frac{\sqrt{N}}{N} = .016$$

$$N = 3906 \text{ counts/pixel}$$

Modern CT units can detect contrast differences of 0.5%.

Changes in Matrix Size

In Example 17.6 if each pixel was 1 mm on a side the system collected 1,000 counts per millimeter^2 with a noise value of 3.2%. By changing the matrix size so each pixel is 2 mm x 2 mm, the number of counts per pixel is increased to 4,000 counts, and the noise per pixel is reduced to 1.6%.

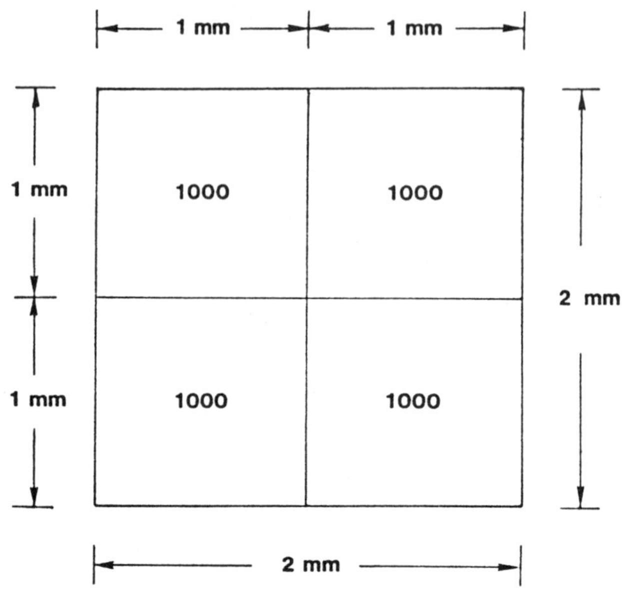

Figure 17.3. Expansion of pixel size from 1 mm x 1 mm to 2 mm x 2 mm with a decrease in noise and resolution by a factor of two.

The contrast of the object is still 8% but now the statistical fluctuations in the surrounding areas have been reduced to the point where this object can be detected. The tradeoff is that the resolution has been degraded by a factor of 2. It is no longer possible to detect objects smaller than 2 mm.

Contrast Scale

The difference between black and white remains constant for a given display screen but the computer can be instructed to place any CT value at the black end of the scale (changing window level) and any other CT number at the white end of the scale (changing window width). This is equivalent to changing the gamma of the display system and often is effective in bringing out areas of diagnostic interest.

Figure 17.4 illustrates the effect of changing the level control on the image appearance.

Figure 17.5 illustrates the effect of changing the window width on image appearance.

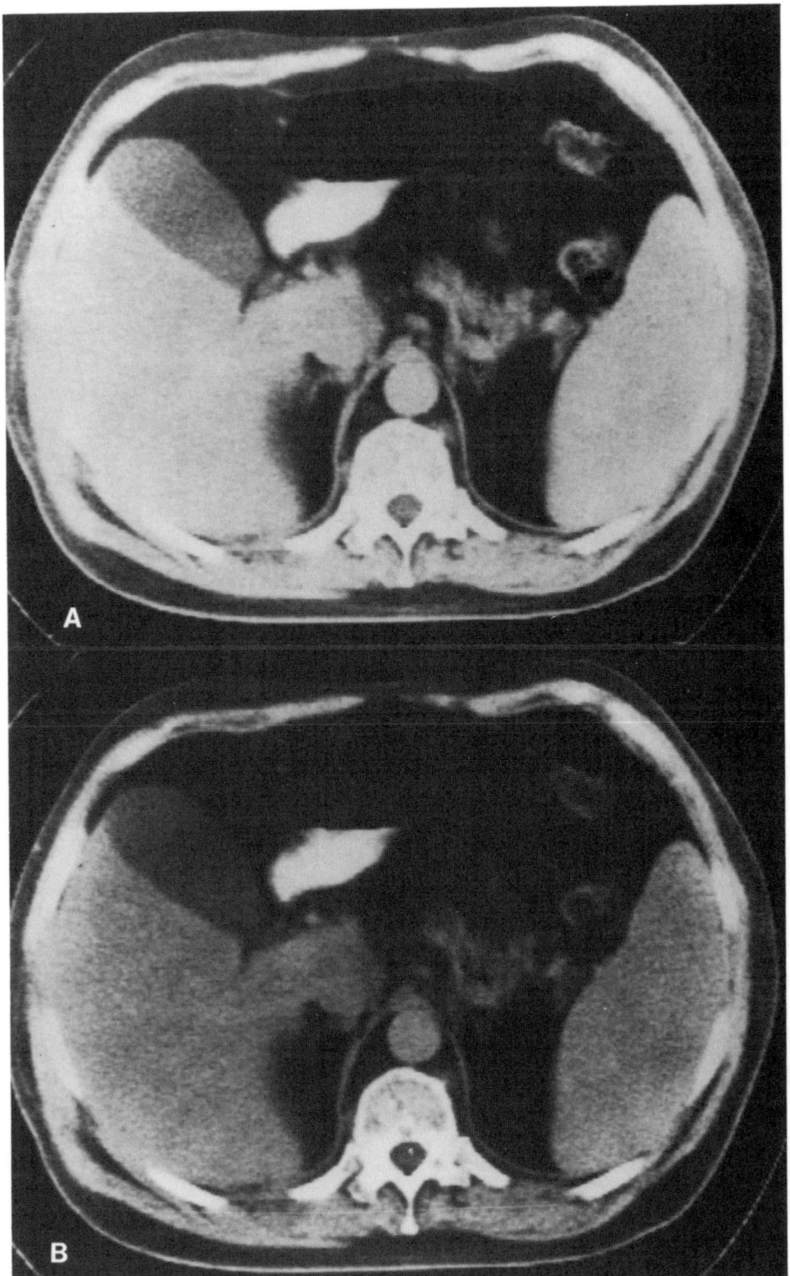

Figure 17.4 (A & B). Changes in image appearance produced by changes in display level. Level values: A = 25, B = 75. Window width = 250.

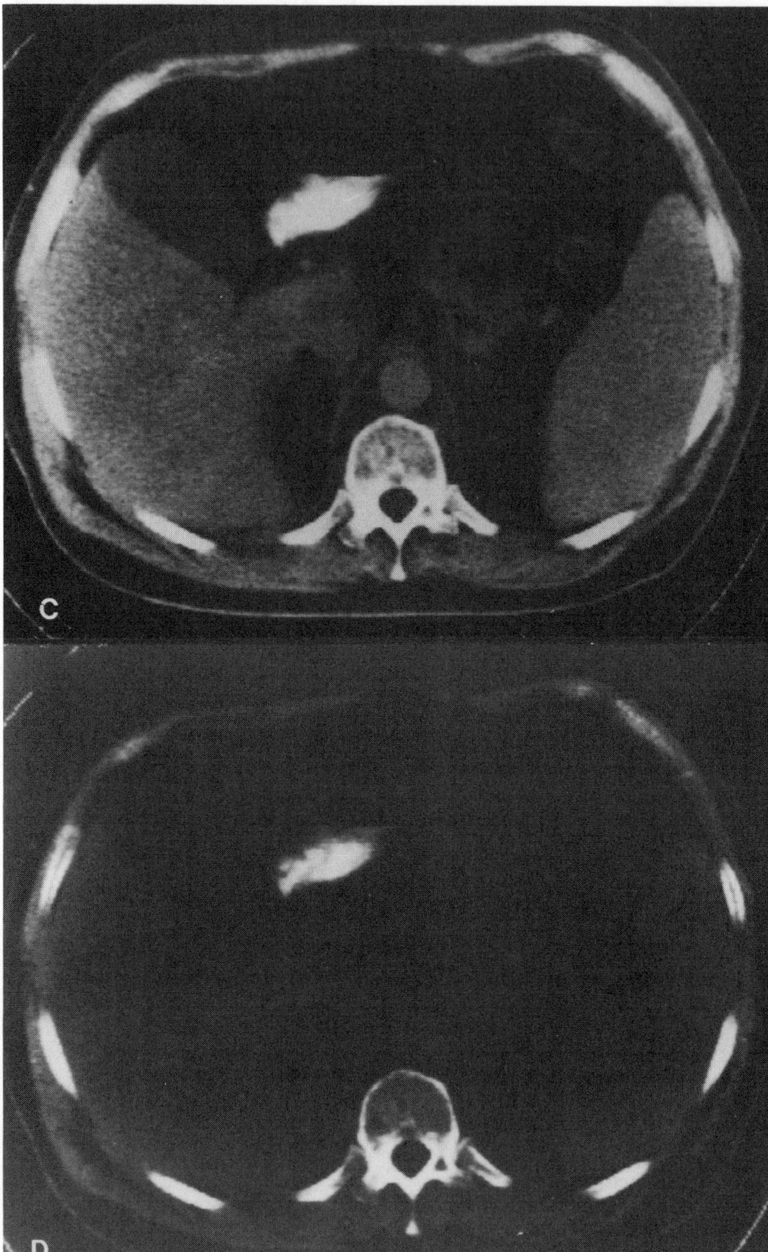

Figure 17.4. (C & D). Changes in image appearance produced by changes in display level. Level values: C = 100, D = 250. Window width = 250.

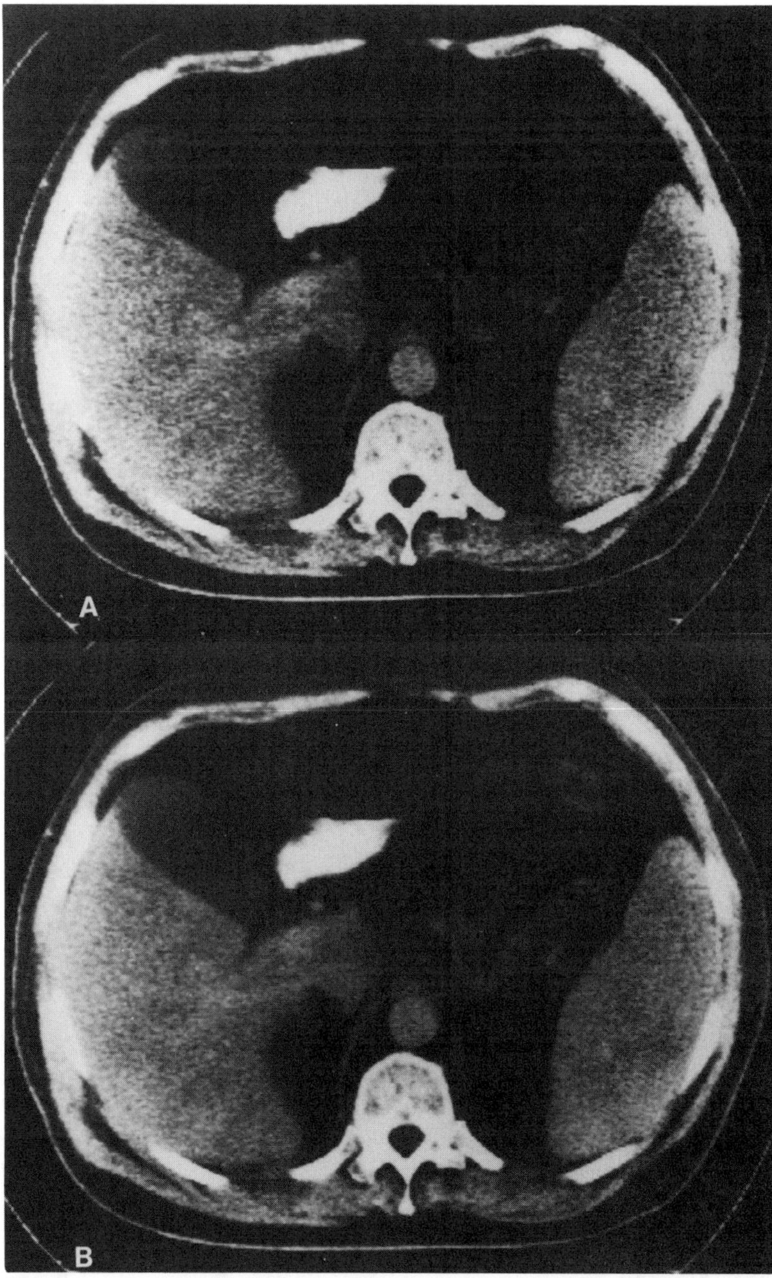

Figure 17.5 (A & B). Changes in image appearance produced by changes in window width. Width values: A = 125, B = 200. Window level = 100.

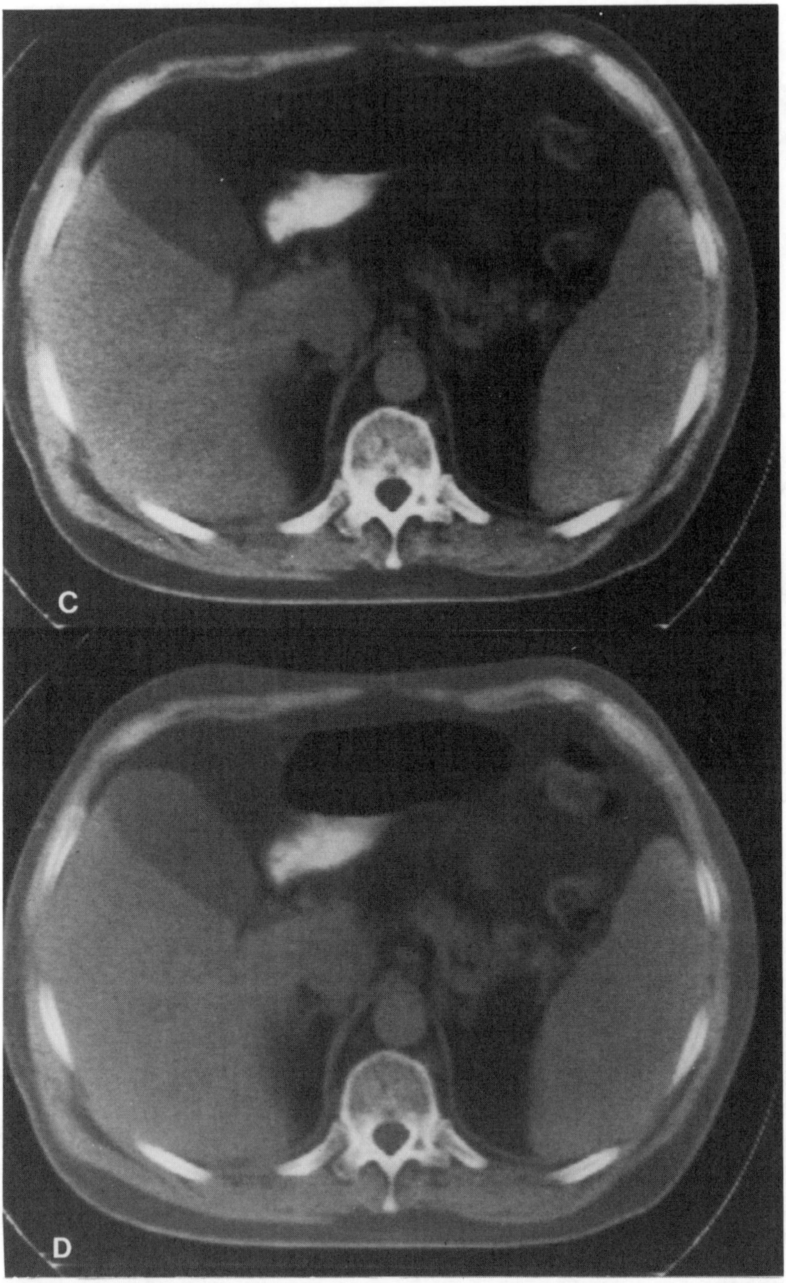

Figure 17.5 (C & D). Changes in image appearance produced by changes in window width. Width values: C = 400, D = 800. Window level = 100.

PARTIAL VOLUME EFFECT

It is possible to have only a part of the pixel in the beam for a particular view.

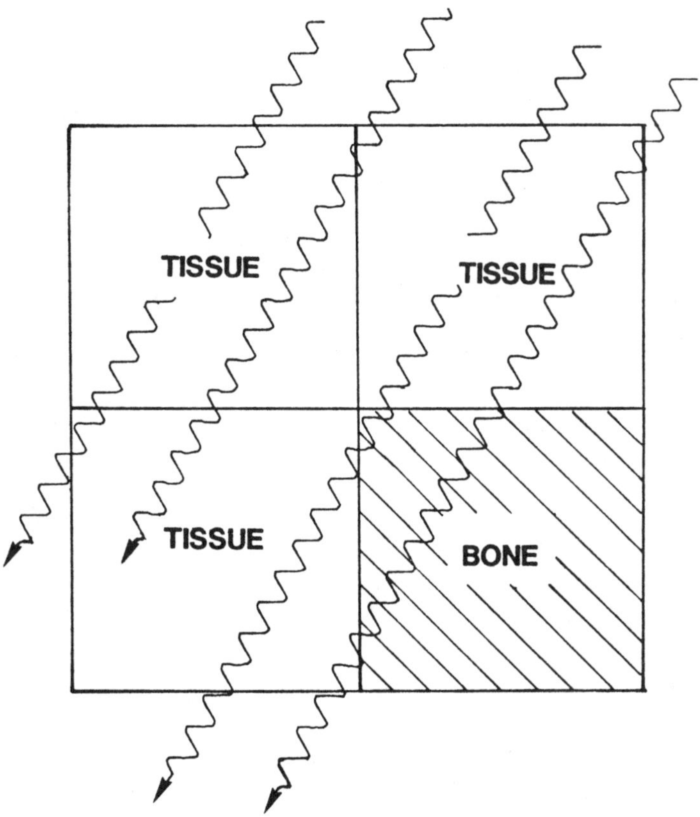

Figure 17.6. Partial volume effect observed when CT beam passes through a mixed group of tissues.

If the partially exposed pixel contains a very different density such as air or bone, the CT number calculated during reconstruction will be in error. Even a small fraction of a voxel containing air or bone will seriously alter the calculated CT numbers. It is possible to correct for the partial volume effect by including a weighting factor in the reconstruction algorithm so that adjacent partially exposed pixels do not get full weight in reconstructing the CT numbers.

CT Artifacts

In addition to being limited by the statistical noise, the picture quality may be degraded even further by artifacts introduced through malfunction of the detectors or problems in the reconstruction artifacts. Several of the more common artifacts are:

- aliasing
- beam hardening
- streak artifacts
- ring artifacts

Aliasing

Aliasing occurs when the signal contains higher frequencies than the CT sampling frequency. Sharp, high contrast boundary edges such as edges of bone (posterior fossa), metal clips or bowel gas contain very high spatial frequencies. If these spatial frequencies are higher than the sampling frequency, the aliasing artifact will be displayed as streaks from the interface edges producing a star-like pattern. These can be reduced by proper choice of the filter function used in the reconstruction algorithm.

A simple cutoff of the high frequencies will not eliminate the aliasing problem because it leads to overshoot at the boundaries between high and low densities. This effect can be seen as a low density ring just inside the skull.

Beam Hardening Artifact

CT algorithms assume a monoenergetic photon beam when they calculate the attenuation coefficients and CT numbers. X-ray tubes, however, produce heterogenous beams containing all photon energies up to the maximum kVp. When such a beam passes through a patient, the low energy photons are selectively absorbed and the average energy of the beam increases with penetration into the patient. Patients are circular or elliptical in shape so x-ray beams passing near the edge of the patient pass through much less material than those passing through the center. The center beams become harder and the CT numbers calculated near the center of the patient are too low. Additional filtration added to the x-ray beam can remove many of the low energy photons before they reach the patient. Filtrations in CT scanners are at least 4 mm Al.

To partially overcome the beam hardening effect, a wedge filter (Figure 17.7) is inserted in the x-ray beam to equalize the path length across the scan field. A different wedge filter must be selected for each different scan diameter.

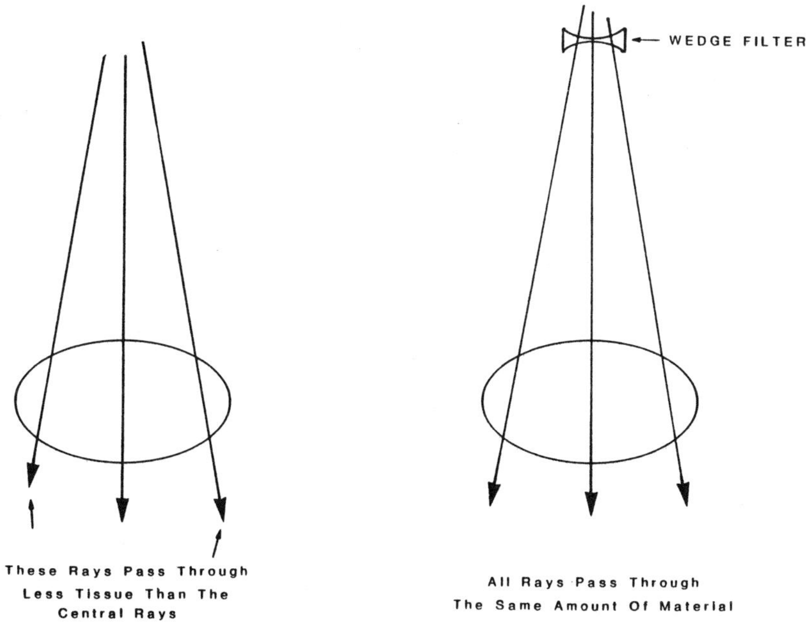

Figure 17.7. Use of a wedge or bow tie filter to reduce beam hardening artifacts.

CT Spatial Resolution

The resolution of modern CT scanners is between 0.5–0.75 lp/mm. This can be compared with image intensifier resolutions from 1–2 lp/mm and film screen resolutions of 2.5–4 lp/mm.

The wedges are designed for a specific scan field size and it is important to use the correct wedge filter with the proper scan field.

Beam hardening effects are reduced by the combination of filtering, and some algorithm corrections. CT scanner x-ray beams have an HVL greater than 4 mm Al. The first approximation of the algorithm corrections is that the patient is a water-filled cylinder. By scanning a water-filled cylinder during machine calibration and setup, it is possible to adjust the reconstruction algorithms so that a uniform cylinder of water will be displayed as a uniform image with the same CT numbers.

Streak Artifacts

Streak artifacts can be caused either by misalignment of the mechanical scanning equipment or by patient motion during the scan. The equipment misalignment is most easily determined by scanning a steel pin or rod in the water phantom. The appearance of such streaks in the calibration image is an indication of misregistration.

Patient motion during the scanning can produce streaks or star patterns especially from high contrast interfaces such as bone interfaces. Motion artifacts are reduced by reducing the scan time.

Ring Artifacts

Ring artifacts are caused by faulty detector calibration or a drift in gain in third generation units. As a worst case example, consider a faulty detector with no response. As illustrated in Figure 17.8, it traces out a ring which the reconstruction algorithm will interpret as blocking out all radiation.

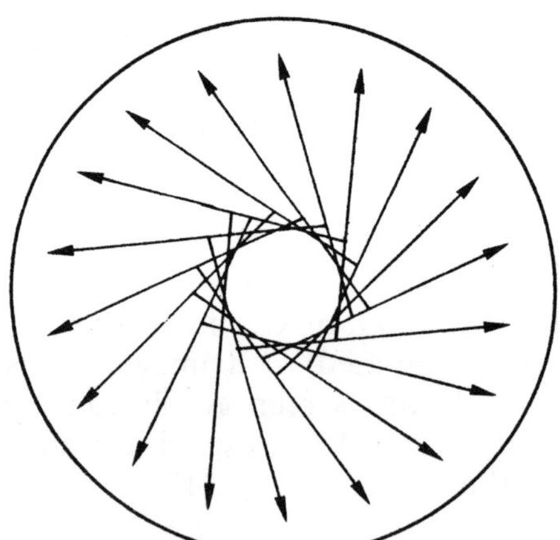

Figure 17.8. Ring artifact caused by miscalibration of one of the detectors in a third generation scanner.

Any miscalibration of the third generation detectors will result in ring artifacts.

Detector Dropout

Detectors which indicate densities greater than bone or less than air are obviously in error. Modern CT scanners are programmed to recognize faulty detector outputs, ignore the faulty data and substitute the average value of the adjacent detectors for the faulty data. Acceptable images can be obtained with as many as 10% of the detectors out of service.

Radiation Dose from CT scans

The radiation dose from a single head scan slice is about 2 rad. The dose from multiple slices is about twice that due to scattered radiation from adjacent slices.

CHAPTER 17 QUESTIONS

1-7, In CT scanning if all other factors remain the same what is the effect on quantum mottle due to the following changes:

A. Increases
B. Decreases
C. Remains the same

1. Decrease in scan time
2. Increase in matrix size
3. Change technique from 50 MA in 2 s to 100 MA in 1 s
4. Increase pixel size
5. Increase slice thickness
6. Increase MA
7. Increase patient thickness

8-13, In CT scanning if all other factors remain the same how is spatial resolution affected by the following changes:

A. Increases
B. Decreases
C. Remains the same

8. Increased matrix size
9. Reduced scan time
10. Increased scan diameter
11. Increased pixel size
12. Increased slice thickness
13. Increased patient thickness

14. How large a memory (in bits) is required to store a 128 x 128 matrix image with 128 shades of gray?

A. 16,384
B. 115,000
C. 131,000
D, 2,100,000

15. Water in Hounsfield units always has the value

A. -1000
B. 0
C. +1000

16. Increasing the ________ will increase the voxel size.
   A. scan time
   B. kVp
   C. MA
   D. slice thickness

17. Increasing the window width control will
   A. decrease the contrast.
   B. decrease the scan diameter.
   C. increase the slice thickness.
   D. decrease quantum mottle.

18. Arrange in order of increasing CT number
   1. Air
   2. Bone
   3. Fat
   4. Muscle
   5. Water

   A. 1, 4, 5, 3, 2
   B. 1, 4, 3, 5, 2
   C. 1, 3, 4, 5, 2
   D. 1, 3, 5, 4, 2

19-22, Match

19.	Pencil Beam Translate Rotate	A. First Generation
20.	Ring Artifacts	B. Second Generation
21.	Stationary Detectors	C. Third Generation
22.	Fan Beam Translate Rotate	D. Fourth Generation

23. What is the pixel size if a 256 x 256 matrix is used to image a 30 cm field?
   A. 0.6 mm
   B. 0.8 mm
   C. 1.0 mm
   D. 1.2 mm

24. An object has 1800 counts per pixel and the surround had 1500 counts per pixel. What is the contrast?
   A. 15%
   B. 20%
   C. 30%
   D. 36%

25. How many counts per pixel must be collected to reliably detect an object with 10% contrast?
    A. 1000
    B. 1500
    C. 2000
    D. 2500

26. The partial volume effect
    A. modifies the adjacent CT numbers because of finite window width.
    B. can be reduced by reducing the patient volume.
    C. increases with increasing kVp.
    D. changes the calculated CT numbers due to partial inclusion of bone in the beam.

27. The beam hardening artifacts
    A. will make the calculated CT numbers too low in the patient center.
    B. will be reduced by decreasing the beam filtration.
    C. will make all CT numbers too low.
    D. cause wedge shaped artifacts in the displayed image.

28. The radiation dose from a CT head examination is:
    A. 0.5 rad
    B. 1.5 rad
    C. 4 rad
    D. 6.5 rad

CHAPTER 18

SPECIAL RADIOGRAPHIC TECHNIQUES

Mammography

Mammography is a special case of low subject contrast high resolution imaging. Fibrous, glandular and connective tissues as well as microcalcifications as small as 0.1 mm must be imaged. This requires high contrast imaging techniques. In mammography the applied voltage is reduced to 25–40 kVp. In this kVp region most of the interactions are photoelectric and the contrast is significantly increased. A molybdenum (Mo) anode x–ray tube with 0.03 mm Mo filtration operated at about 30 kVp produces almost monoenergetic 19 KeV x–ray beam. The 17.5 and 19.5 KeV characteristic x–rays (average energy 19 KeV) pass through the Mo filter but much of the other energies are removed from the beam. Tungsten anode tubes with alumunum filtration, which are also used in mammography, have higher average beam energies. As the average beam energy increases the proportion of Compton scattering interactions increases. Mammographic tubes with focal spots of 0.3 to 1 mm are commonly used.

Film Screen Systems in Mammography

Early mammographic systems which used no–screen industrail film for good resolution resulted in doses of 5 to 10 rads per film to the patient. In the early 1970's several types of film–screen systems were introduced to achieve high resolution mammographic images with significantly lower doses. These systems use a single emulsion film and a rare earth screen for good resolution with higher efficiency. Modern mammographic film screen systems require about 5mGy (500 mrad) per film.

The film–screen combination is packed in a vacuum cassette. When evacuated, atmospheric pressure presses the film and screen together for excellent contact. The emulsion side of the film should always face the screen. There is a slight improvement in resolution when the x-rays first pass through the film and then strike the screen.

Breast Compression

Adequate breast compression is important during mammography because it produces a more uniform exposure, reducing the thickness fo the breast near the chest wall and reducing the overall thickness of the breast by spreading it over a larger area. The reduced thickness results in less scatter and an image with better contrast. Antiscatter girds used in mammography improve contrast but increase the dose to the breast.

Xeroradiography

Xeroradiography is used in mammography because of its wide latitude and **edge enhancement** characteristics. The latent image in Xeroradiography is a charge distribution on a selenium photoconductive plate. Selenium is a good insulator in the dark but becomes a conductor when exposed to light or x-rays. When a charged selenium plate is exposed to x-rays it becomes conductive. The amount of charge leaking off an area of the plate depends on the x-ray intensity striking the area. Table 18.1 and Figure 18.1 present the steps in forming a Xeroradiographic image.

TABLE 18.1
THE STEPS IN MAKING A XEROGRAPH

1) Charge the selenium plate to +1500 volts.
2) Make an x-ray exposure.
3) The charge distribution on the selenium plate reflects the x-ray distribution transmitted through the breast.
4) Add a back bias and spray a charged powder (toner) over the selenium plate to develop the image.
5) Transfer the toner pattern to a special heat sensitive paper.
6) Heat the paper to make the image permanent.

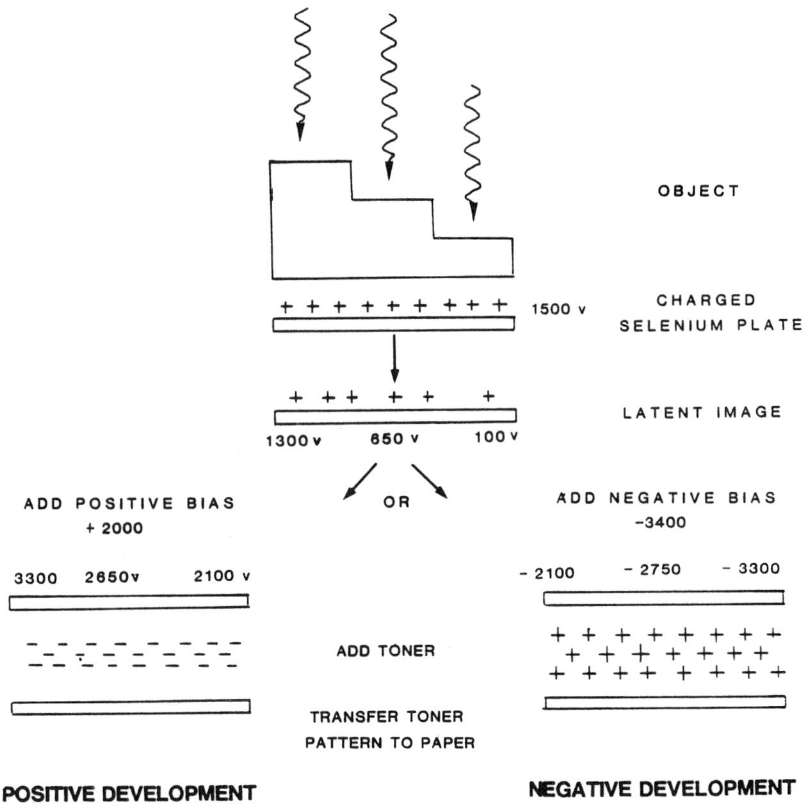

Figure 18.1. Steps in forming a xeroradiograph.

Edge Enhancement

In the vicinity of an edge the charge distribution sets up an electric field parallel to the selenium plate. Figure 18.2 illustrates the field lines above the selenium plate in the vicinity of an edge after an x-ray exposure. When the charged toner powder is sprayed over the charged selenium plate, the electric field forces the powder away from the edge and concentrates it in the regions near the edges. This **halo** around edges visually enhances the edges. Xeroradiographs have a wide latitude because only the edges are enhanced.

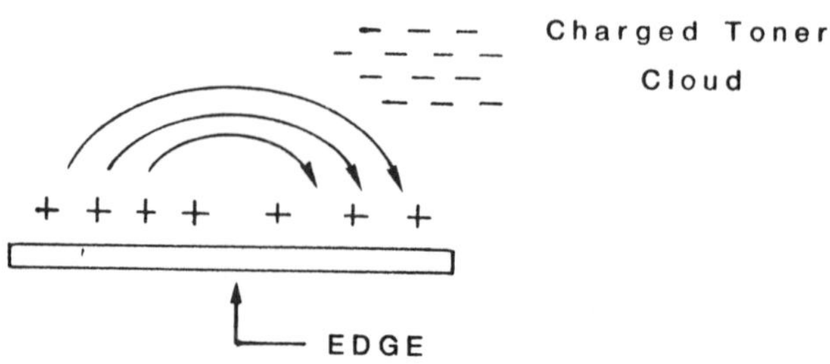

Figure 18.2. Xerographic field lines near an edge produce a collection of toner powder near the edge.

Positive or Negative Development

The Xerographic latent image can undergo either positive or negative development depending on whether a positive of negative charge is applied to the plate during the development process. Figure 18.1 illustrates the steps in both positive and negative development together with representative voltages. Negative development is more efficient than positive development and requires about 25% less dose to the patient. Table 18.2 presents the appearance of various portions of the Xerographic image under positive and negative development.

TABLE 18.2
XERORADIOGRAPHIC IMAGE APPEARANCE UNDER POSITIVE AND NEGATIVE DEVELOPMENT

Area	*Positive*	*Negative*
Unexposed	Dark	Light
Exposed	Light	Dark
Calcification	Dark	Light
Soft Tissue	Medium Dark	Medium Light
Halo	Thin Side	Thick Side

MTF of Xerographic Systems

Figure 18.3 presents the MTF of a typical Xerographic system. Because of the wide latitude, edge enhancement characteristics of Xerography, low spatial frequency objects are not imaged as well as smaller high frequency objects.

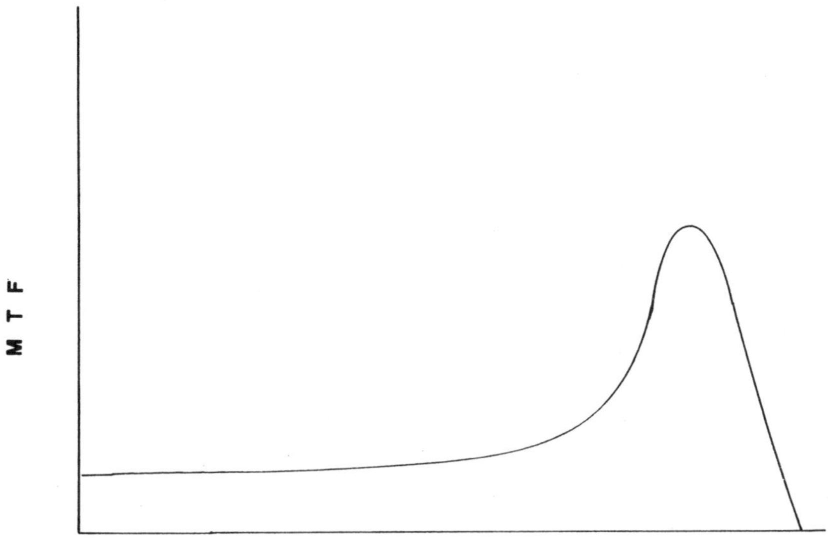

Figure 18.3. MTF of xerographic system.

Typical radiation doses in mammography are given in Table 18.3.

TABLE 18.3
TYPICAL MAMMOGRAPHIC RADIATION DOSES

Technique	*Radiation Dose Per Film*
No Screen	10 rads
Low Dose Film Screen	400-800 mrad
Xerography	1200-1500 mrad

Risk Benefit of Mammography

The risk of radiation induced breast cancer is approximately 3.5×10^{-6}/yr/cGy (3.5×10^{-6}/yr/rad) with a low dose film screen imaging system. The risk of dying from a radiation induced cancer from a mammographic examination is about the same as dying from driving 200 miles in a car. The benefit of mammography is the early detection and cure of breast cancer. As much as a 50% reduction in breast cancer mortality could be expected from annual mammographic screening of all women over age 40.

Conventional Tomography

Conventional tomography or body section radiography makes use of **motion blurring** to selectively blur out unwanted images by moving both the x-ray source and the film during the exposure. The eye-brain combination considers objects with less than about 0.5 mm blur to be in-focus and objects with greater than 0.5 mm blur to be out-of-focus. Thus objects within the "plane of focus" above and below the fulcrum plane appear in focus. Objects lying outside the "tomographic cut" are blurred to a greater or lesser extent. Figure 18.4 illustrates how objects located in the fulcrum plane (II) are imaged without blurring but objects above or below (I and III) the "tomographic cut" are blurred across the entire detector.

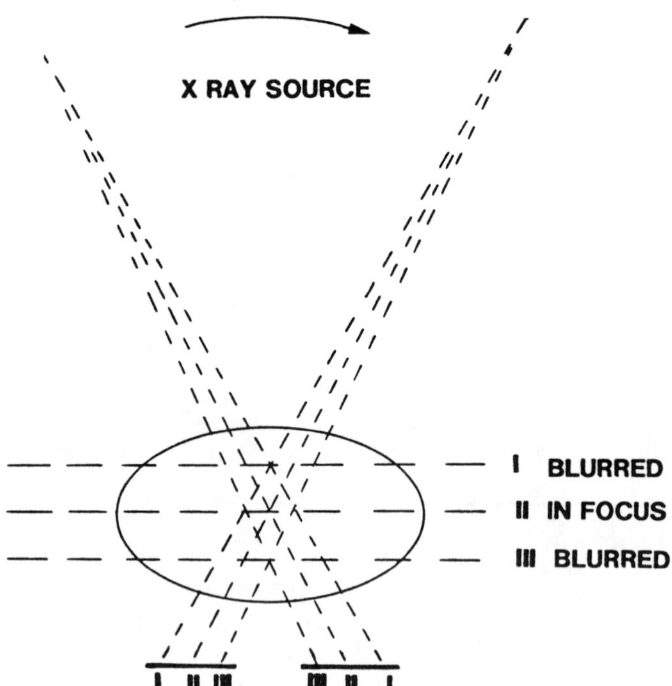

Figure 18.4. Tomographic blurring.

The thickness of the tomographic layer or "cut" can be changed by changing the amount of tube and film motion. The amount of tube motion is often described by the angle through which the tube and detector move. Larger angles result in thinner layers. Table 18.4 gives representative angles and the resulting thickness.

TABLE 18.4
TOMOGRAPHIC CUT THICKNESS vs TUBE MOTION ANGLE

Angle	*Thickness*
4°	15 mm
7°	9 mm
10°	6 mm
20°	3 mm

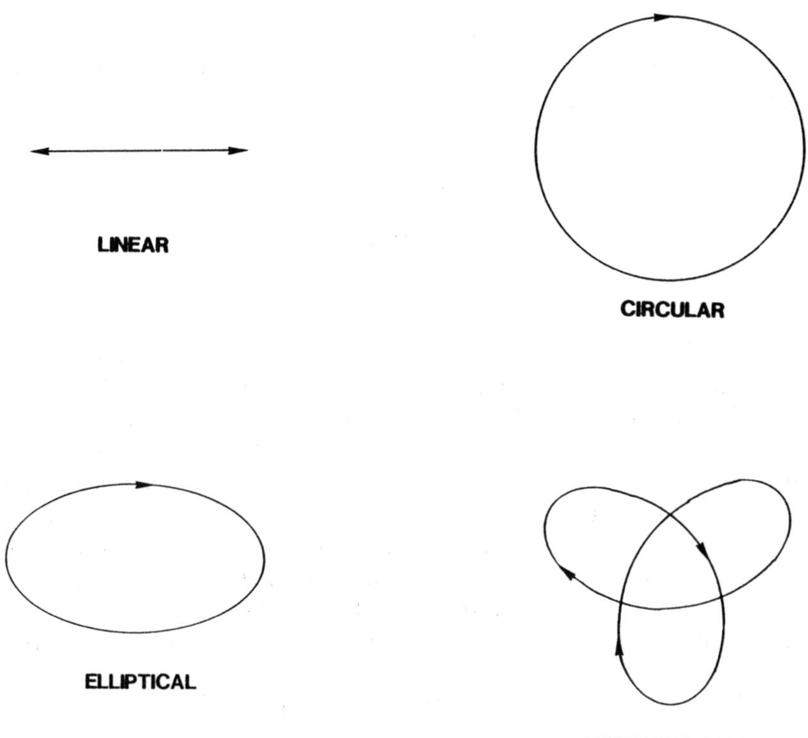

Figure 18.5. Types of tomographic motion.

Types of Tomographic Motion

Motion perpendicular to linear objects will blur the objects but motion parallel to a linear object blurs only the ends and leaves the rest of the object unblurred. With linear tomographic motion, only two sides of circular objects are effectively blurred. This can give rise to confusing linear streaks and so other types of motion are often used. Figure 18.5 illustrates **linear, circular, elliptical and hypocycloidal** motions. The more complex tube motions are used to reduce or eliminate different artifacts. Circular and elliptical motions can produce phantom or "ghost" images. Hypocycloidal motion eliminates all artifacts but suffers from long exposure times and large tube loads.

Magnification Radiography

Magnification radiography is used to study extremely small objects by increasing the source image distance (SID) while maintaining the same source object distance (SOD). The magnification factor, m, is given by:

$$m = \frac{\text{image size}}{\text{object size}} = \frac{\text{SID}}{\text{SOD}} \qquad 18.1$$

Magnification radiography is often used in angiography to study small vessels. The focal spot penumbra is magnified as well as the object size. For this reason, small focal spots are used in magnification radiography. Figure 18.6 illustrates a typical magnification geometry. The source image distance is twice the conventional radiographic SID. This would require a factor of four increase in tube load and patient dose. However the **magnification geometry** is effectively an **air gap geometry** so that the antiscatter grid can be eliminated. This almost cancels out the need for an increased exposure factor and tube load so the exposure factors with magnification radiography without a grid are about the same as with conventional radiography with a grid.

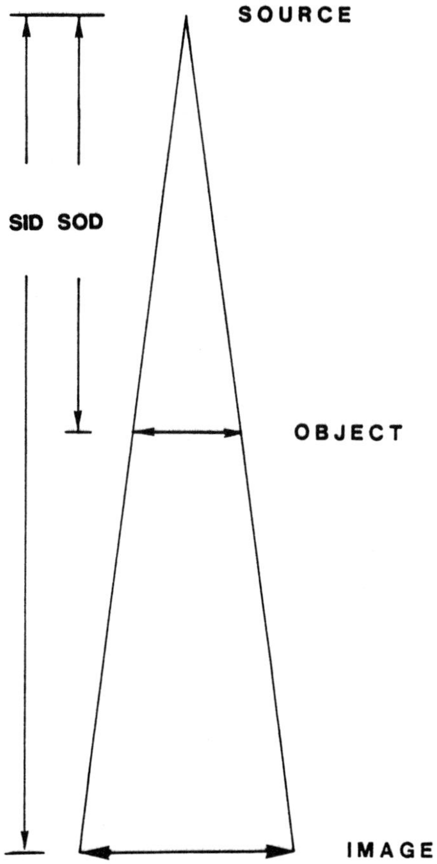

Figure 18.6. Magnification geometry.

Resolution in Magnification Radiography

The resolution requirements on detector systems are less stringent with magnification radiography because small objects undergo significant magnification. Figure 18.7 illustrates how an object of four line pairs per millimeter requires a detector resolution of only two line pairs per millimeter under a factor of two magnification.

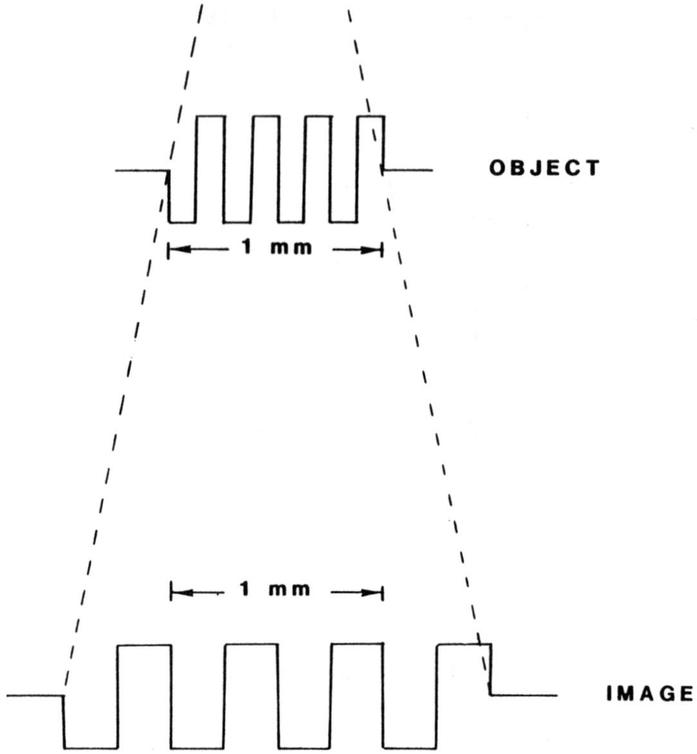

Figure 18.7. Magnification reduces detector resolution requirements.

Stereoscopic Radiography

Stereoscopic radiography utilizes a shift of the x–ray source to produce two images with different amounts of parallax. Parallax is the relative shifting of position of objects at different distances from an observer when viewed at different angles. The amount of tube shift required for stereoscopic viewing is approximately 10% of the SID, i.e., a 72" SID would require a 7" tube shift. A stereoscopic tube has two cathode cups arranged to produce two focal spots on opposite sides of the anode axis.

Stereoscopic Viewing

Viewing of stereoradiographs can be accomplished by viewing the shifted radiographs side by side through a stereoscope. The two images, one from each eye are adjusted until they fuse together into one three dimensional image. The observer appears to be located inside the x-ray tube. Some observers can form a three dimensional image by crossing their eyes and observing a third three dimensional image between the two single eye images. Stereoradiography allows lesions or foreign bodies to be localized relative to other anatomical structures, to gain insight into the relationship between the various anatomical structures and to eliminate confusing overlapping overlying sturctures. The major disadvantages of stereoradiography are the added expense and exposure of the second radiograph. Since the patient is already in position, and the additional technician and room time is minimal, the major added expense is the cost of the x-ray film and the small cost of the developing chemicals. The added exposure doubles the patient dose in stereoradiography.

CHAPTER 18 QUESTIONS

1. Mammographic examinations
   - A. use high KVP to emphasize the photoelectric effect.
   - B. use low KVP to reduce Compton scattering.
   - C. use molybdenum tubes to reduce the heat load.
   - D. use high KVP to enhance the contrast.

2. Xeroradiographs
   - A. add toner to increase x-ray detection efficiency.
   - B. transfer charge patterns to paper for later viewing and toner powder addition.
   - C. use x-rays to cancel out the selenium plate latent image.
   - D. can be developed with either positive or negative charge.

3. Breast compression in mammography
   - A. improves image contrast.
   - B. reduces the charge collected in Xerography.
   - C. spreads the radiation grid over a larger area.
   - D. increases scatter.

4. Edge enhancement in Xerography
   - A. is produced only by negative development.
   - B. refelcts the charge distributions under large uniform subject areas.
   - C. is produced by field lines near different subject areas.
   - D. increases the low contrast detectability of large objects.

5. A vacuum cassette is used in film screen mammography
   A. to hold the cassette close to the breast.
   B. to hold the cassette close to the anti-scatter grid.
   C. to eliminate air scatter between the screen and the film.
   D. to hold the screen and film in good contact.

6-9, How will these changes affect the thickness of the cut in conventional tomography if all other factors remain the same?

A. Increase
B. Decrease
C. Stay the same

6. Increase tube angle.
7. Use high speed screens.
8. Decrease linear motion.
9. Increase circumference of the circular motion.

10-12, Match the characteristics of the tomographic motions.

A. Linear
B. Circular
C. Hypocycloidal

10. Highest Tube Load
11. Ghost Images
12. Streak Artifacts

13. What is the magnification of an object if the source object distance is 30" and the source image distance is 50"?
   A. .6
   B. 1.2
   C. 1.5
   D. 1.7

14. Stereoradiographs

A. produce a stereoscopic image by shifting the patient during the x-ray exposure.
B. produce a stereoscopic image by shifting the x-ray source during the x-ray exposure.
C. can provide a three dimensional image of patient anatomy.
D. can blur out unwanted images above and below the stereo plane.

15. Viewing of stereoradiographs

A. can be done with one eye closed.
B. is best accomplished in a darkroom with the light boxes turned off.
C. must be done at 72".
D. can be done with crossed eyes.

CHAPTER 19

NUCLEAR DECAY

Isotopes

Isotopes of an element have the same number of protons (same Z) but different atomic weights (different A). The stability of an isotope depends on the relative number of neutrons and protons in the nucleus. The electrostatic repulsion between the protons is counteracted by the attractive nuclear forces between all nucleons. For light elements a neutron to proton ratio of about 1.2 is the most stable ratio. For heavy elements, the ratio rises to about 1.5.

Isotopes which significantly deviate from these ratios are unstable, decay spontaneously and are said to be **radioactive.** Isotopes with an even number of protons and an even number of neutrons are the most stable and isotopes with an odd number of protons and an odd number of neutrons are least stable. All isotopes heavier than ^{209}Bi are unstable. Nuclear forces hold the nucleus together. Most nuclei have a binding energy of about 8 MeV per nucleon (i.e., Carbon 12 has a binding energy of about 8 x 12 = 96 MeV).

Types of Decay

The principle modes of nuclear decay are:

- alpha decay
- beta decay
- gamma decay
- isomeric transitions
- internal conversion
- positron decay
- electron capture

Alpha Decay

In alpha particle decay, an alpha particle (nucleus of helium) is emitted. An alpha particle has an atomic number of 2 and an atomic weight of 4. The decay of ^{226}Ra is an example of alpha decay.

$$^{226}_{88}\mathrm{Ra} \rightarrow {}^{222}_{86}\mathrm{Rn} + {}^{4}_{2}\alpha + \gamma \qquad 19.1$$

Alpha decay occurs when the parent nucleus has too many positive charges.

In alpha decay:
Z decreases by 2
Z decreases by 4

Nuclear decay is often presented in a schematic representation. The decay of ^{226}Ra could be indicated as in Equation 19.1 or shown schematically as in Figure 19.1.

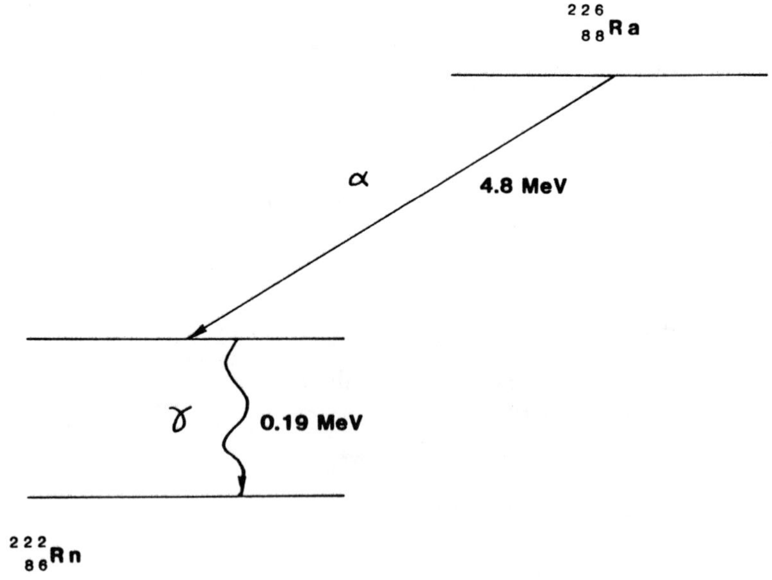

Figure 19.1. Radium-226 decay via alpha emission.

The alpha particles and gamma rays each have specific energies in nuclear decay. $^{222}_{86}Rn$ is written to the left of Radium because the atomic number Z has decreased. In a decay which increases Z the daughter would be written to the right of the parent.

Example 19.1:
What is the energy of the alpha particle in the decay scheme shown at the right?

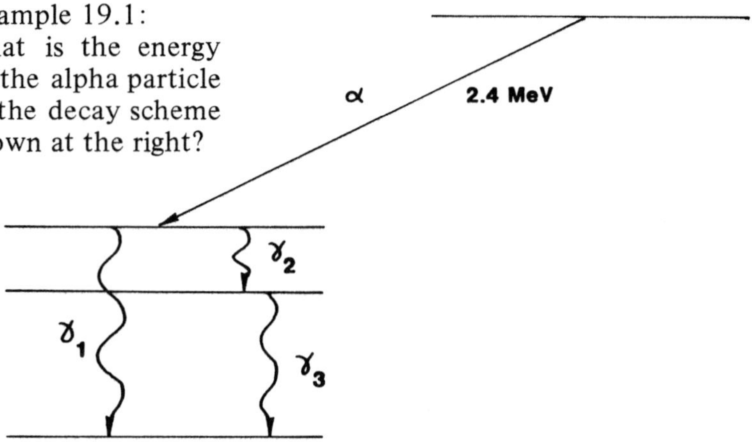

$$E_\alpha = 2.4 \text{ MeV}$$

$$\gamma_1 = 1.4 \text{ MeV}$$

$$\gamma_2 = 0.6 \text{ MeV}$$

What is the total decay energy?

$$\text{Total decay energy} = E_\alpha + E_{\gamma_1}$$

$$= 2.4 + 1.4$$

$$= 3.8 \text{ MeV}$$

What is the energy of γ_3?

$$E_{\gamma_1} = E_{\gamma_2} + E_{\gamma_3}$$

$$1.4 = 0.6 + E_{\gamma_3}$$

$$E_{\gamma_3} = 0.8 \text{ MeV}$$

Beta Decay

Beta decay occurs when the parent nuclei has too few positive charges. The decay of Cs–137 is an example of beta decay.

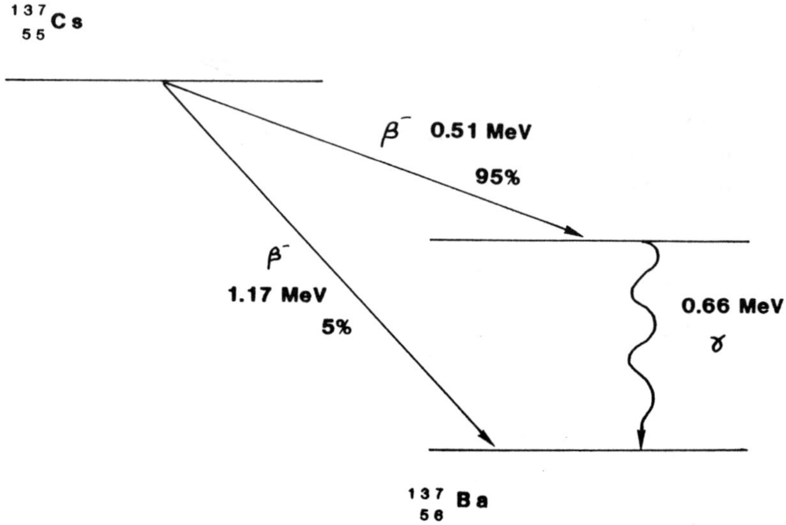

Figure 19.2. Beta minus decay of Cesium–137.

The decay scheme indicates that in 95% of the decays a beta minus particle with a maximum energy of .51 MeV is emitted followed by a 660 keV gamma ray. In 5% of the decays, a beta particle with 1.17 MeV maximum energy is emitted with no accompanying gamma ray. Notice that both branches of decay have a total decay energy of 1.17 MeV.

Example 19.2:
What is the total decay energy and the energy of γ_3 in this decay scheme?

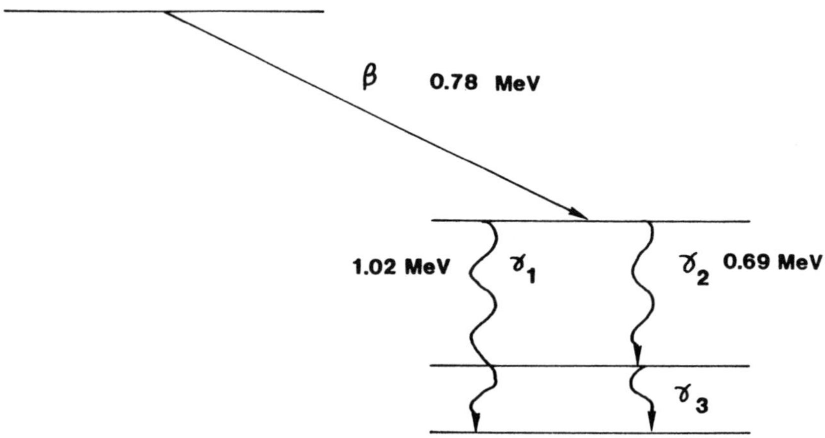

$$\text{Total Decay Energy} = \beta + \gamma_1$$

or

$$\beta + \gamma_2 + \gamma_3 = E_{Total}$$

$$\text{Total Decay Energy} = 0.78 + 1.02 = 1.80 \text{ MeV}$$

$$\gamma_3 \text{ Energy} = \text{Total Energy} - \beta - \gamma_2$$

$$= 1.80 - (.78) - (.69)$$

$$= .33 \text{ MeV}$$

Energy Spectra of Decay Particles

The energy spectra of the beta particles and gamma rays from Cs–137 decay are presented in Figure 19.3.

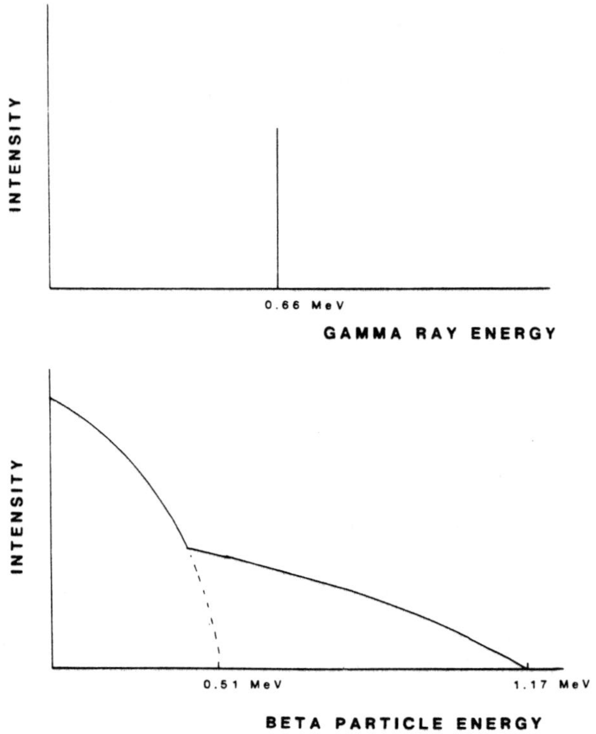

Figure 19.3. Energy spectra of gamma and beta particles from Cesium–137 decay.

All gamma rays emitted from Cs–137 decay have 660 keV. The beta particle spectra shown in Figure 19.4 is quite different. Most of the beta particles have less than the total decay energy.

Gamma Decay

In gamma decay, all the energy is accounted for. Each gamma ray has the same energy which is the total transition energy.

In beta decay, some energy appears to be missing. If all the beta particles had the maximum beta energy all the decay energy **would** be accounted for. But they don't! The average energy of the beta particles in only one third the maximum energy. Where does the rest of the energy go?

The "missing" energy is carried away by a new particle – the **anti-neutrino, ν^***. The decay of Cs–137 is written:

$$^{137}_{55}Cs \rightarrow {}^{137}_{56}Ba + \beta^- + \nu^*$$

An anti-neutrino has no mass and no charge; it just carries off energy. Because it has no mass or charge it is almost impossible to detect. Every nuclear decay by beta emission also emits an anti-neutrino.

Isomeric Transitions

In most nuclear decays, the emission of the decay product is followed by gamma ray emissions so rapidly that the events are almost simultaneous. In some cases however, the decay products exist longer than 10^{-12} seconds before the gamma ray is emitted. In such cases, the decay product is called an **isomer** and the subsequent gamma emission is termed an **isomeric transition.** The decay of Molybdenum–99 is an example of isomeric transition. The daughter $^{99}Tc^m$ has a half life of six hours.

$$^{99}_{42}Mo \rightarrow {}^{99}_{43}Tc^m + \beta^- + \nu^*$$

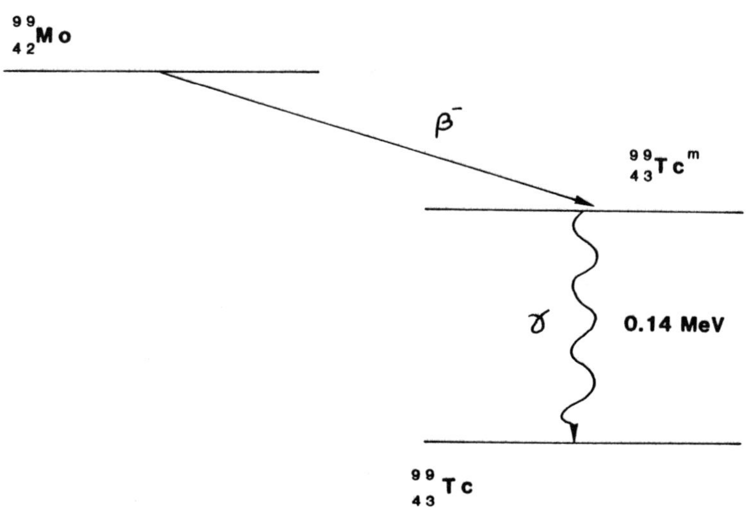

Figure 19.4. Molybdenum–99 decay to Technecium–99^{mg}.

The daughter product $^{99}Tc^{m}$ exists long enough to undergo chemical separation. It is a long lived **isomer.**

Radioactive Decay

Radioactive decay is a random process. The rate of radioactive decay cannot be changed by any chemical or physical process. The number of atoms present at any time is given by:

$$N = N_o e^{-\lambda t}$$

where λ is the **decay constant** which is specific for each isotope.

Half Life

The **half life** of an isotope is the time required to reduce the amount remaining to one half the original amount.

The half life of an isotope is related to the decay constant

$$T_{1/2} = \frac{.693}{\lambda}$$

or

$$T_{1/2} = \frac{\ln 2}{\lambda}$$

because

$$\ln 2 = .693$$

Example 19.3:
What is the half life of an isotope whose decay constant is 2.6 x 10^{-6}/sec?

$$T_{1/2} = \frac{.693}{2.6 \times 10^{-6}}$$

$$= 260{,}000 \text{ sec.}$$

$$= 3 \text{ days}$$

The **average life** is defines as:

$$T_{Avg} = 1.44\ T_{1/2}$$

Example 19.4:
What is the average life of an isotope with a four day half life?

$$T_{Avg} = 1.44 \text{ x } T_{1/2}$$

$$= 1.44 \text{ x } 4$$

$$= 5.8 \text{ days}$$

Effective Half Life of an Isotope

If an isotope is injected into a patient, some of it will decay and some of it will be excreted. The processes reduce the amount of isotope in the body. The **effective half life** is a combination of the **physical** and **biological half life.** The biological half life is the time required to reduce the amount of isotope to half the original amount through excretion.

Effective half life of an isotope is given by:

$$\frac{1}{T_{eff}} = \frac{1}{T_b} + \frac{1}{T_p}$$

where T_{eff} is the effective half life, T_p is the physical half life and T_b is the biological half life.

Example 19.5:
What is the effective half life of an isotope whose physical half life is 6 days and whose biological half life is 4 days?

$$\frac{1}{T_{eff}} = \frac{1}{4} + \frac{1}{6}$$

$$\frac{1}{T_{eff}} = \frac{10}{24}$$

$$T_{eff} = 2.4 \text{ days}$$

The effective half life is always shorter than either the physical or biological half life.

Activity

Activity of a radioactive material is defined as the number of disintegrations per second and is measured in **becquerels** or **curies.**

$$1 \text{ curie} = 3.7 \times 10^{10} \text{ dps}$$

$$1 \text{ m Ci} = 3.7 \times 10^{7} \text{ dps}$$

$$1 \ \mu \text{ Ci} = 3.7 \times 10^{4} \text{ dps}$$

$$1 \text{ becquerel} = 1 \text{ dps}$$

$$1 \ \mu \text{ Ci} = 3.7 \times 10^{4} \text{ Bq}$$

The activity is given by:

$$A = N\lambda$$

where N is the number of atoms present and λ is the decay constant.

The activity at any time t is given by:

$$A = A_o e^{-\lambda t}$$

where A_o is the original activity and λ is the decay constant. The units of λ and time must be the same, if λ is in seconds, t must be in seconds; if t is in hours, λ must be in hours.

Example 19.6:
What is the activity of an isotope with a 3 day half life 24 hours after a 100 mCi shipment is received?

$$\lambda = \frac{.693}{3 \times 24}$$

$$\lambda = 9.6 \times 10^{-3}/\text{hr}$$

$$A = A_o e^{-\lambda t}$$

$$A = 100 \exp\text{-}(9.6 \times 10^{-3} \times 24)$$

$$= 100 \exp\text{-}(.231)$$

$$= 100 \times .794$$

$$= 79.4 \text{ mCi}$$

Activity to be Shipped

We can also calculate the amount of isotope that must be shipped to ensure a specific amount arrives.

Example 19.7:
How much activity must be shipped on Monday at 0800 (8 am) to deliver 100 mCi on Wednesday morning at 0800 if the isotope's half life is 3 days?

$$\lambda = \frac{.693}{3 \times 24}$$

$$\lambda = 9.6 \times 10^{-3}/\text{hr}$$

Monday at 0800 to Wednesday at 0800 is 48 hours

$$A = A_o e^{-\lambda t}$$

$$100 = A_o \exp\text{-}(9.6 \times 10^{-3} \times 48)$$

$$= A_o \exp\text{-}(.46)$$

$$= .63 A_o$$

$$A_o = 100/.63$$

$$= 159 \text{ mCi}$$

159 mCi should be shipped Monday morning to have 100 mCi delivered Wednesday morning.

Specific Activity

Specific activity refers to the amount of activity per gram of sample. In some isotope preparation methods, it is necessary to add nonradioactive isotopes of the same element to act as a carrier during the chemical preparation of the isotope. The higher the specific activity the less volume is required to inject a given activity. Isotopes produced in a reactor by adding a neutron to the nucleus usually have lower specific activities. Isotopes obtained from fission products have higher specific activities.

Example 19.8:
What is the specific activity of a 200 gm sample containing 450 μCi?

$$\text{Specific Activity} = \mu\text{Ci/gm}$$

$$= 450/200$$

$$= 2.25\ \mu\text{Ci/gm}$$

Internal Conversion

Internal conversion is an alternate to gamma emission. Internal conversion is illustrated schematically in Figure 19.5 where the excess nuclear decay energy is transferred directly to an orbital electron which is ejected. Internal conversion is the nuclear analog of Auger electron emission. Characteristic x–rays follow internal conversion as the orbital vacancy is filled.

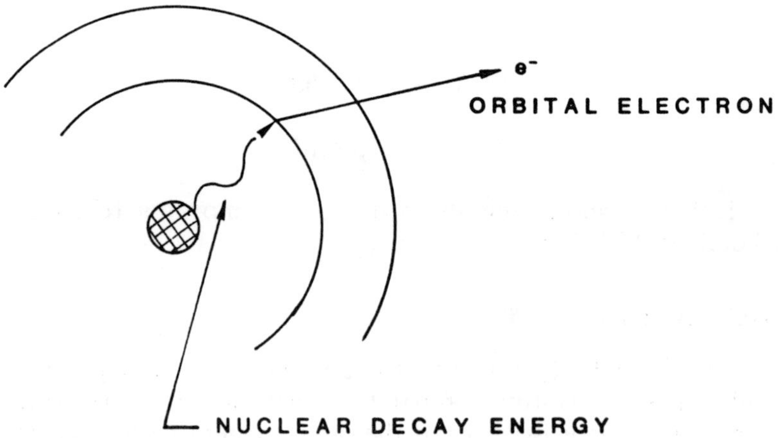

Figure 19.5. Internal conversion.

Positron Decay

Positron decay occurs when the parent nucleus has too many protons and too few neutrons. **In positron decay Z decreases by 1 and A remains the same.** The positron decay of Na-22 is:

$$^{22}_{11}Na \rightarrow {}^{22}_{10}Ne + \beta^{+} + \gamma + \nu$$

A neutrino is emitted with the positron. The decay of ^{22}Na can be represented schematically as shown in Figure 19.6.

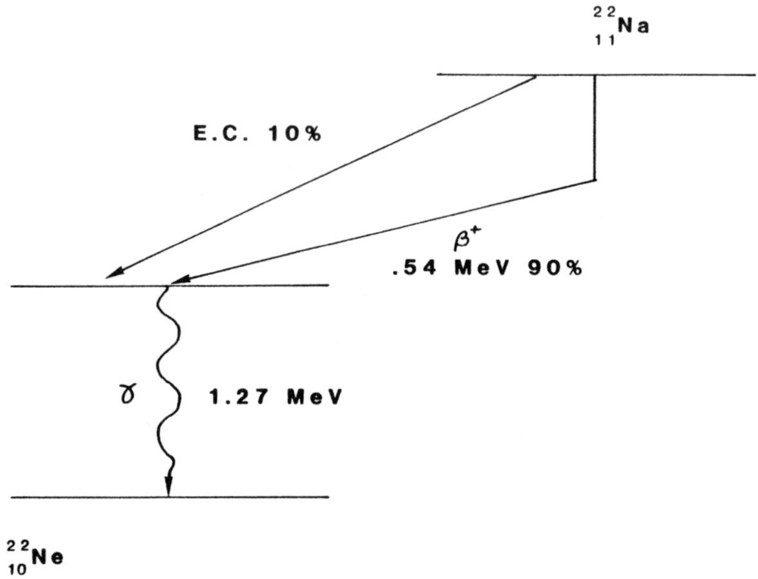

Figure 19.6. Positron decay of Na-22.

The vertical line represents the **minimum decay energy** (1.022 MeV) required before positron decay can occur. This energy will reappear as annihilation radiation. The decay arrow goes to the left because the Z decreases by one with the emission of a positive charge. The excess decay energy above 1.022 MeV is shared between the positron and the neutrino.

Positron Annihilation

After emission, a positron loses its energy in tissue by collisions with the surrounding atoms and comes to rest within a few millimeters of the decay site. The positron then annihilates with an ordinary electron producing two .511 MeV photons which are emitted in opposite directions. The two electrons taking part in the annihilation process have rest energies of 0.511 MeV, their charges cancel and the resulting annihilation photons share the rest mass energy (1.022 MeV) of the electrons.

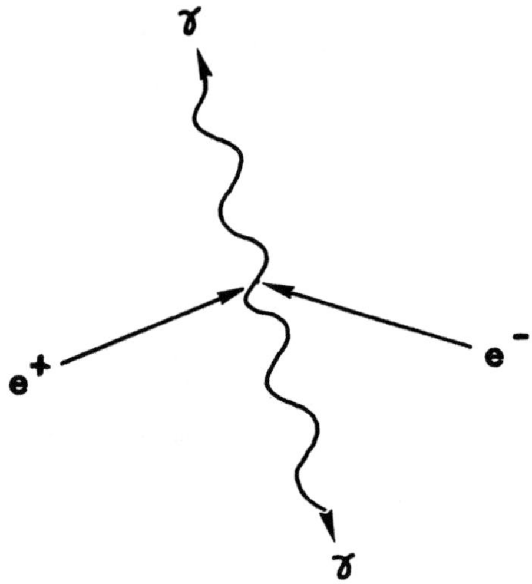

Figure 19.7. Positron annihilation resulting in two .511 MeV annihilation photons.

Electron Capture

Electron capture is an alternate to positron decay. Capturing a negative electron is an alternate way to reduce the positive charge in the nucleus. Electron capture involves the capture of an orbital electron into the nucleus. There is no minimum energy required for electron capture. **Z decreases by 1 and A remains the same in electron capture decay.**

The decay of Mn-25 is an example of electron capture.

$$^{54}_{25}Mn + e^- \rightarrow\ ^{54}_{24}Cr + \gamma$$

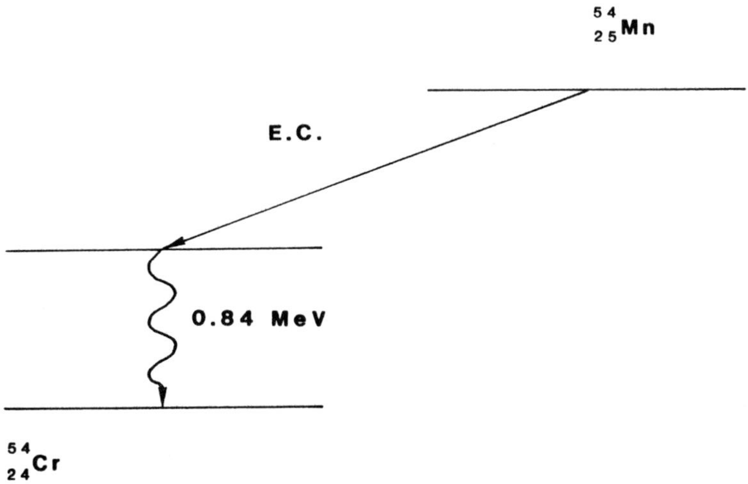

Figure 19.8. Decay of Mn-25 to Cr-24 via electron capture.

The decay scheme of Na–22 shown in Figure 19.6 indicates that 10% of the decays proceed via electron capture and 90% decay through the emission of 0.54 MeV positrons. In both cases, the final step is an emission of a 1.27 MeV gamma ray. Electron capture can be distinguished from positron decay because no beta particles are emitted in electron capture.

Radioactive Equilibrium

In some decay schemes, it is possible for the daughter product to have approximately the same activity as the parent activity. Such cases are known as radioactive equilibrium. Two cases are of special interest: **transient equilibrium**, when the daughter half life is approximately equal to the parent half life; **secular equilibrium**, when the daughter half life is much shorter than the parent half life.

Figure 19.9 gives an example of transient equilibrium. In transient equilibrium, the activity of the daughter is the same as the activity of the parent a short time ago.

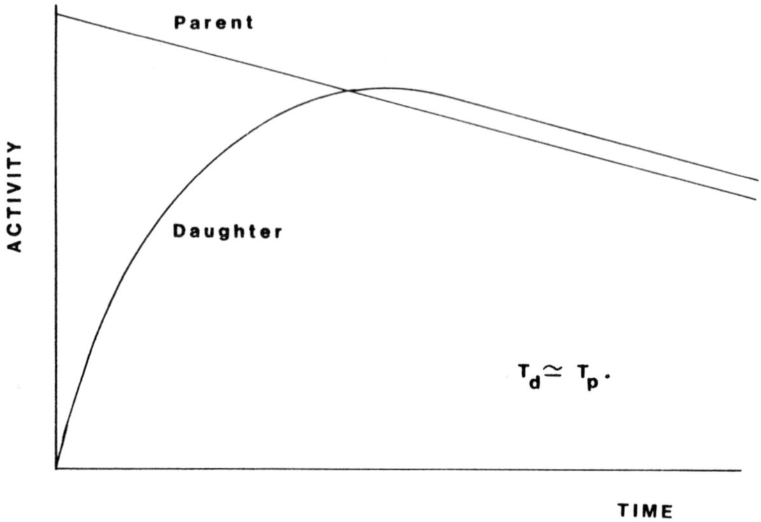

Figure 19.9. Transient equilibrium where the daughter and parent half lives are almost equal.

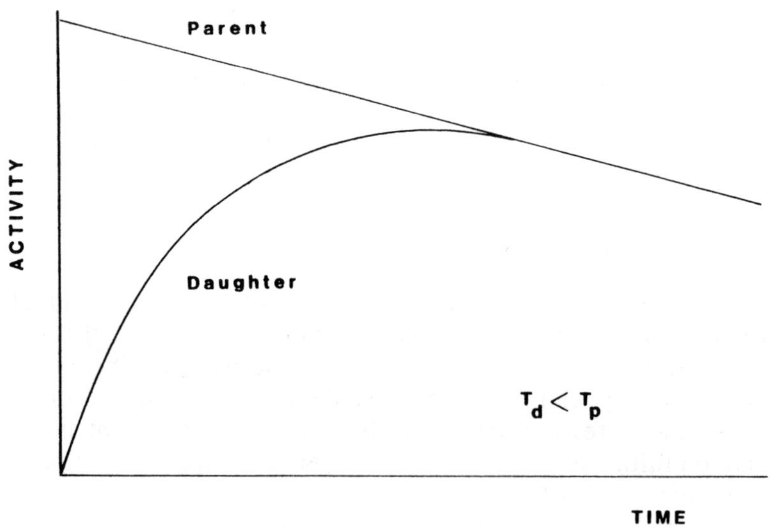

Figure 19.10. Secular equilibrium.

Secular Equilibrium

If the daughter has a much shorter half life than the parent half life, then the isotopes are in secular equilibrium. The activity of the daughter is the same as the activity of the parent because the daughter half life is so much shorter than the parent half life. In this case, every daughter nucleus decays "immediately" after being produced from a parent nucleus.

Relation of Activity and Exposure

The gamma factor Γ relates the amount of activity to the exposure rate in R/hr at a distance d from the source.

$$E = \frac{n\,\Gamma}{d^2} \qquad 19.2$$

where E is the exposure in R/hr, n is the number of millicuries, d is the distance to the source in cm and Γ is the gamma factor of the isotope. Typical gamma factors are given in Table 19.1.

TABLE 19.1

Γ in R - cm^2/hr -mCi i.e., R/hr. 1 cm from 1 mCi source

Isotope	Γ *Factor*
Br - 82	14.6
Cs - 137	3.3
Cu - 64	1.2
Co - 60	13.0
Ga - 67	1.1
Au - 198	2.3
I - 125	0.7
I - 131	2.2
Ir - 192	4.8
Fe - 59	6.4
Kr - 85	0.04
Mo - 99/Tc - 99	1.8

The gamma factor is only used for exposure rates due to gamma rays and not for beta particles.

Example 19.9:
Consider Technetium 99–m. What is the exposure rate 10 cm from a 5 mCi (5×10^7 Bq) source of Technetium 99–m?

$$E = \frac{n\Gamma}{d^2}$$

$$n = 5 \text{ mCi}$$

$$d = 10 \text{ cm}$$

$$\Gamma = 1.8 \text{ R–cm}^2/\text{mCi–hr}$$

$$E = \frac{5 \times 1.8}{(10)^2}$$

$$= \frac{9}{100}$$

$$= .09 \text{ R/hr}$$

$$= 90 \text{ mR/hr}$$

Isotope Production

Radioisotopes can be produced using either reactors or accelerators. Two processes in reactors can produce radioisotopes; fission production and neutron bombardment. **Fission products** result from the breakup (fission) of the nuclear fuel. These fission products are isotopes of different elements than the fuel and are readily separated chemically. Fission produced radioisotopes have a high specific activity and can be either beta positive or beta negative emitters.

Neutron bombardment adds a neutron to a nonradioactive nucleus creating an isotope with too many neutrons which is a beta minus emitter. Radioisotopes created by neutron bombardment have lower specific activity because initial and final nuclei are isotopes of the same element. They cannot be separated chemically.

Accelerator produced radioisotopes result from the proton ($^1_1H^+$), deuteron ($^2_1H^+$) or alpha particle ($^4_2H_e{}^{++}$) bombardment of target nuclei. The product nucleus is an isotope of a different element than the target nucleus. The radioactive product can be separated from the target material by chemical means resulting in a high specific activity. Accelerator produced isotopes have too many protons and are beta plus emitters.

CHAPTER 19 QUESTIONS

1. Nuclei are unstable
   - A. when electron capture is energetically impossible.
   - B. when the nuclear binding energy is above 8 MeV.
   - C. if they have an odd number of neutrons or protons.
   - D. when the neutron to proton ratio is greater than 1.6.

2–8, Match: Answers can be used more than once.

2. Alpha Decay
3. Positron Decay
4. Isomeric Transition
5. Beta Decay
6. Gamma Ray Decay
7. Electron Capture
8. Internal Conversion

- A. Z increases by 1 and A remains the same.
- B. Z decreases by 1 and A remains the same.
- C. Z decreases by 2 and A decreases by 4.
- D. Z and A remain the same.

Use this figure for Questions 9–11.

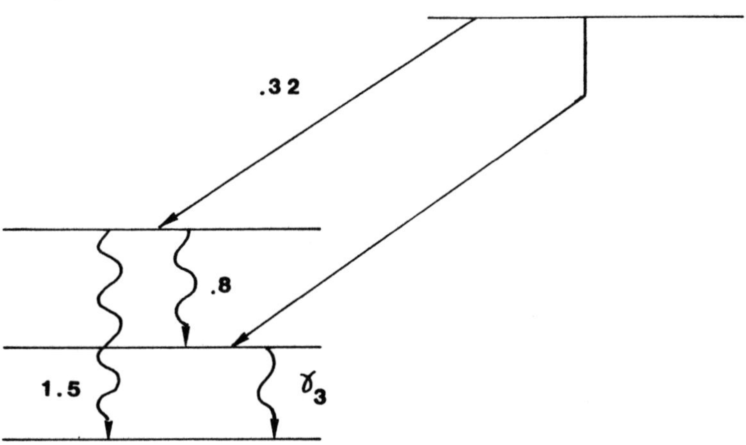

9. In the decay scheme above, the total decay energy is:
   - A. 1.34 MeV
   - B. 1.52 MeV
   - C. 1.82 MeV
   - D. 2.12 MeV

10. In the decay scheme above, the maximum energy of the positron is:
    A. 0.1 MeV
    B. 0.8 MeV
    C. 1.02 MeV
    D. 1.12 MeV

11. In the decay scheme above, the energy of γ_3 is:
    A. 0.5 MeV
    B. 0.7 MeV
    C. 0.8 MeV
    D. 1.5 MeV

12. The half life of an isotope with a decay constant of 2×10^{-6} s is:
    A. 2 days
    B. 3 days
    C. 4 days
    D. 6 days

13. What is the average life of an isotope whole half life is 6 days?
    A. 4.2 days
    B. 5.4 days
    C. 8.6 days
    D. 9.3 days

14 An isotope with a physical half life of 8 days and a biological half life of 6 days has an effective half life of:
    A. 3.4 days
    B. 4.8 days
    C. 7.2 days
    D. 14 days

15. An isotope with a physical half life of 4 days and a biological half life of 5 days has an effective half life of:
    A. 1.8 days
    B. 2.2 days
    C. 4.8 days
    D. 9 days

16. The effective half life

A. is the reciprocal of the sums of the reciprocal of the physical and biological half lives.
B. is the sum of the reciprocal of the physical and biological half lives.
C. is the reciprocal of the sum of the physical and biological half lives.
D. is always longer than either the physical or biological half lives.

17. An activity of 7.4×10^7 Bq corresponds to:

A. 2 μCi
B. 2 mCi
C. 3 mCi
D. 2 Ci

18. An activity of 3 mCi corresponds to

A. 3.7×10^7 Bq
B. 9×10^7 Bq
C. 11×10^4 Bq
D. 11×10^7 Bq

19. What is the activity Wednesday at 1500 (3 pm) of an isotope whose half life is four days if the activity on Monday at 0800 is 200 mCi?

A. 67 mCi
B. 71 mCi
C. 134 mCi
D. 141 mCi

20. What activity should be shipped on Friday at 1700 (5 pm) in order for 150 mCi of an isotope (half life 5 days) to arrive at 0800 Monday morning?

A. 104 mCi
B. 170 mCi
C. 216 mCi
D. 222 mCi

21–25, Match

21.	Positron Decay	A. Alternate to Gamma Decay
22.	Gamma Decay	B. Alternate to Positron Emission
23.	Electron Capture	C. Requires at least 1.022 MeV Decay Energy
24.	Internal Conversion	
25.	Isomeric Transition	D. Zero mass, zero charge

26. Annihilation radiation
    A. results from a combination of a positron and an electron.
    B. results from a combination of two 511 keV gamma rays.
    C. results from a combination of a 511 keV gamma ray and a positron.
    D. is an alternate to positron decay.

27. A daughter is in transient equilibrium with its parent nucleus.
    A. The daughter activity can be greater than the parent activity.
    B. The parent activity is always greater than the daughter.
    C. The daughter activity is equal to the parent activity.
    D. The daughter half life is much shorter than the parent half life.

28. The initial activity of a parent ($T_{1/2}$ = 60 hr) is 200 mCi. What is the daughter activity ($T_{1/2}$ = 1.6 hr) 120 hours later?
    A. 100 mCi
    B. 50 mCi
    C. 25 mCi
    D. 12.5 mCi

29. What is the exposure rate 40 cm from a 7 mCi source whose Γ factor is 3.7 R-cm^2/mCi hr?
    A. 647 mR/hr
    B. 162 mR/hr
    C. 67 mR/hr
    D. 16.2 mR/hr

30. What is the exposure rate 10 cm from a 3 mCi source whose Γ factor is 4.2 R-cm^2/mCi hr?

A. 1260 mR/hr
B. 126 mR/hr
C. 12.6 mR/hr
D. 1.3 mR/hr

CHAPTER 20

NUCLEAR MEDICINE IMAGING

Nuclear imaging consists of introduction of radioactive material into a patient and subsequent measurement of the distribution of the radioactivity in the patient. The distributions are displayed as nuclear medicine images.

Early nuclear medicine images were formed by moving a NaI (Tl) crystal across a patient in a back and forth scanning motion. Such **linear scanners** produced adequate images but required a long time to build up the image line by line.

Nuclear Camera Imaging

The **gamma camera** or **anger camera** forms a simultaneous image of a wide field of view with relatively good efficiency and resolution. The gamma camera consists of a **collimator**, a **sodium iodide crystal** and a group of **photomultiplier tubes** arranged to detect both energy and position. Figure 20.1 illustrates the operation of a gamma camera.

The NaI crystal is a single crystal 6.4 mm (0.25") thick. The thickness is a compromise between resolution and detection efficiency. A thicker crystal will have improved efficiency and degraded spatial resolution. The photomultiplier tubes are packed side by side. Increasing the number and decreasing the size of the photomultiplier tubes increases the camera resolution.

An analog position signal for both the X and Y coordinates is obtained from each photomultiplier tube. All the X signals are combined to form the final X position signal to be displayed. The Y position signals from each photomultiplier tube are combined to obtain the final Y position to be displayed. For example, a gamma ray detected at the center of the NaI crystal would have the Y signals from the upper photomultiplier tubes cancel the Y signals from the lower photomultiplier tube. Similar cancellation would occur with the X position signals and the position would be

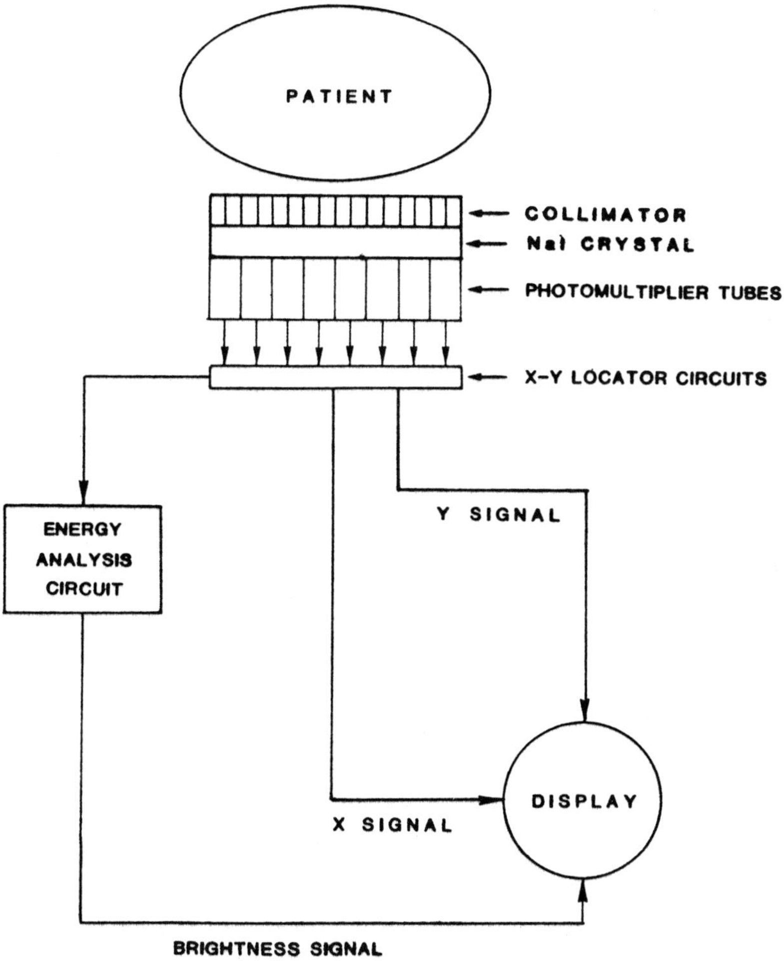

Figure 20.1. Operation of a gamma camera.

displayed in the center of the display screen. The display screen is usually a cathode ray tube (CRT).

The energy analysis circuit can be set to accept only pulses in the photo peak to assist in the rejection of scattered gamma rays. If the pulse doesn't fall in the photo peak, a dot is not displayed. The energy of the pulses accepted is controlled by the **level** control, the range of pulses is set by the **window width** control. Figure 20.2 illustrates the settings of the level and window width controls. Accepting more pulses by operating with a wider window will increase the efficiency but decrease the resolution because more scattered photons will be accepted.

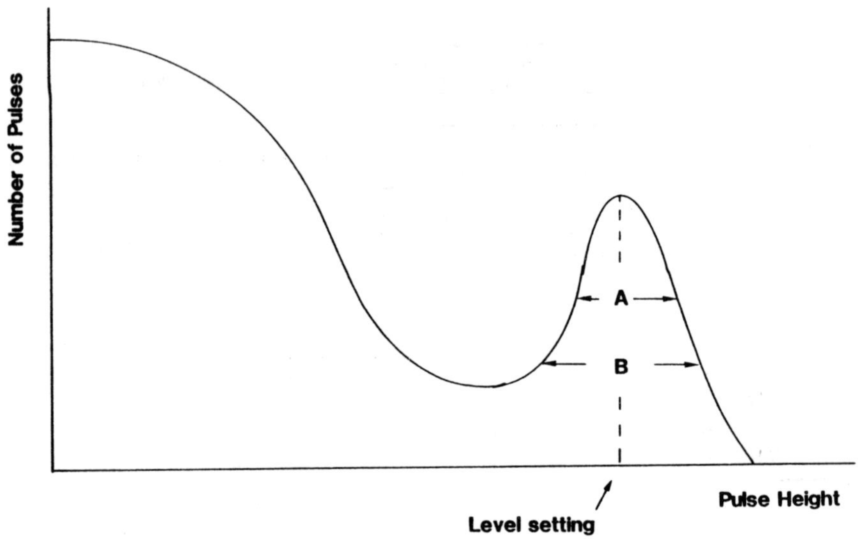

Figure 20.2. Adjustments of level and window setting control the portion of the pulse height spectrum accepted.

Collimator Designs

The four types of collimators used in nuclear medicine imaging are:

Pinhole
Parallel Hole
Diverging
Converging

Collimator efficiency depends on whether the radiation source is a point source or a large area extended radiation source covering the entire camera field of view. Efficiency is **independent** of distance to a **large area full field source** for all these collimators. Questions about collimator efficiency which do not specify the type of source assume a **point source.**

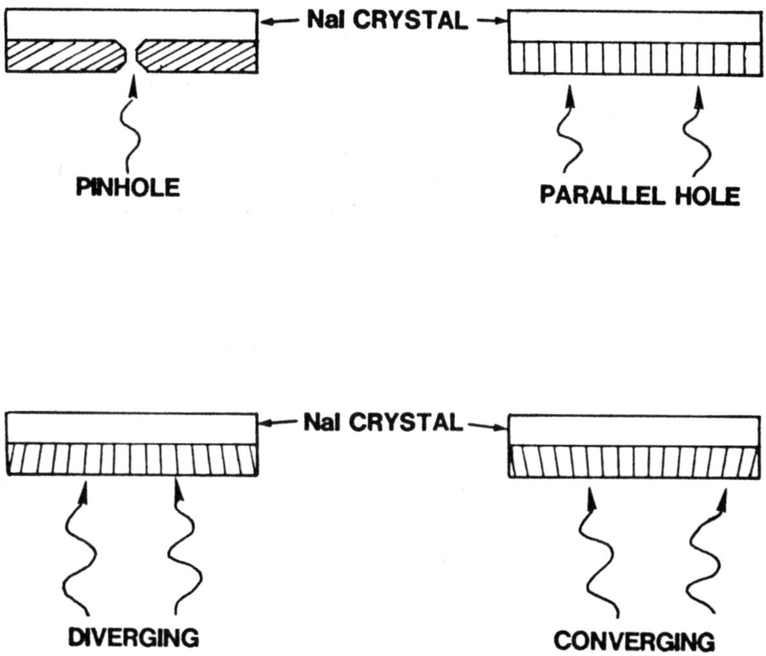

Figure 20.3. Types of nuclear camera collimators.

Pinhole Collimators

Pinhole collimator efficiency **decreases** with increasing source-detector distance from a point source. Pinhole collimators provide good resolution with poor efficiency for imaging of small organs relatively close to the collimator face. They can provide magnified or minified views depending on whether the source is close to, or far from the collimator face respectively.

Multihole Collimators

Multihole collimators are used to provide greater efficiency than pinhole collimators in gamma ray collection. Efficiency and resolution of multihole collimators depends on the hole size, septal thickness, and geometry of the holes. The walls between the collimator holes are called **septa**. Gamma camera collimators can be obtained as low energy, medium energy or high energy collimators. Higher energy collimators have greater septal thickness to prevent interseptal penetration of scattered gamma rays. High energy collimators have decreased efficiency and resolution compared to lower energy collimators. High energy collimators have thicker septa which decrease their efficiency and wider holes which decrease their resolution. Low energy collimators are most effective when used with gamma emitters with energies between 100 and 200 keV.

Multihole Collimator Resolution and Efficiency

Multihole collimator resolution increases with:
- increased collimator thickness
- decreased hole size
- increased septal thickness

Multihole collimator efficiency increases with:
- decreased collimator thickness
- increased hole size
- decreased septal thickness

Interseptal Penetration

If the septal thickness is too thin, the gamma rays can reach the crystal by penetrating through the septal walls. Scattered radiation will not be rejected and image contrast will be degraded.

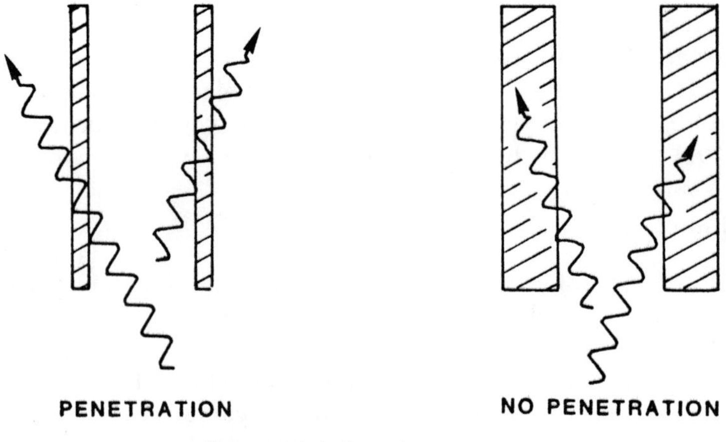

Figure 20.4. Septal penetration.

Parallel Hole Collimators

Parallel hole collimators neither magnify nor minify the object size. The resolution of parallel hole collimators decreases with increasing source detector distance. Parallel hole collimator efficiency is independent of source–collimator distance for both point and large area sources.

Converging Collimators

Converging collimators are so named because the sensitivity converges on a point. For point sources of radiation, the **sensitivity** or efficiency of a converging collimator increases with increasing distance from the collimator face up to the focal plane about 40 cm in front of collimator. Efficiency is maximum at the focal plane and then decreases for distances greater than the focal distance. The sensitivity is independent of distance for a large area radiation source. The **resolution** of a converging collimator **decreases** with increasing source-to-collimator distance. Converging collimators provide a magnified image. They trade improved resolution and efficiency for a more limited field of view.

Diverging Collimators

A diverging collimator has septa that diverge from an imaginary point approximately 40 cm behind the crystal face. This results in a minified image. For point sources, the diverging collimator **resolution decreases** with increasing distance from the collimator face. Its sensitivity also decreases with increasing source–collimator distance.

Count Densities

The contrast resolution of a nuclear image depends on the statistical noise; the more counts collected, the lower the noise. To ensure that different views have the same statistics, most nuclear images are collected until a preset number of counts is collected. The information density is related to the statistical noise and is measured in counts per cm^2.

Example 20.1:
What is the information density if a 30 cm diameter image collects 400,000 counts?

$$\text{Area of image} = \pi D^2/4$$

$$= \pi \text{ x } 1/4 \text{ x } (30)^2$$

$$= \pi/4 \text{ x } 900$$

$$= 707 \text{ cm}^2$$

$$\text{Information Density} = \frac{400{,}000 \text{ counts}}{707 \text{ cm}^2}$$

$$= 566 \text{ c/cm}^2$$

Often, the organ image does not completely fill the display. In that case, only the organ image area should be used in calculating the information density.

Example 20.2:
What is the information density in a bladder which covers 50% of a 30 cm diameter camera if 450,000 counts have been collected?

$$\text{Area of Camera Face} = \pi D^2/4$$

$$= \pi/4 \text{ x } (30)^2$$

$$= 707 \text{ cm}^2$$

$$\text{Area of bladder} = 707 \text{ x } .5$$

$$= 354 \text{ cm}^2$$

Assume almost all the recorded counts came from the bladder.

$$\text{Information Density} = \frac{450{,}000 \text{ counts}}{354 \text{ cm}^2}$$

$$= 1270 \text{ c/cm}^2$$

Overall Resolution of Cameras

The resolution of the camera without a collimator is the **intrinsic resolution** of the camera. It can be combined with the resolution of the collimator to give the total resolution of the camera plus collimator, R_T, by:

$$R_T = \sqrt{R_i^2 + R_c^2}$$

where R_i is the intrinsic resolution of the crystal and electronics and R_c is the collimator resolution.

If the MTF values of camera and collimator have been measured, the overall MTF is the product of the individual MTF values.

Emission Computed Tomography (ECT)

Single photon emission computed tomography, **SPECT**, involves the use of a camera at different angles around the patient to collect data from different emission angles. Data from these multiple views are processed in the same manner that radiographic CT scans are processed to provide tomographic slices through the patient. A modification of this tomographic approach is PET, (positron emission tomography) which uses positron emission and annihilation photons which are emitted at 180° from each other.

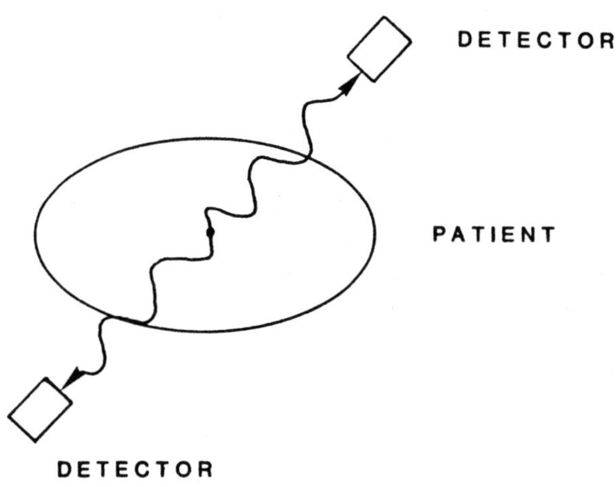

Figure 20.5. Coincidence detection of positron annihilation photons.

Annihilation photons are collected in **coincidence.** A photon is simultaneously detected in each of two detectors on opposite sides of the patient. If the photons are not detected **in coincidence**, the electronics reject the event. The coincidence requirement makes the background very low. Most PET detectors employ a ring of detectors around the patient.

Internal Dosimetry

The dose to an organ due to internal radioisotopes can be calculated using the **absorbed fraction method.** The dose to the **target** organ is calculated by adding up the contributions to the dose from all the **source** organs. In many cases, the target organ is also the only source organ. For example, we might want to know the dose to the bladder from a beta emitter concentrated in the bladder. In this case, the bladder would be both the source and target organ.

To calculate the dose to the target organ we must know

I. The amount of radiation.
II. The energy of the radiation.
III. The fraction of the source organ energy that reaches the target organ.

Cumulative Activity

The cumulative activity, $\tilde{A}$, is measured in μCi–hr. It depends on the initial activity and the effective half life of the isotope.

Cumulative activity is given by:

$$\tilde{A} = 1.44\ T_{eff}\ A_o \qquad 20.1$$

where T_{eff} is the effective half life and A_o is the initial activity. The average effective life of the isotope is given by 1.44 T_{eff}. The cumulative activity is a measure of the total number of disintegrations in the source organ.

Example 20.3:
What is the cumulative activity in a liver which initially contains 35 μCi of an isotope whose effective half life is 1.2 days?

$$\text{Effective half life} = 1.2 \times 24 \text{ hr}$$

$$= 28.8 \text{ hr}$$

$$\text{Cumulative Activity} = 1.44\, T_{eff}\, A_o$$

$$\tilde{A} = 1.44 \times 28.8 \times 35$$

$$\tilde{A} = 1452\ \mu\text{C-hr}$$

If there is no biological excretion, then

$$T_{eff} = T_p$$

Example 20.4:
What is the cumulative activity in a thyroid which has trapped 0.75 μCi of I-131 (T_p = 8.1 days)?

If the iodine is trapped in the Thyroid $T_b = \infty$ and

$$T_{eff} = T_p$$

$$= 8.1 \times 24$$

$$= 194.4 \text{ hr}$$

$$\tilde{A} = 1.44 \times 194.4 \times .75$$

$$= 210\ \mu\text{Ci-hr}$$

If the physical half life is much longer than the biological half life then:

$$T_{eff} = T_{bio}$$

Example 20.5:
What is the cumulative activity due to 100 μCi of Tritium (H-3) whose physical half life is 12.6 years and whose biological half life is 10 days?

$$\tilde{A} = 1.44\, T_{eff}\, A_o$$

$$T_{eff} \simeq 10 \text{ days}$$

$$= 240 \text{ hours}$$

$$\tilde{A} = 1.44 \text{ x } 240 \text{ x } 100$$

$$= 34560\ \mu\text{Ci–hr}$$

Equilibrium Absorbed Dose Constant

To calculate the energy per disintegration we must add up the contributions from all the radiations from each disintegration. From one disintegration there may be one beta particle and several gamma rays.

The equilibrium absorbed dose constant for the ith radiation, Δ_i, is given by:

$$\Delta_i = 2.13\, n_i\, E_i \text{ gm rad}/\mu\text{Ci–hr} \qquad 20.2$$

where 2.13 is a conversion factor, n_i is the fraction of times a disintegration produces the ith radiation and E_i is the mean energy of the ith radiation in MeV.

Example 20.6:
What is the equilibrium absorbed dose constant for Xe–133 if an E_{max} = 350 keV beta particle is emitted in 98% of the disintegrations?

$$\Delta_\beta = 2.13\, n_\beta \overline{E}_\beta$$

$$\overline{E}_\beta = 1/3\, E_{max}$$

$$= 117 \text{ keV}$$

$$= 117 \text{ MeV}$$

$$\Delta_\beta = 2.13 \text{ x } .98 \text{ x } 117$$

$$= .24 \text{ g–rad}/\mu\text{Ci–hr}$$

Absorbed Fraction

The absorbed fraction ϕ_i (t ← s) is the fraction of energy emitted from the source organ for the ith radiation which is absorbed by the target organ. It is very complicated to calculate absorbed fractions but tables are available if needed. There are some simplifications for beta particles and low (<10 KeV) energy photons. Their range is so short that none of the radiation leaves the source organ. Thus ϕ = **1 if the source organ is the target organ** and ϕ = **0 if the source organ is not the target organ for beta particles.**

The **dose reciprocity** theorem states that the absorbed fraction for an organ pair does not depend on which organ is the source and which is the target.

Total Energy Absorbed

The total energy absorbed in the target organ is given by:

$$\text{Energy absorbed} = \tilde{A} \, \Sigma \, \phi_i \, \Delta_i \qquad 20.3$$

where the equilibrium absorbed dose constant and the absorbed dose fractions are added up over all the radiations.

Average Absorbed Dose

The average absorbed dose is obtained by dividing the total energy absorbed in the target organ by the mass M_t of the target organ. The average dose D is given by:

$$\overline{D} = \frac{\tilde{A}}{M_t} \sum_i \phi_i \, \Delta_i \qquad 20.4$$

Mean Dose per Cumulative Activity

The mean dose per μCi–hr, S, is a combination of all the factors in equation 20.4 except the cumulative activity. S can be written:

$$S = \frac{1}{M_t} \sum_i \phi_i \, \Delta_i$$

S has units of rad/μCi–hr and the mean dose to an organ is given by:

$$\overline{D} = \tilde{A} \times S$$

Example 20.7:
What is the dose to the liver due to 2 mCi Tc–99 sulfur colloid trapped in the liver if:

$$S = 5 \times 10^{-5} \text{ rad}/\mu\text{Ci–hr} \quad (T_{1/2} = 6 \text{ hr})$$

$$\tilde{A} = 1.44 \times 6 \times 2000$$

$$= 17280 \ \mu\text{Ci–hr}$$

The dose to the liver is:

$$\overline{D} = \tilde{A} \times S$$

$$= 17280 \times 5 \times 10^{-5}$$

$$= .864 \text{ rad}$$

$$= 864 \text{ mrad}$$

Dose to the Bladder Wall

The absorbed dose to the surface of an organ is one half the dose inside the organ because the surface only receives radiation from inside the organ. This is important in calculating the dose to the bladder wall.

CHAPTER 20 QUESTIONS

1. A gamma camera

   A. forms simultaneous images of the before and after distribution of radioisotopes.
   B. can image an entire organ in one view.
   C. detects gamma rays interacting in a group of photomultiplier tubes.
   D. is slower than the rectilinear scanner but has better resolution.

2-5, Using a thicker NaI crystal in a gamma camera will make the following changes on _________.

A. Increases
B. Decreases
C. Remains the same

2. Sensitivity
3. Spatial Resolution
4. Septal Penetration
5. Efficiency

6. Increasing the number of photomultiplier tubes will result in the spatial resolution of a gamma camera _____________.

   A. increasing
   B. decreasing
   C. remaining the same

7. The position of the display in a gamma camera

   A. is calculated by the microcomputer.
   B. depends on the energy of the gamma ray.
   C. is recalibrated after every gamma ray is detected.
   D. is obtained from the position signals from all the photomultiplier tubes.

8. The energy analysis signal

A. determines the activity injected in the patient.
B. is the sum of the x and y signals.
C. determines whether a dot will be displayed on the image.
D. is the difference of the x and y signals.

9-13, Match the collimators and their characteristics.

9. Provides a minified image.
10. Near the collimator face the sensitivity increases with distance from the collimator.
11. Can provide either magnified or minified views depending on distance to the source.
12. Provides a 1:1 image.
13. Provides a magnified image.

A. Pinhole
B. Parallel Hole
C. Diverging
D. Converging

14. Single photon emission computed tomography (SPECT)

A. provides stereoscopic views of the 3-D distribution of radioisotopes in the body.
B. provides computed tomographic views of the 3-D distribution of radioisotopes in the body.
C. provides a 3-D distribution of the MTF values in the body.
D. provides sequential views around the 3-D distribution of radioisotopes in the body.

15. A 30 cm diameter collimator image contains 300,000 counts. What is the count density?

A. 10,000 c/cm^2
B. 3,180 c/cm^2
C. 425 c/cm^2
D. 110 c/cm^2

16. A 30 cm diameter camera images a liver which fills 70% of the display which contains 550,000 counts. What is the count density?
    A. 110 c/cm^2
    B. 425 c/cm^2
    C. 780 c/cm^2
    D. 1,100 c/cm^2

17. The overall resolution of a camera system with intrinsic resolution R_i and collimator resolution R_c is:
    A. $R_i + R_c$
    B. $\sqrt{R_i + R_c}$
    C. $R_i^2 + R_c^2$
    D. $\sqrt{R_i^2 + R_c^2}$

18. The overall MTF of a camera system with collimator $(MTF)_c$ and intrinsic $(MTF)_i$ is:
    A. $(MTF)_c + (MTF)_i$
    B. $(MTF)_c \times (MTF)_i$
    C. $(MTF)^2 + (MTF)_i^2$
    D. $\sqrt{(MTF)_c^2 \times (MTF)_i^2}$

19. The cumulative activity $\tilde{A}$ is given by
    A. the average life times the initial activity.
    B. the effective half life times the initial activity.
    C. the biological excretion coefficient times the initial activity.
    D. the absorbed dose constant times the initial activity.

20. The cumulative activity in a 1800 gm liver is ___________ if the initial activity of a 1.8 day half life isotope is 800 μCi.
    A. 28 μCi hr
    B. 1,440 μCi hr
    C. 50,000 μCi hr
    D. 2,600,000 μCi hr

21. What is the cumulative activity of an isotope with a 3 day half life and an initial activity of 2 mCi?

A. 6 μCi hr
B. 1,940 μCi hr
C. 144,000 μCi hr
D. 207,000 μCi hr

22. The equilibrium absorbed dose constant

A. measures the energy given off per disintegration.
B. is a measure of the total number of disintegrations.
C. measures the fraction of energy absorbed by the target organ.
D. coverts the energy per disintegration into number of disintegrations.

23. The absorbed fraction is

A. the fraction of disintegrations in the target organ which remains inside the target organ.
B. 1 for the beta particles if the source organ is the target organ.
C. measures the total number of disintegrations in the target organ.
D. is 0 for low energy ($\langle$10 keV) photons if the target organ is the source organ.

24. The mean dose per cumulative activity S in a 1 gm organ is _______ rad/μCi-hr if the absorbed fraction is 0.8, the cumulative activity is 15,000 μCi hr and the equilibrium absorbed dose constant is 0.18 gm rad/μCi hr.

A. .14
B. .98
C. 2,160
D. 12,000

25. The dose to a 20 cm diameter bladder wall is ________ mrad if the cumulative activity is 12,000 μCi hr and S is 3×10^{-5} rad/μCi-hr.

A. 180
B. 360
C. 1,150
D. 7,200

26. Thinner septal walls in a nuclear medicine collimator will

A. improve the resolution by allowing more scattered radiation through the collimator.
B. improve image contrast by packing the holes closer together.
C. degrade image contrast by allowing more scattered radiation through the collimator.
D. degrade camera efficiency by reducing the amount of lead between collimator holes.

CHAPTER 21

DIAGNOSTIC ULTRASOUND IMAGING

Sound consists of increases and decreases in pressure in a medium. Sound radiation is **not** electromagnetic radiation. Sound frequencies above 20,000 cycles per second (Hertz) are classified as ultrasound because they are beyond normal human hearing range. Electrical energy is converted to sound energy by means of a **transducer.** Figure 21.1 plots the pressure as a function of time at some point in front of a transducer.

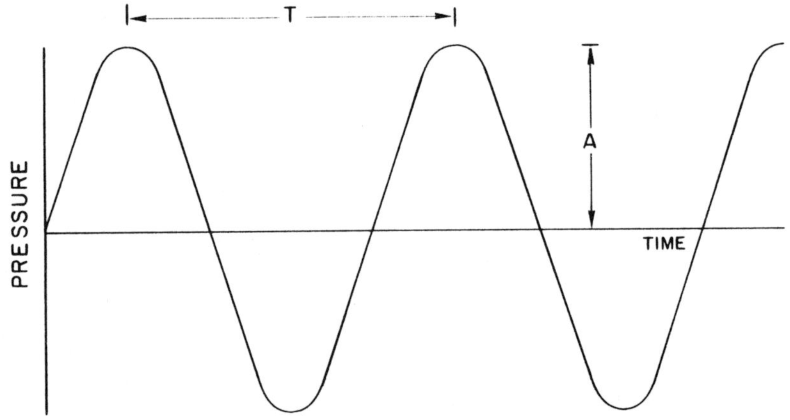

Figure 21.1 Ultrasonic wave pressure at a point in front as a function of time.

The **frequency** is defined as the number of cycles which pass a point per second. The **period** of the wave is the time required for one cycle. The period is related to the frequency by:

$$T = 1/f \text{ (seconds)} \qquad 21.1$$

The **amplitude** is 1/2 the peak to peak pressure variations.

Figure 21.2 represents a snapshot at some time of the pressure distribution as a function of distance. The **wave length** is the distance between adjacent peaks or valleys in the waves. The **velocity** of a wave measures how fast the signal (i.e., the changes in pressure) moves from one place to another. It is **not** equal to the velocity of the particles in the medium. The velocity v of a wave is related to its frequency f and wavelength λ by:

$$v = f\lambda \qquad 21.2$$

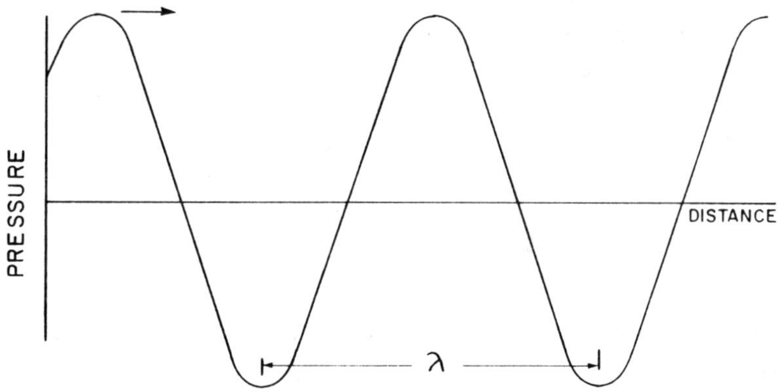

Figure 21.2. Distribution of pressure in front of a transducer as a function of distance.

Although Figure 21.1 and 21.2 appear similar, they focus on different properties of the ultrasound wave. Figure 21.1 concentrates on the time characteristics of the wave, Figure 21.2 concentrates on the distribution of the wave in space.

Example 21.1:
What is the wavelength of a 3 MHz ultrasonic wave if its velocity in tissue is 1500 m/sec?

$$v = f\lambda$$

$$\lambda = v/f$$

$$\lambda = 1500 \text{ m/s} / 3 \times 10^6 \text{ Hz}$$

$$\lambda = 5 \times 10^{-4} \text{ m}$$

$$\lambda = .5 \text{ mm}$$

Ultrasound Transducers

A **transducer** converts electrical energy into sound energy. Ultrasound beams are formed by transducers made of piezoelectric crystals. The piezoelectric effect describes certain crystals - quartz, barium titanate or lead zirconium titanate (PZT) which both change shape when a voltage is applied to them and produce a voltage when their dimension is changed by an applied pressure. Figure 21.3 illustrates how a piezoelectric crystal changes shape under the application of voltage.

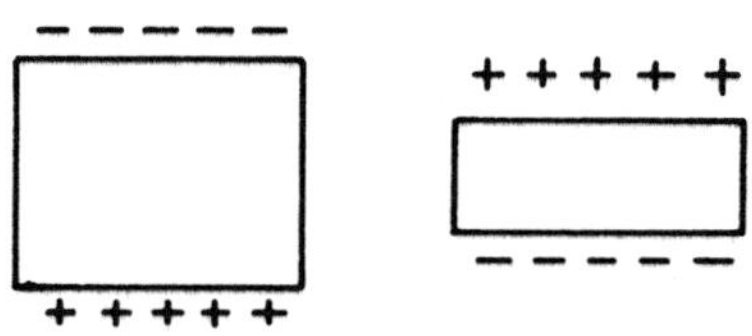

Figure 21.3. Piezoelectric crystal changes shape with changes in applied voltage.

The **frequency** of sound produced by the transducer depends on the **thickness** of the transducer. Thinner transducers produce higher frequencies. Diagnostic medical ultrasound uses frequencies between two and twenty MHz (1 Hz = 1 cycle/s). At frequencies much lower than 2 MHz the wavelength of the ultrasound waves is so large the spatial resolution is poor.

The attenuation of ultrasound increases with frequency so that at frequencies greater than about 20 MHz the returning signals are so small they are hidden in the noise. Ophthalmological applications can use the higher frequency range ($\geq$15 MHz) because their depth of interest is so small.

The same transducer can be used to both send and receive signals. The transducer holder contains a piezoelectric crystal, the electrical connections and a damping material used to prevent reflections from the back of the holder and to rapidly stop the crystal vibrations (ringing) so it will be ready to detect the returning echoes.

The response of the piezoelectric crystal and holder as a function of frequency is described by the **Q value** of the system. Q is defined as the ratio of the resonant frequency divided by the system band width. **High Q** transducers have high sensitivity to a narrow range of frequencies. They are excellent transmitters but have little damping and a **long ring-down** time. They are insensitive to echoes for a long time after the transmit pulse.

Low Q transducers have a lower sensitivity to a wide range of frequencies. They are **highly damped** with a **short ring-down** time. They can respond to echoes which return immediately after the transmit pulse. Ultrasound systems with only one transducer use highly damped low Q transducers.

Figure 21.4 illustrates the basic pulse echo technique used in ultrasound imaging. An ultrasound pulse is sent into the body and the time for the echo return is related to the distance to the reflecting interface.

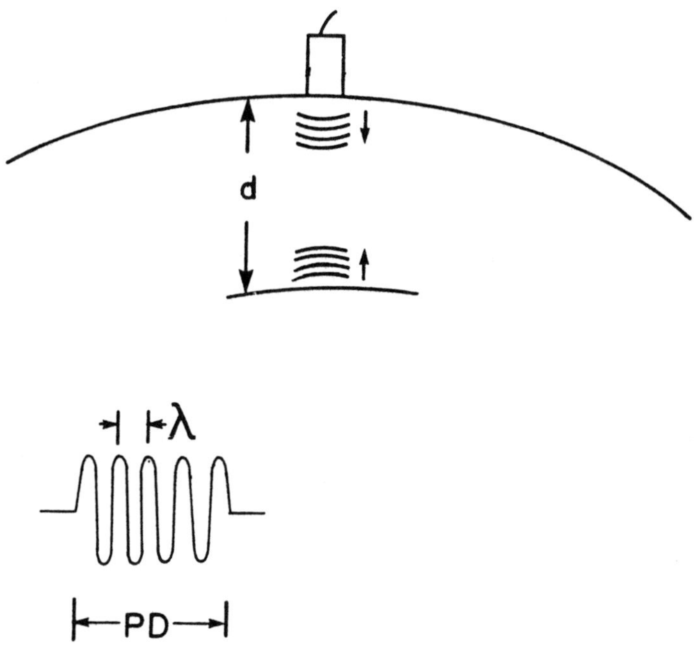

Figure 21.4. Pulse echo technique.

By measuring the time for echo return t and assuming a constant sound velocity v in tissue, the distance d to the reflecting interface is given by:

$$2d = v\,t$$

$$d = \frac{v\,t}{2}$$

The product vt is divided by 2 because the time measured is the time for the ultrasound signal to travel to the reflecting interface and return.

Pulse Duration

Typical ultrasound pulses contain two to five cycles in each pulse as shown in Figure 21.4. The **pulse duration, PD** is the number of cycles in the pulse times the period of the wave. The pulse duration is given by:

$$PD = N \times T$$

or

$$PD = {}^{N}/_{f}$$

N is the number of cycles in the pulse and where T is the period of the ultrasound wave and f is the frequency of the wave.

The pulse duration is sometimes referred to as the **pulse length,** i.e., how long is the pulse "on."

Example 21.2:
What is the pulse duration (pulse length) if four cycles of a 6 MHz ultrasound signal are contained in the pulse?

$$PD = N \times T$$

Period of Ultrasound Wave

$$T = 1/f$$

$$T = 1/6 \times 10^{6}$$

$$T = .17 \times 10^{-6} \text{ s}$$

$$PD = 4 \times .17 \times 10^{-6}$$

$$PD = .66 \times 10^{-6} \text{ s}$$

$$= 6.6 \times 10^{-7} \text{ s}$$

$$= .66 \,\mu\text{s}$$

Example 21.3
What is the pulse duration (pulse length) of a pulse containing 5 cycles of a 4.5 MHz ultrasound wave?

$$PD = N \times T$$

Period of Ultrasound Wave

$$T = 1/f$$

$$= 1/4.5 \times 10^{6}$$

$$= .22 \times 10^{-6} \text{ s}$$

$$PD = 5 \times .22 \times 10^{-6}$$

$$= 1.1 \times 10^{-6} \text{ s}$$

$$= 1.1 \ \mu\text{s}$$

Pulse Repetition Frequency

The **pulse repetition frequency, (PRF)**, measures how often the ultrasound beam pulse is sent out by the transducer. PRF is measured in pulses per second. A 5 MHz pulse containing 5 cycles (PD = 1 usec) could be sent into the body twice each second (PRF = 2 per second); or 30 times per second (PRF = 30 per second); or 400 times each second (PRF = 400 each second). The PRF is independent of the ultrasound frequency. On some ultrasound units it can be set by the operator. The PRF must be adjusted so that all echoes from distant reflecting surfaces have returned before the next ultrasound pulse is sent out.

Example 21.4:
What is the pulse duration (pulse length) and the pulse repetition frequency of a 3.5 MHz pulse containing 4 cycles which is sent out 200 times each second?

$$PRF = 200/\text{s}$$

$$PD = N \times T$$

$$T = 1/f$$
$$= 1/3.5 \times 10^6$$
$$= .29 \times 10^{-6} \text{ s}$$
$$PD = 4 \times .29 \times 10^{-6} \text{ s}$$
$$= 1.1 \times 10^{-6} \text{ s}$$
$$= 1.1\ \mu\text{s}$$

The Duty Factor

The **duty factor** is the fraction of time the ultrasound beam is "on." Duty factor is calculated from:

$$DF = PD \times PRF \qquad 21.3$$

Example 21.5:
What is the duty factor when an ultrasound beam has a pulse repetition frequency of 200 per second and a pulse duration of 1 microsecond?

$$DF = PD \times PRF$$
$$DF = \frac{200 \text{ pulses}}{\text{s}} \times \frac{1\ \mu\text{s}}{\text{pulse}}$$
$$= 200 \times 10^{-6}$$
$$= 2 \times 10^{-4}$$

Example 21.6:
If the frequency of the ultrasound beam is five megahertz, how many cycles are contained in the 1 μs pulse?

$$PD = N \times T$$
$$PD = N/f$$
$$N = PD \times f$$

$$= 1 \times 10^{-6}\ \text{s} \times 5 \times 10^{6}\ \text{cycles/s}$$

$$= 5\ \text{cycles/pulse}$$

Ultrasound Power and Intensity

Ultrasound beam power is measured in watts (joule per second). Intensity is the power per area. Medical ultrasound beams are measured in milliwatts per square centimeter (mw/cm^2).

Typical intensities for different forms of ultrasound beams are shown in Table 2.1.

TABLE 21.1
TYPICAL INTENSITY LEVELS OF ULTRASOUND BEAMS

Purpose		*Intensity*
Diagnostic		
	Average	$10 mw/cm^2$
	Peak	$20 mw/cm^2$
Therapy		$1 - 5\ w/cm^2$

Therapy ultrasound beams are used in Physical Therapy to treat strained and aching muscles.

Ultrasound Attenuation

Attenuation of ultrasound in tissue is a complex process which includes scattering, absorption and reflections. Attenuation is measured in db per centimeter. Attenuation increases **linearly** with frequency for most tissues.

Decibel Scale

The decibel scale is a logarithmic scale designed to compare signals with widely different intensities.

The strength in db of a reflected signal is:

$$\text{db} = 10 \log \frac{I_r}{I_o} \qquad 21.4$$

where I_r is the reflected signal intensity and I_o is the surface intensity.

TABLE 21.2
REPRESENTATIVE INTENSITY RATIOS AND CORRESPONDING db VALUES

I/I_o *Ratio*	*db Value*
1	0
1/2	-3
1/10	-10
1/50	-17
1/100	-20
1/500	-27
1/1000	-30

Table 21.2 gives intensity ratios and db values for some representative intensity ratios.

Example 21.7:
What is the signal strength in db of a reflected echo whose intensity is 1/2000 the incident signal?

$$\text{db} = 10 \log \frac{I_r}{I_o}$$

$$\text{db} = 10 \log (1/2000)$$

$$= -33$$

The reflected signal intensity is -33 db or "33db down" from the original signal intensity.

Table 21.3 gives attenuation values in db for several representative tissues for a 1MHz ultrasound beam. A useful rule of thumb is that ultrasound attenuation in soft tissue is about 1 db/cm/MHz. Notice that the attenuation in muscle depends on whether the sound beam is directed along or across the muscle fibers. If the attenuation of an ultrasound beam is 2 db/cm, only 10% of the intensity of the ultrasound beam is transmitted through a 5 cm thick tissue layer.

Ultrasound Velocity

Ultrasound velocity increases with the density of the medium.

TABLE 21.3
ATTENUATION VALUES IN db/cm
FOR SOME REPRESENTATIVE BODY MATERIALS

Tissue	*Attenuation at 1 MHz db/cm*
Air	11
Blood	0.15
Bone	18
Brain	0.7
Fat	0.6
Kidney	0.9
Liver	0.8
Muscle	
Along Fibers	1.1
Across Fibers	3
Water	0.002

Ultrasound Reflections

Ultrasound reflections occur wherever there is a change in accoustic impedence, Z. The accoustic impedence, Z, is defined as:

$$Z = \rho v \qquad 21.5$$

where ρ is the physical density in g/cm^3 and v is the velocity of sound in cm/s. The accoustic impedence Z is measures in rayls, (1 rayl = 1 gm/cm^2–s). Table 21.4 presents some representative tissues together with their physical density, velocity and accoustic impedence.

Ultrasonic Reflection Coefficient

When an ultrasound beam passes from medium one to medium two as shown in Figure 21.5, the reflection coefficient is given by:

$$R = \frac{\text{Reflected Intensity}}{\text{Incident Intensity}} \qquad 21.6$$

$$= \left(\frac{Z_2 - Z_1}{Z_2 + Z_1}\right)^2$$

TABLE 21.4
PHYSICAL DENSITY AND VELOCITY OF SOME REPRESENTATIVE TISSUES

Material	*Density g/cm³*	*Velocity m/sec*	*Acoustic Impedence Z Rayls x 10⁵*
Air	.001293	330	.00042
Average Soft Tissue	1.0	1540	1.63
Blood	1.05	1550	1.62
Bone	1.8	4100	7.4
Brain	1.03	1540	1.59
Fat	0.92	1450	1.33
Kidney	1.05	1560	1.64
Liver	1.05	1570	1.65
Lung	0.3	1550	0.46
Muscle	1.06	1580	1.67
Spleen	1.06	1570	1.66
Water	1.00	1480	1.48

The reflection coefficient doesn't depend on which is medium 1 and which is medium 2.

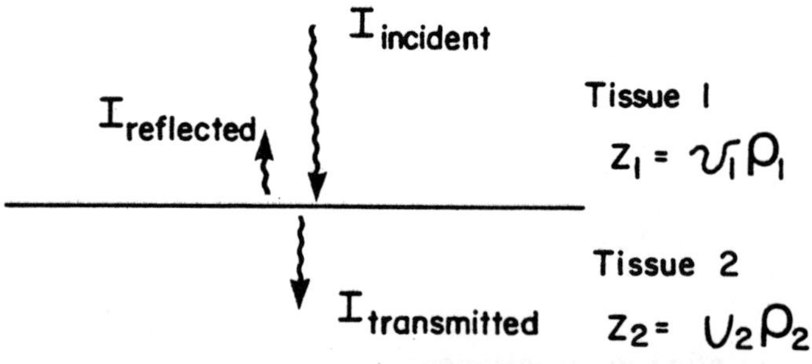

Figure 21.5. Reflection and transmission from a tissue interface.

Reflections from a muscle–fat and a fat–muscle interface are the same. It doesn't matter which is the incident and which is the transmitted medium. If either the velocities or the physical densities are **very different** between the two media, the reflection coefficient will be near 100%. Tissue–air and muscle–bone interfaces give large reflections. The reflection coefficients are large because of the large differences in densities and velocities. Typical tissue–tissue reflection coefficients in the body are approximately

1%. The transducer–air interface also will produce nearly a 100% reflection. For this reason, a coupling fluid or gel must be used between the transducer and the skin surface. Air spaces between the transducer and the skin reflect the ultrasound energy back to the transducer.

Refraction

If the sound beam is not perpendicular to the reflecting interface, **refraction** and **reflection** occur as the beam passes from medium 1 to medium 2. Figure 21.6 shows examples of reflection and refraction. The transmitted beam doesn't continue in the same direction as the incident beam. It is **refracted** to a new direction.

In Figure 21.6, θ_i is the angle of the incident beam, θ_r is the angle of the reflected beam measured relative to the perpendicular to the reflecting surface and θ_t is the transmitted beam which has been refracted.

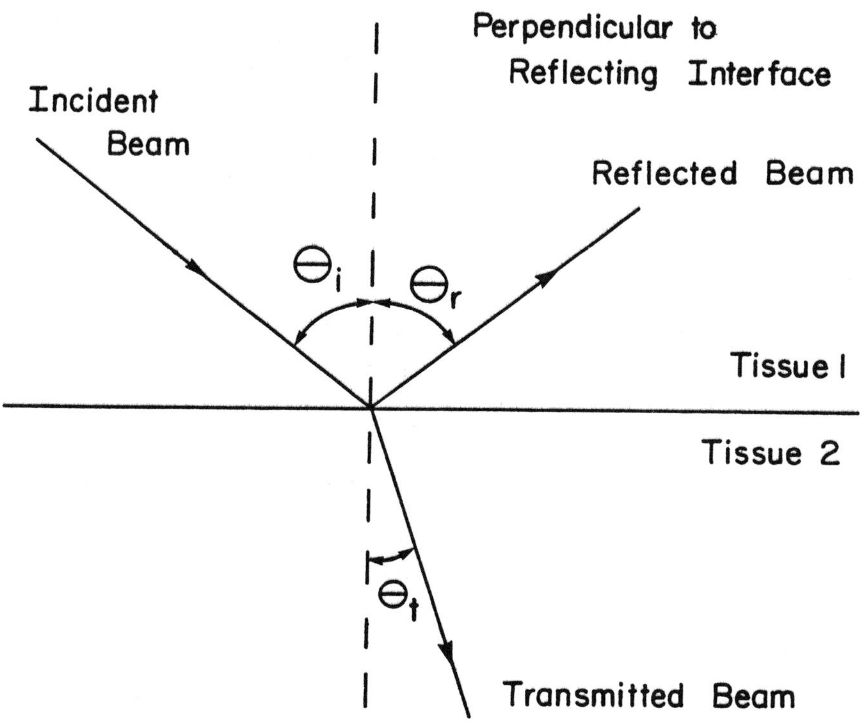

Figure 21.6 Oblique incidence results in reflection and refractions.

Snell's Law

Snell's Law relates the transmitted beam angle to the incident beam angle and the ratio of the two velocities.

Snell's Law is given by:

$$\frac{\sin \theta_i}{\sin \theta_t} = \frac{v_1}{v_2} \qquad 21.7$$

where v_1 is the velocity in the first (incident) medium and v_2 is the velocity in medium 2. In Figure 21.6, the velocity in medium 2 is less than the velocity in medium 1.

The angle of incidence is equal to the angle of reflection. Unless the angle of incidence is close to 0° (perpendicular incidence) the reflected beam will be directed away from the transducer and the reflected signal will be very small. For single transducer application, the angle must be within a few degrees of 90° incidence.

Example 21.8:
What are the reflected and transmitted angles if an ultrasound beam with incident angle 30° passes from medium 1, v_1 = 1540 m/s to medium 2, v_2 = 1420 m/s?

Reflected Angle:
The reflected angle is equal to the incident angle.

$$\theta_r = \theta_i$$

$$\theta_r = 30°$$

Transmitted Angle:
The transmitted angle is calculated from Snell's Law.

$$\frac{\sin \theta_i}{\sin \theta_t} = \frac{v_1}{v_2}$$

$$\sin \theta_t = \frac{v_2}{v_1} \sin \theta_i$$

$$= \frac{1420}{1540} \sin 30°$$

$$= 0.922 \sin 30°$$

$$= 0.922 \times .5$$

$$\sin \theta_t = .46$$

$$\theta_t = 27.4°$$

Depth Compensation Circuits

The large attenuation by tissue can cause signals from the same kinds of interfaces at different depths to be very different. A signal from a deeper interface will be much smaller. This could present difficulties in imaging organs because the far side interface may be attenuated so much it may not be recognized.

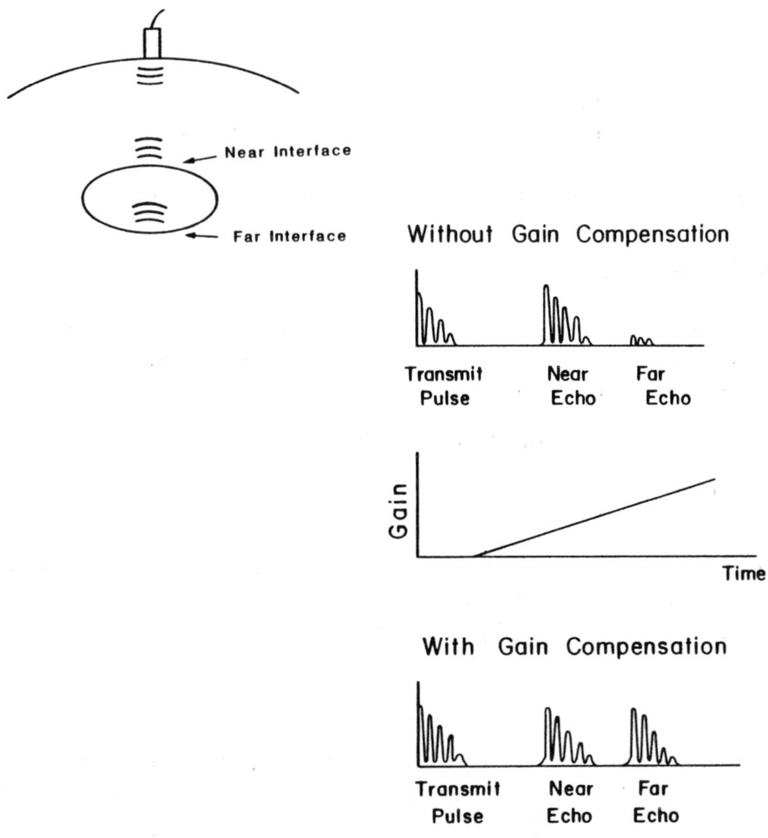

Figure 21.7. Depth compensation circuits.

To compensate for this attenuation, the amplifier gain is increased so the echoes from the deeper interfaces have more amplification, Depth Compensation Circuits, called, Time Gain Compensation (TGC) or Time Varied Gain (TVG), display echoes from the same interfaces at different depths with the same amplitude.

Resolution in Ultrasound Scanning

There are two types of resolution in ultrasound scanning:

Direction Parallel to Beam	Direction Perpendicular to Beam
Axial or Depth or Longitudinal Resolution	Azmuthal or Width or Lateral Resolution

The resolution in the two directions is not the same.

Axial Resolution

Axial or **depth** resolution depends upon the frequency and pulse duration. Higher frequencies allow shorter pulse durations. The minimum separation detectable is:

$$\text{Minimum Separation} = d_m \qquad 21.8$$

$$2d_m = v\,t$$

where t is the time to travel twice the separation distance. The pulse duration PD must be less than t, or the first part of the reflected pulse will overlap with the last part of the incident pulse.

Recall

$$\text{Pulse duration} = N/f$$

so the time for pulse to travel back and forth between the two interfaces at a minimum separation is related to the Pulse Duration by:

$$PD = t$$

or

$$PD = \frac{2d_m}{v}$$

$$t = N/f$$

or Resolution Distance $d_m = \frac{v}{2}\frac{N}{f}$

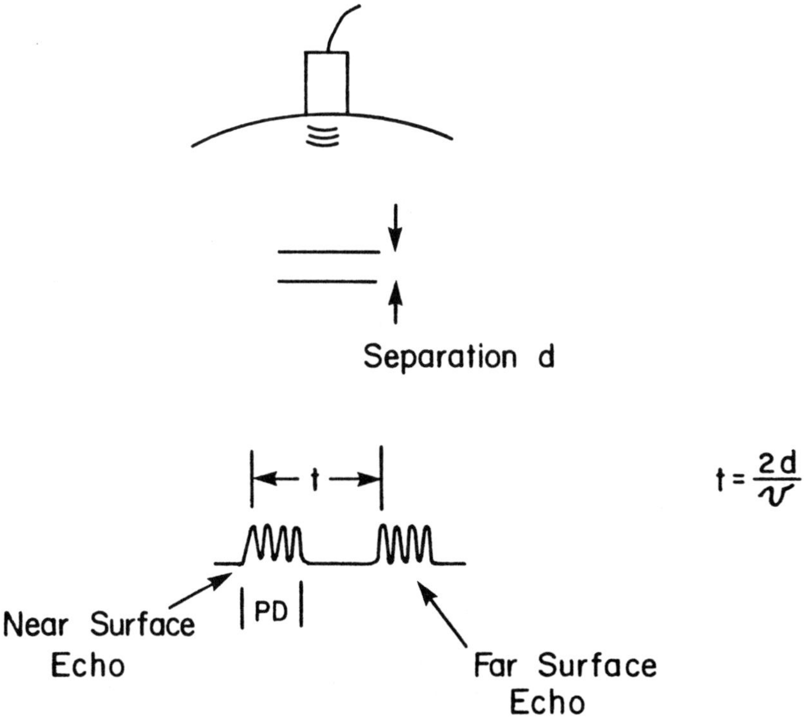

Figure 21.8. The minimum separation distance between reflection interfaces depends on the pulse duration, the number of cycles in the pulse and the frequency of the ultrasound beam.

Higher frequencies and shorter pulse durations (smaller N) yield better depth resolution. Typical resolution values as a function of frequency are given in Table 21.5.

TABLE 21.5
DEPTH RESOLUTION IN SOFT TISSUE FOR TYPICAL ULTRASOUND FREQUENCIES

Frequency (MHz)	*Depth Resolution (mm)*
1	3
2.5	1.2
5	0.6
10	0.3

Example 21.9:
What is the minimum interface separation that can be resolved with a 1.5 μs pulse of frequency 3 MHz?

$$d_m = \frac{PD \times v}{2}$$

$$v = 1500 \text{ m/sec}$$

$$d_m = \frac{1.5 \times 10^{-6} \text{s} \times 1.5 \times 10^{3} \text{m}}{2}$$

$$= 1.1 \times 10^{-3} \text{m}$$

$$= 1.1 \text{ mm}$$

Increasing the frequency improves the depth resolution at the expense of tissue penetration. Penetration **decreases linearly** with increasing frequency for most tissues except bone. Attenuation in bone increases as the square of the frequency.

Azmuthal or Lateral Resolution

The sound beam in front of a transducer can be conveniently divided into a **near** or **Fresnel zone** and a **far** or **Fraunhoffer zone.** The **azmuthal resolution** depends on the **beam diameter,** the **frequency** and the **distance from the transducer** to the objects. Figure 21.9 illustrates the relation between the Fresnel and Fraunhoffer zones.

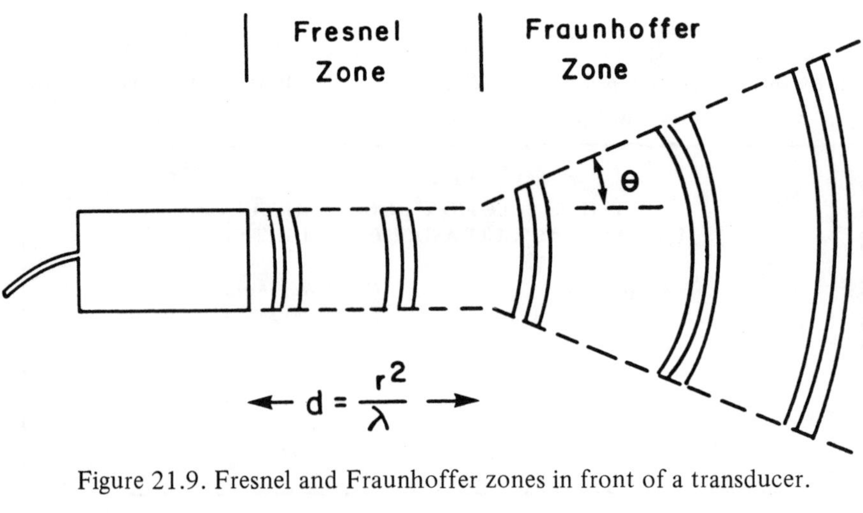

Figure 21.9. Fresnel and Fraunhoffer zones in front of a transducer.

Fresnel Zone or Near Zone

Near the transducer, the ultrasound beam has a diameter about the same size as the transducer. This region is called the **Fresnel** or **Near Zone.** The Fresnel zone or focal length extends to a distance in front of the transducer:

$$d = r^2/\lambda \qquad 21.9$$

where r is the radius of the transducer and λ is the wavelength of the ultrasound beam. Higher frequency transducers have a longer Fresnel zone. In the Fresnel zone, the intensity undergoes large fluctuations. Medical transducers are generally about 20 λ in diameter. By shaping an ultrasonic transducer, it is possible to focus the beam so in the focal region it has a smaller diameter than the transducer. Ultrasound beams can be focused **ONLY** in the Fresnel zone. The Fresnel zone is also called the **focal** zone.

Example 21.10:
How far in front of a 3 MHz 1.5 cm diameter transducer does the focal zone (Fresnel zone) extend?

$$d = r^2/\lambda$$

$$r = 0.75 \text{ cm}$$

$$\lambda = \nu/f$$

$$v = 1500 \text{ m/s}$$

$$f = 3 \times 10^6/\text{s}$$

$$\lambda = 1500/3 \times 10^6 \text{ m}$$

$$\lambda = .5 \times 10^{-3} \text{ m}$$

$$\lambda = 0.5 \text{ cm}$$

$$d = (0.75)^2/.05$$

$$= 0.56/.05$$

$$d = 11.25 \text{ cm}$$

Fraunhoffer or Farfield Zone

Beyond the Fresnel zone, the beam begins to spread out. The divergence angle is given by:

$$\sin \theta = 0.61 \lambda/r \qquad 21.10$$

Beams from smaller diameter transducers spread more rapidly in the Fraunhoffer region.

Variation of Fresnel and Fraunhoffer Zones With Transducer Diameter and Ultrasound Frequency

Figure 21.10 illustrates how the Fresnel zone **increases** and the angle of divergence of the ultrasound beam **decreases** in the Fraunhoffer zone as the transducer diameter **increases** for the same ultrasonic frequency.

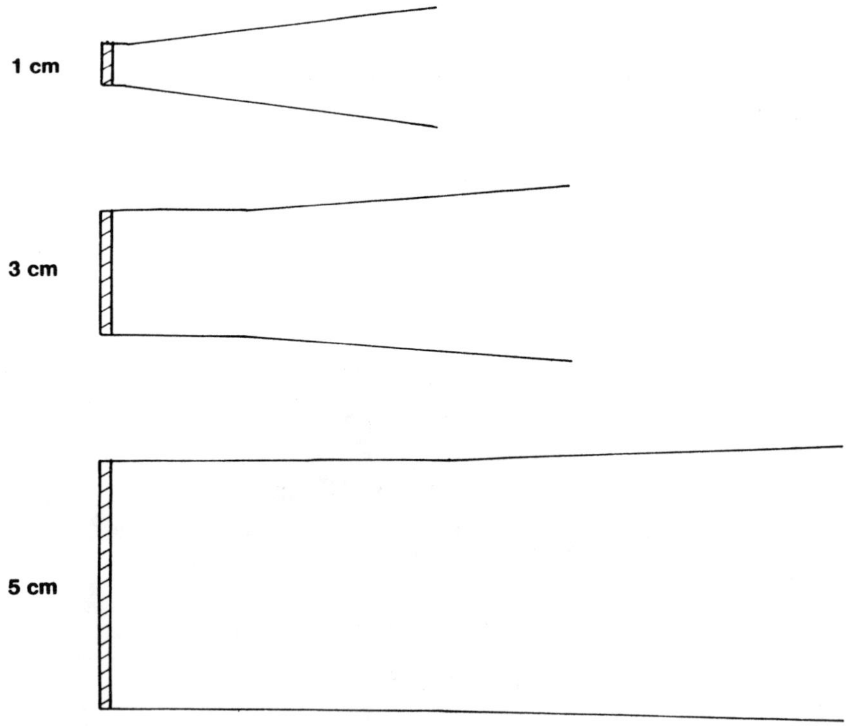

Figure 21.10. Variation of Fresnel zone length and divergence angle in the Fraunhoffer zone for ultrasound beams of the same frequency but different transducer diameters.

Figure 21.11 illustrates the variation of Fresnel zone length and beam divergence in the Fraunhoffer zone as a function of ultrasound frequency for the same transducer diameter.

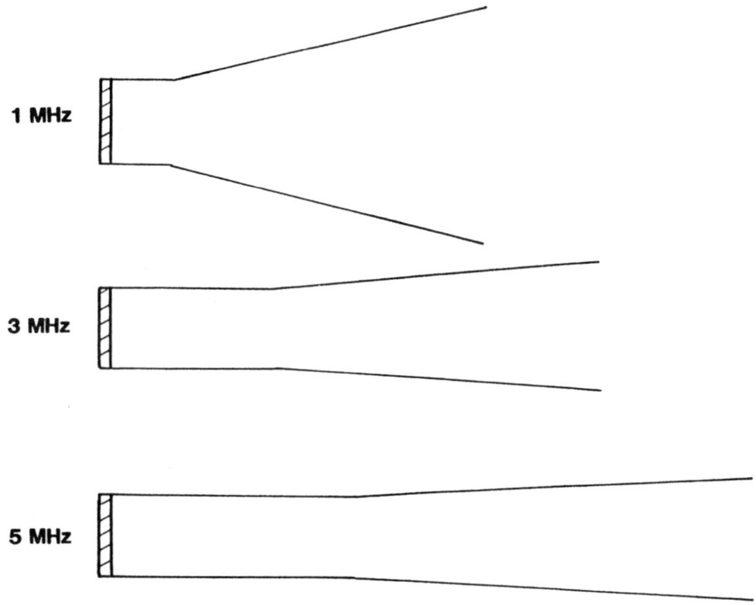

Figure 21.11. Variation of Fresnel zone length and beam divergence in the Fraunhoffer zone for different ultrasound frequencies with the same diameter transducer.

Display Techniques

The simplest display technique, known as A mode display, displays the amplitude of the reflected signal as a function of time. The B mode display converts the amplitude to an intensity signal which is displayed only if the amplitude is above a threshold value. For compound B mode scanning, the position of the displayed dot is displayed at the middle of the ultrasound beam. Thus, a point reflector will be displayed as a line whose width depends on the width of the ultrasound beam.

M Mode Display

M mode display is the ultrasound equivalent of a strip chart recorder. The B mode display is slowly swept across the screen to produce a trace which yields the relative positions of two moving interfaces. Figure 21.12 illustrates the three display modes.

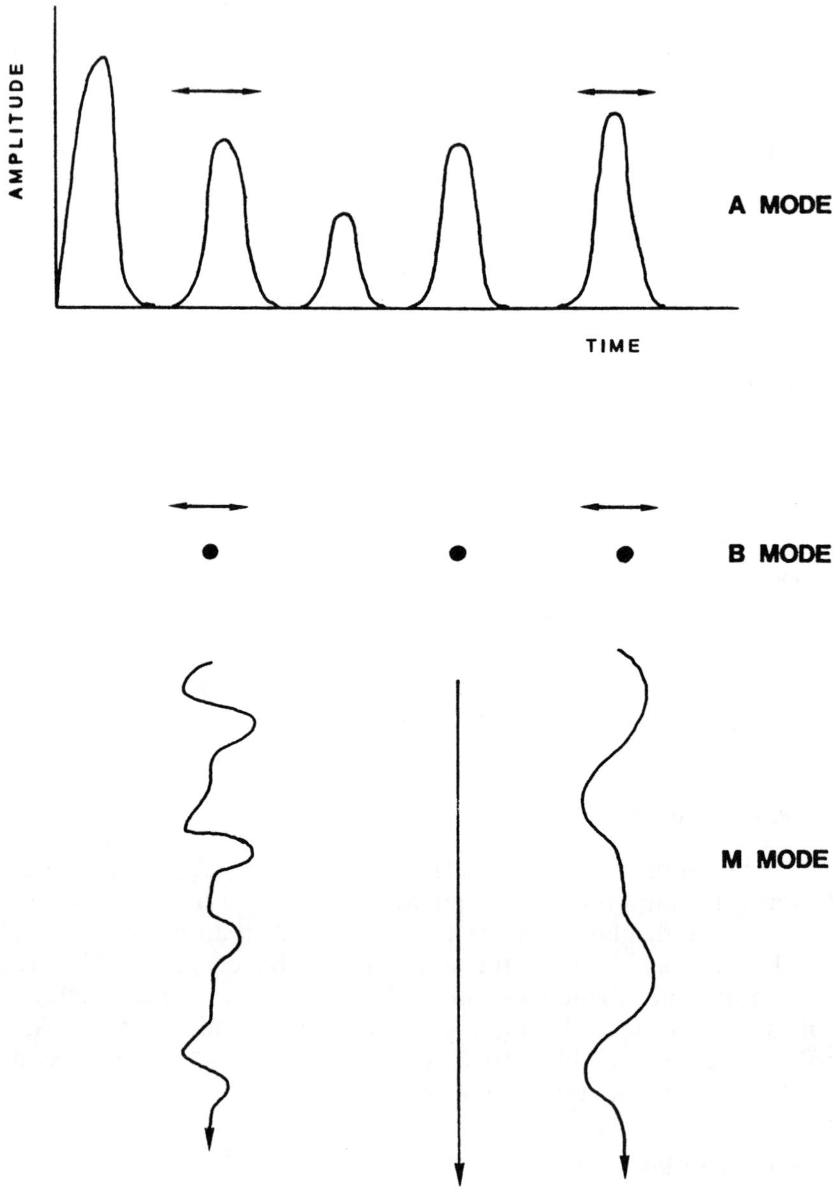

Figure 21.12. A mode, B mode and M modes of ultrasonic display.

Doppler Ultrasound

The doppler ultrasound examination uses continuous rather than pulsed ultrasound beams to detect the presence and measure the velocity of moving interfaces. Doppler examinations detect the frequency shift in echoes from moving objects. The doppler shift produces the familiar rise in pitch of an automobile horn from a rapidly approaching car. The same horn moving away will appear to have a decreasing pitch. This change in frequency is known as the doppler effect and is given by:

$$f = f_o \frac{2v}{C} \cos \theta$$

where f_o is the original frequency of the source, C is the **ultrasound** velocity, v is the velocity of the reflecting object and θ is the angle between the sound beam and the direction of motion. Doppler examinations usually monitor blood motion. Blood particles produce a return signal by scattering rather than reflection as illustrated in Figures 21.13.

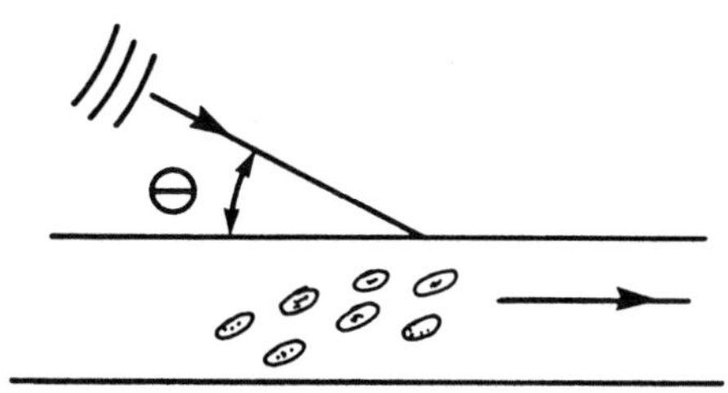

Figure 21.13. Doppler scattering from moving blood vessels.

Notice that the scattering of ultrasound from blood particles moving perpendicular to the sound beam will produce zero doppler shift.

A pulsed doppler unit can measure both the velocity and the position of the moving interfaces by measuring the frequency shift of the reflected pulse as well as the time of echo return.

Array Transducers

Array transducers can be used to produce a scanning ultrasound beam without moving the transducer. Array transducers can produce a "real time" image of internal structures including moving interfaces. An array of transducers consists of ten to fifty narrow transducers mounted on the same transducer head. If all the transducers are pulsed at once, a plane wave of ultrasound is sent out perpendicular to the array face. When the individual transducers are pulsed in sequence the direction of the ultrasound beam depends on which transducer was pulsed first and the delay between the pulses. A phased array allows rapid scanning of patient anatomy without moving the transducer on the skin surface. Resolution with array scanners is limited by the interdector spacing and is worse than with single transducers.

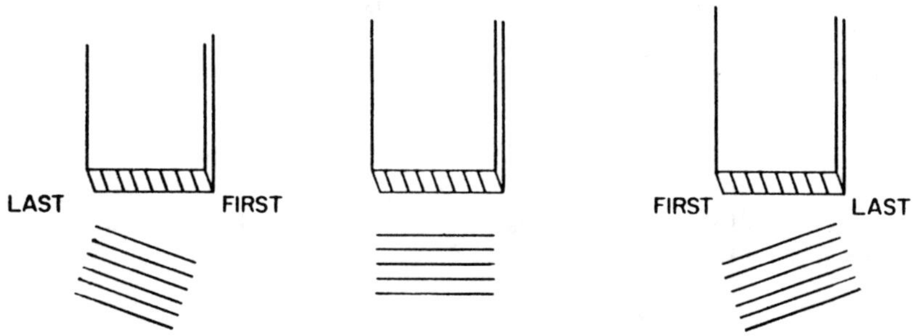

Figure 21.14. An array transducer

Cavitation

Cavitation is the formation of tiny bubbles in the medium which collapse producing intense shock waves. Cavitation occurs at intensity levels of hundreds of watts/cm^2 and can break cellular bonds and kill cells. Cavitation does not occur at diagnostic ultrasound intensities.

CHAPTER 21 QUESTIONS

1. Ultrasound consists of
   A. frequencies below 20,000 Hz.
   B. increases and decreases in distance in front of the transducer.
   C. electromagnetic radiation.
   D. increases and decreases in pressure in front of the transducer.

2. The frequency of an ultrasound beam
   A. is equal to the period of the wave.
   B. depends on how long the transducer is energized.
   C. depends on the transducer thickness.
   D. depends on the transducer diameter.

3. The amplitude of an ultrasonic wave
   A. is equal to half the peak to peak pressure variation.
   B. is equal to the peak to peak pressure variation.
   C. depends on the crystal thickness.
   D. depends on the transducer diameter.

4. The period of an ultrasound wave
   A. is one over the wavelength.
   B. is one over the velocity.
   C. is one over the frequency.
   D. is the time required for one half cycle.

5. The velocity of an ultrasonic wave
   A. is equal to the velocity of the particles in the medium.
   B. depends only on the frequency.
   C. depends only on the wavelength.
   D. depends both on the frequency and the wavelength.

6. The wavelength of an ultrasound beam
   A. is the distance between positive and negative peaks in the amplitude.
   B. is the velocity divided by the frequency.
   C. is the velocity divided by the period.
   D. is the frequency divided by the velocity.

7. The wavelength of a 2.5 MHz beam in tissue (v = 1500 m/s) is
   A. 1.6 mm
   B. .6 mm
   C. 6 mm
   D. 1.6 cm

8. The wavelength of a 4 MHz beam in tissue (v = 1500 m/s) is
   A. .27 mm
   B. .38 mm
   C. 2.7 mm
   D. 3.8 mm

9. The piezoelectric effect
   A. describes the change in dimensions of a crystal when a voltage is applied.
   B. describes the change in electrical charge on a crystal when a voltage is applied.
   C. describes the change in dimensions of a crystal when a pressure is applied.
   D. describes the change in frequency of a crystal when a voltage is applied.

10. Changing the thickness of a transducer
   A. changes the diameter of the sound beam.
   B. changes the period of the sound beam.
   C. changes the amplitude of the sound beam.
   D. changes the velocity of the sound beam.

11. The damping material behind the crystal in the transducer holder
 A. protects the transducer from moisture.
 B. amplifies reflections from the back of the holder.
 C. reduces the time of echo return.
 D. reduces the "ring down" time of the transducer.

12. The Q of a transducer
 A. describes the resonant frequency of the crystal.
 B. describes the spreading of the ultrasound beam in the far field.
 C. describes the frequency response of the crystal.
 D. describes the length of the focal zone.

13. A high Q transducer
 A. has a high response over a narrow range of frequencies.
 B. has a low response over a wide range of frequencies.
 C. has a short focal zone.
 D. has a long focal zone.

14. A low Q transducer
 A. has a high response over a narrow range of frequencies.
 B. has a low response over a wide range of frequencies.
 C. has a short focal zone.
 D. has a long focal zone.

15. The pulse duration
 A. depends on the period of the wave.
 B. depends on the velocity of the wave.
 C. depends on the Q of the transducer.
 D. depends on the diameter of the transducer.

16. A short pulse duration ultrasound beam
    A. has a short focal length.
    B. has better azimuthal resolution.
    C. has better axial resolution.
    D. has no Fraunhoffer zone.

17. A 5 MHz ultrasound pulse whose pulse length is 0.8 s contains ____ cycles.
    A. .16
    B. .4
    C. 1.6
    D. 4

18. A 4 MHz ultrasound pulse contining 6 cycles has a pulse duration of:
    A. .15 s
    B. .24 s
    C. 1.5 s
    D. 2.4 s

19 The pulse repetition frequency (PRF) of a 5 MHz beam which repeats 250 times per second with a pulse duration of 3 μs is
    A. 15
    B. 50
    C. 250
    D. 750

20. What is the duty factor of an ultrasound beam which has a PRF of 300 per second and a pulse duration of 1.5 μs?
    A. .00020
    B. .00045
    C. .0020
    D. .0045

21. A reflected signal that is 3 db down from the incident signal has an intensity of _______ the incident signal.
    A. .001
    B. .2
    C. .3
    D. .5

22. If a reflected signal is 20 db down from the incident signal the incident signal has _______ times the reflected signal intensity.
    A. 10
    B. 20
    C. 100
    D. 500

23. If the attenuation of a 2 MHz sound beam by muscle is about 2 db/cm, the attenuation of a 1 MHz sound beam will be about
    A. 1 db/cm
    B. 2 db/cm
    C. 3 db/cm
    D. 4 db/cm

24. If the attenuation of a 2 MHz sound beam is about 1 db/cm in tissue the attenuation of a 5 MHz sound beam will be about
    A. 1 db/cm
    B. 2.5 db/cm
    C. 4 db/cm
    D. 5 db/cm

25. If the accoustic impedence of muscle for a 2 MHz sound beam is about 1.7×10^5 rayls, what will it be at 4 MHz?
    A. 1.7×10^3 rayls
    B. $.8 \times 10^5$ rayls
    C. 1.7×10^5 rayls
    D. 3.4×10^5 rayls

26. Place in order of increasing reflection coefficient:
    1. Muscle-Fat Interface
    2. Bone-Brain Interface
    3. Muscle-Air Interface
    4. Muscle-Blood Interface

    A. 4, 1, 2, 3
    B. 4, 2, 1, 3
    C. 4, 1, 3, 2
    D. 3, 2, 1, 4

27. Refraction is

A. the change of direction of the reflected sound beam.
B. the change of velocity of the transmitted beam.
C. the equality of incident and transmitted angles.
D. the change in direction of the transmitted sound beam.

28. The angle of reflection

A. equals the angle of incidence.
B. depends on the velocity of the second medium.
C. is smaller than the incidence angle if $v_2 > v_1$.
D. is greater than the incidence angle if $v_2 > v_1$.

29. Snell's Law describes

A. the relation between the angles of incidence and reflection.
B. the length of the focal region.
C. the ratio of transducer diameter to divergence angle.
D. the relation between the angles of incidence and transmission.

30. Depth gain compensation

A. adjusts the depth as the gain increases.
B. decreases the gain as the depth increases.
C. increases the gain as the time of echo return increases.
D. increases the gain as the transducer diameter increases.

31-35, Axial resolution ________ with

A. increases
B. decreases,
C. remains the same

31. Increasing period.
32. Increasing wavelength.
33. Increasing transducer diameter.
34. Increasing frequency.
35. Increasing pulse length.

36. The depth of penetration for most tissues

A. is independent of frequency.
B. increases linearly with increasing frequency.
C. decreases linearly with increasing frequency.
D. decreases with transducer diameter.

37. An ultrasound beam can be focused

A. only in the Fresnel zone.
B. only in the Fraunhoffer zone.
C. in both the Fresnel and Fraunhoffer zones.
D. only in the Twilight zone.

38. The focal zone extends a distance _______ in front of a transducer with Diameter D.

A. πD^2
B. D^2/λ
C. $D^2/2\lambda$
D. $D^2/4\lambda$

39. The focal zone extends _______ cm in front of a 4 MHz, 2 cm diameter transducer.

A. .38
B. 2.7
C. 3.8
D. 27

40. The focal zone extends _______ in front of a 3 cm diameter 2 MHz transducer.

A. 6 cm
B. 9 cm
C. 15 cm
D. 30 cm

41. A smaller diameter transducer

A. has a longer focal zone but spreads more rapidly in the far zone.
B. has a shorter focal zone but spreads more rapidly in the far zone.
C. has a longer focal zone but spreads less rapidly in the far zone.
D. has a shorter focal zone but spreads less rapidly in the far zone.

Match display modes.

42. Adjusting TVG	A. A mode
43. Cardiac examination	B. B mode
44. Placental localization	C. M mode

45. A 2 MHz ultrasound beam passes through 2 cm muscle tissue (along the fibers) and 3 cm liver tissue. Using the values from Table 21.3, the total attenuation is approximately

A. 3 db
B. 5 db
C. 9 db
D. 12 db

46. Doppler ultrasound examinations

A. can measure distances in the near zone.
B. use continuous waves to measure velocities.
C. must have the sound beam direction perpendicular to the interface to detect motion.
D. can only be used in the pulsed mode.

47. Array scanning

A. can produce real time images of moving surfaces.
B. can produce better resolution than single transducer scanning.
C. eliminates the Fresnel zone.
D. eliminates the Fraunhoffer zone.

48. Cavitation

A. enhances diagnostic echoes.
B. occurs at frequencies higher than those normally used in diagnostic ultrasound.
C. is caused by the formation and collapse of tiny bubbles at high intensities.
D. occurs at intensities too low for use in diagnostic ultrasound.

CHAPTER 22

MAGNETIC RESONANCE IMAGING

Magnetic Resonance Imaging, also called Nuclear Magnetic Resonance (NMR), imaging, forms images of different tissues by recording the resonance frequencies of their nuclear spins.

Magnetic Resonance Imaging

The technique of magnetic resonance imaging consists of placing the patient in a magnetic field, adding an RF signal to alter the nuclear spins and detecting the resulting signal. A computer processes the detected signals and produces a display whose intensity depends on the MR signal.

Figure 22.1 presents a block diagram of MR Imaging System.

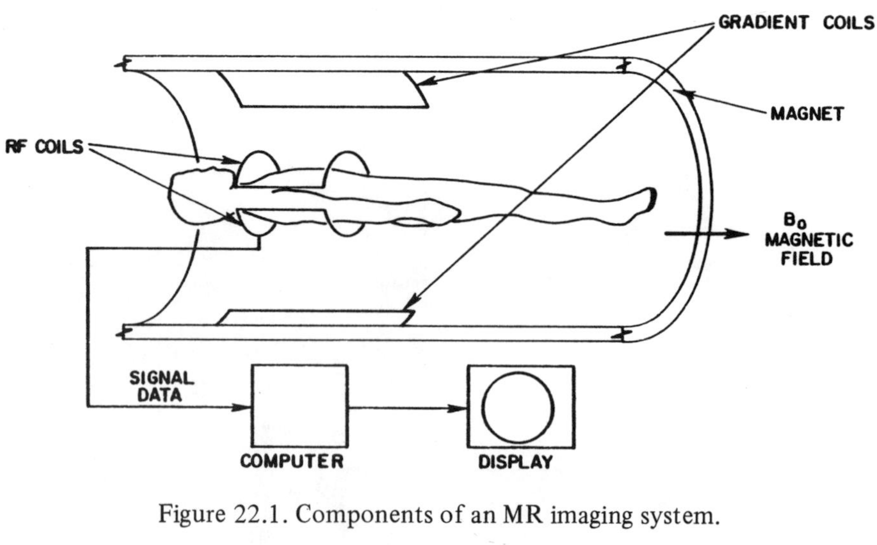

Figure 22.1. Components of an MR imaging system.

The components of an MR Imaging System are:

Magnet
Gradient System
RF Coils
Surface Coils
Computer
Display System

Before discussing the components of the MR Imaging System, it is worthwhile to understand where the various signals come from. Basically MR imaging:

a. places the tissues of interest in a strong uniform magnetic field.
b. rotates the nuclear spins with an rf pulse or pulses.
c. measures the rf signal given off as the spins relax back to their original directions.
d. forms an image using a rapid computer.

Almost all images are formed by measuring proton spin signals because hydrogen is present in almost all body tissues.

Nuclear Spins

Most nuclei have a spin and a magnetic moment. They act as if they were tiny magnets with a north and south pole. Only nuclei with even numbers of protons and even numbers of neutrons (even–even nuclei) have zero magnetic moment. In the absence of a magnetic field, the nuclear spins point in all directions. If the nuclei are placed in an external magnetic field B_O, a few more will align themselves in the same directions as the magnetic field than opposite to the magnetic field (about 1 out of 10^6 more). This is shown in Figure 22.2.

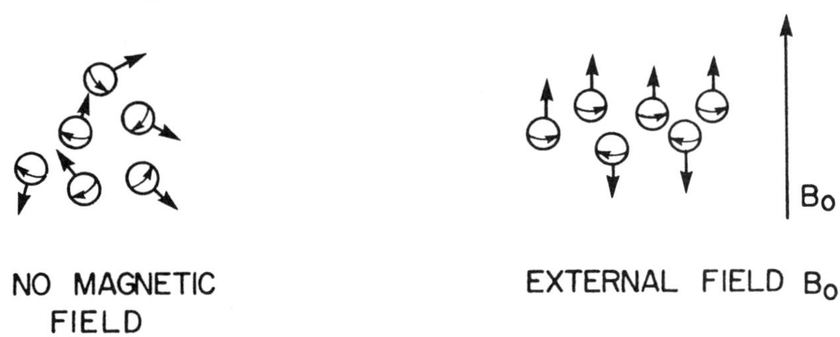

Figure 22.2 Alignment of nuclear spins in a magnetic field B_O.

All the nuclear spins can be averaged together to form a net magnetization M as shown in Figure 22.3.

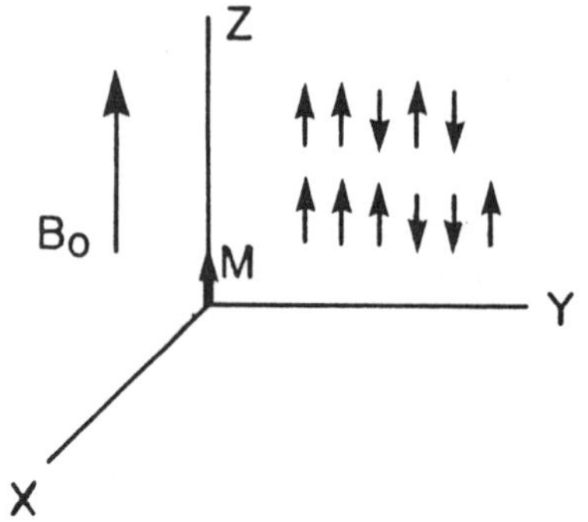

Figure 22.3. The magnetization M is the average of all the spin values.

The energies of the nuclei pointing along and against the magnetic field are not exactly the same. The nuclei aligned **against** the magnetic field have slightly higher energy than those aligned with the field as shown in Figure 22.4.

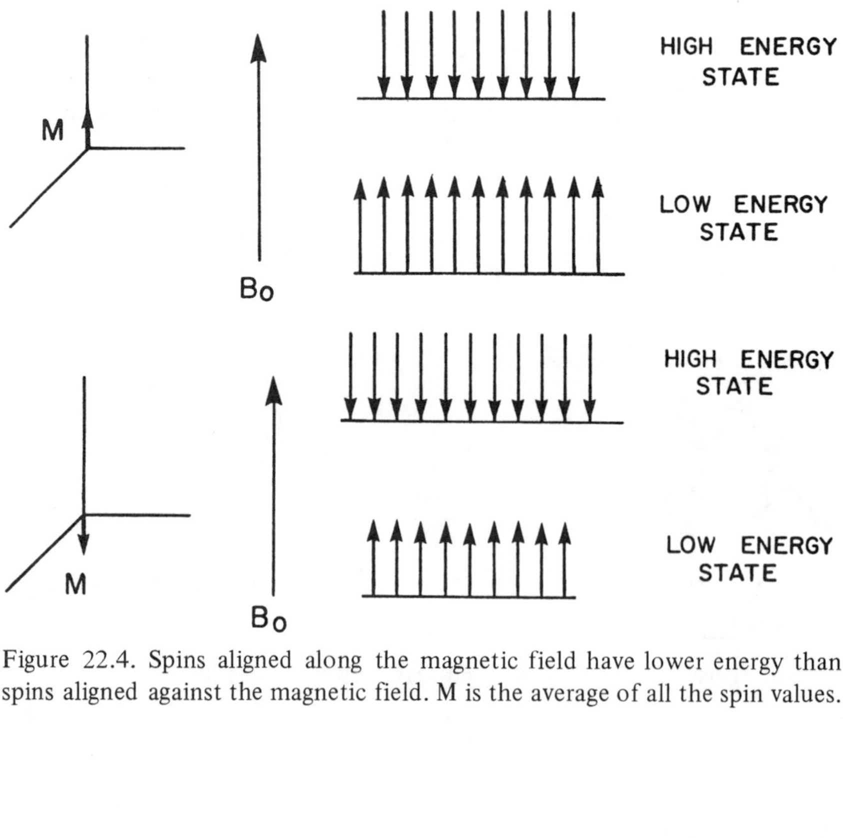

Figure 22.4. Spins aligned along the magnetic field have lower energy than spins aligned against the magnetic field. M is the average of all the spin values.

If one of the higher energy nuclei flips its spin to become aligned with the magnetic field, it will give up its extra energy as an rf (radio frequency) photon.

Similarly, an rf input pulse can cause the spins to change their orientation so that more spins are pointed against B_O than along B_O. The magnetization M will point against the magnetic field direction.

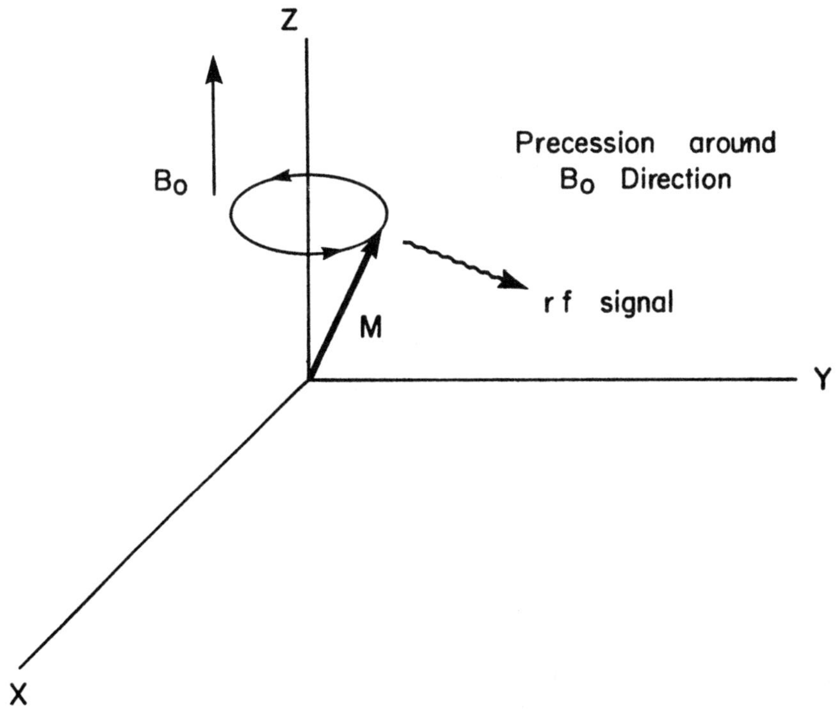

Figure 22.5. Precession of magnetization M around the external magnetic field direction.

Spin Lattice – T_1 Relaxation

If all the spins are flipped through 90° by an external rf pulse, the net magnetization will precess around the B_O direction.

The nuclei in this tissue sample will eventually realign (relax) themselves so that most of them, and the net magnetication M, point along the external magnetic field B_O. Figure 22.5 illustrates the precession of M around the magnetic field direction. As the M realigns with B_O, it **precesses** around the external field B_O direction with an angular frequency ω which is related to B_O and, γ, the gyro magnetic ratio by:

$$\omega = \gamma B_O$$

ω is known as the Larmor precessional frequency which is the frequency the magnetization M precesses or rotates around the direction of B_O. The precession produces an rf signal which can be detected by an rf detection coil.

Each different kind of nucleus has its own gyromagnetic ratio. The Free Induction Decay (FID) measures the time for the magnetic moment to relax back to its original direction. The signal strength depends on the number of nuclei and the magnetic field strength.

Fourier Transform

The detected rf signal can be converted from a time dependent signal to a frequency dependent signal by a **Fourier Transform.** Figure 22.6 illustrates how a time dependent signal can be converted into a frequency signal through a Fourier Transform.

Spin Lattice Relaxation Time

When a 90° pulse rotates the magnetization, M, 90° from the direction of B_O, there is a strong rf precessional signal, but no magnetization in the direction of B_O.

The magnetization in the B_O direction builds up after the 90° pulse with a characteristic time T_1, the spin lattice relaxation time. T_1 is the time for the magnetization M to build up to 63% of its final value. Figure 22.7 presents the magnetization M which is proportional to signal strength, as a function of time.

T_1 is known as the **Spin Lattice** or **Longitudinal Recovery Time.** It depends on the magnetic field strength and the number of protons present. T_1 measures the proton density. Some authors refer to the 90° pulse as the $\pi/2$ pulse.

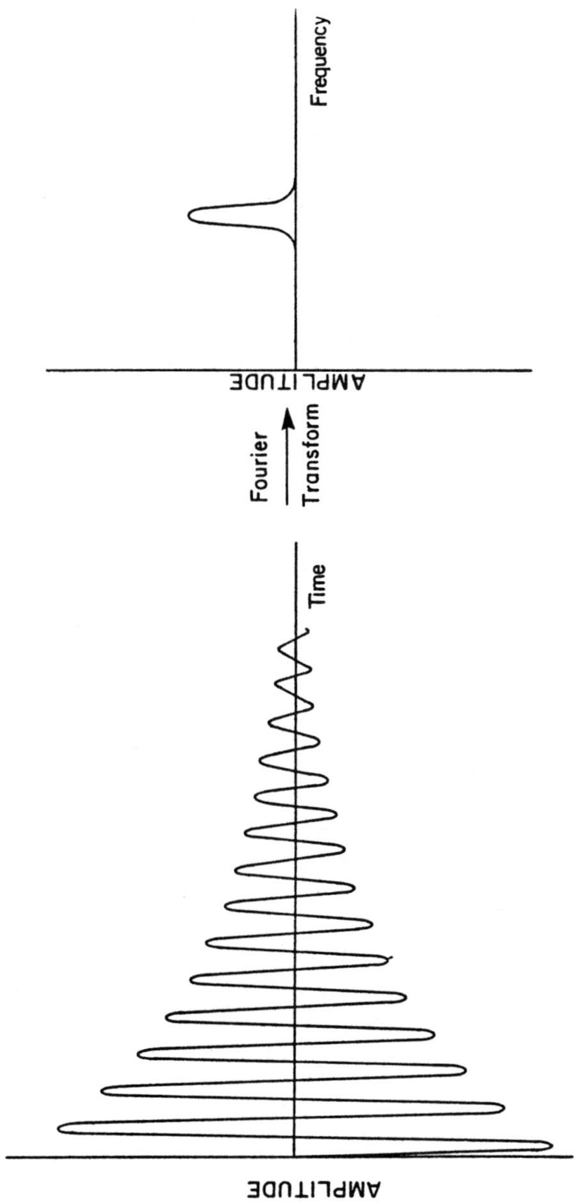

Figure 22.6. Fourier transform of a time dependent signal to a frequency dependent signal.

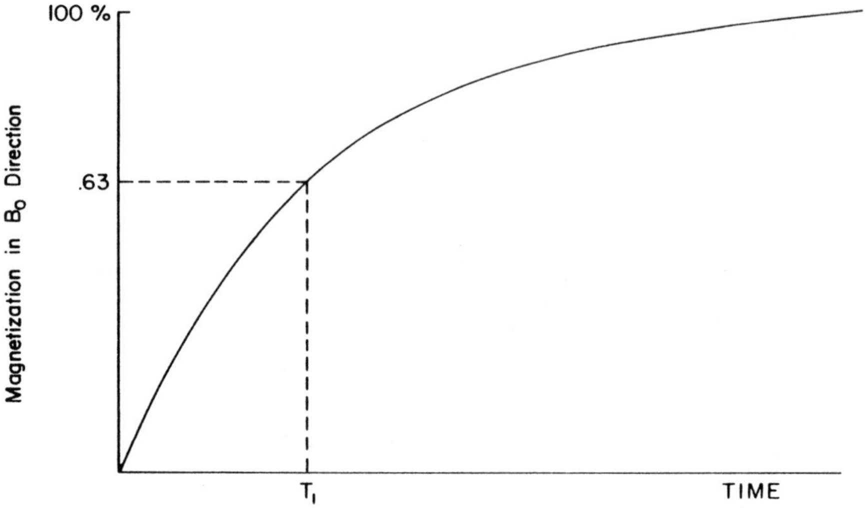

Figure 22.7. Recovery of magnetization along B_O after a 90° rf pulse.

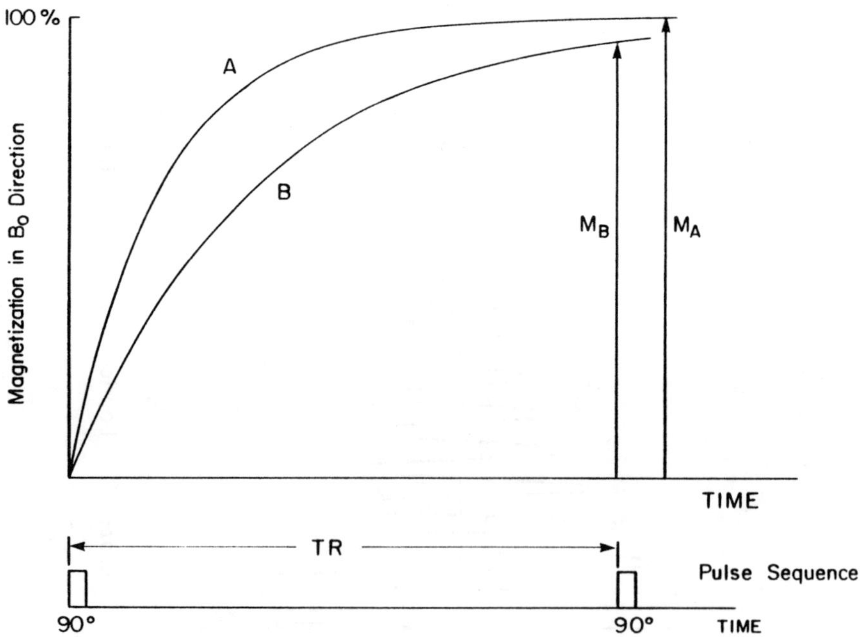

Figure 22.8. Magnetization of two tissues as a function of time after 90° rf pulse.

Partial Saturation Recovery Sequence

If two tissues with different T_1 values are examined, the image contrast (signal difference) will depend on TR, the **pulse repetition** time.

If TR the pulse repetition time is long, there will not be much difference between the magnetization of A and B as shown in Figure 22.8. The signal strength from A and B is proportional to their magnetization.

If TR is shortened, the recovery or saturation of M_A and M_B will not be complete and the signal difference (contrast) will be greater. Figure 22.9 illustrates the pulse sequence for partial saturation recovery. Figure 22.10 illustrates the magnetization in the B_O direction, or signal strength, as a function of time.

In this pulse sequence, known as **Partial Saturation Recovery**, the contrast between different tissues is dependent on TR.

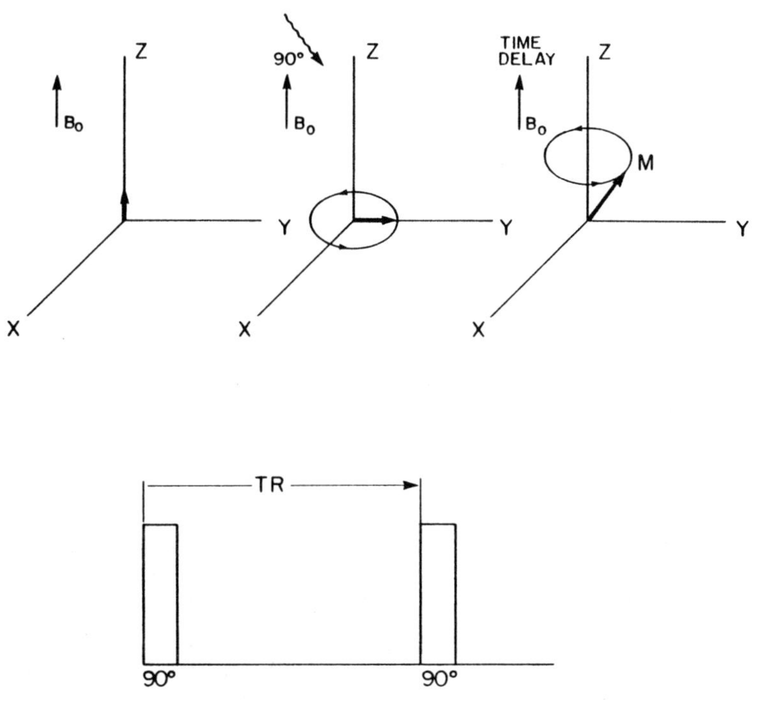

Figure 22.9. Partial saturation recovery pulse sequence.

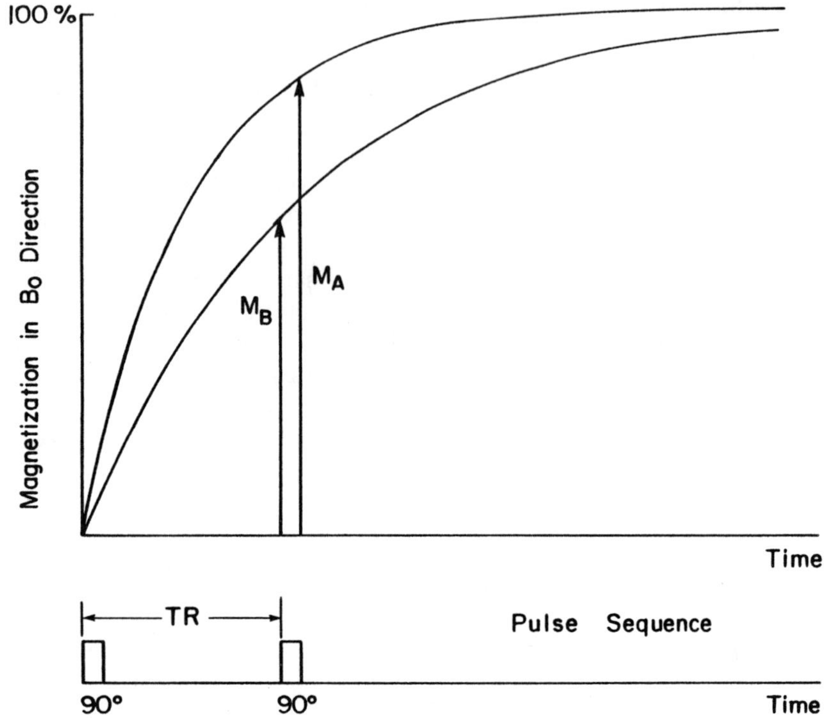

Figure 22.10. Partial saturation recovery signal as a function of time.

Inversion Recovery Sequence

Even greater contrast differences can be obtained by first rotating the spins through 180°. No signal will be detected because M is aligned in a direction against B_O.

After waiting a time τ after the first 180° pulse, called the **prepare pulse,** a second 90° pulse, called the **observe pulse,** is applied, M will precess about the B_O direction and an rf signal can be detected. The **inversion time TI** is the time delay between the prepare and observe pulses. Figure 22.11 illustrates the pulse sequence and signal strength in Inversion Recovery.

With selection of a short TI, the contrast between the two tissues can even be reversed. Figure 22.12 illustrates how the contrast can be reversed by changing TI.

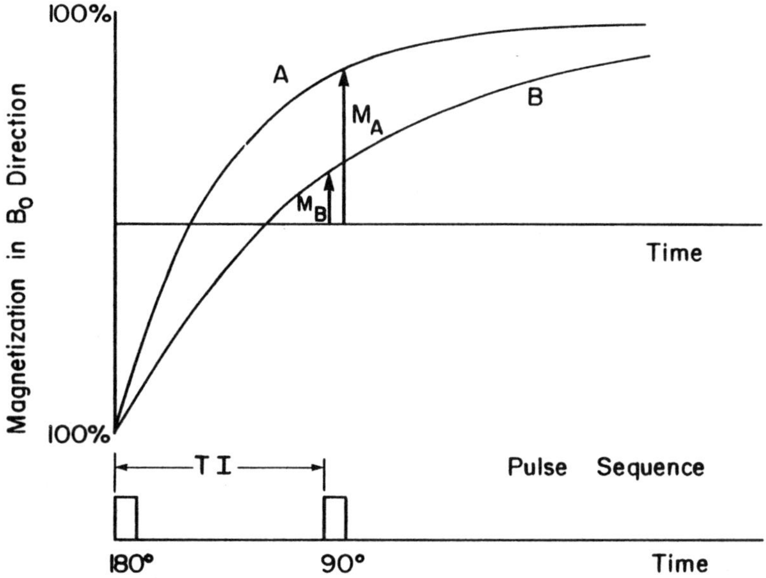

Figure 22.11. Inversion recovery pulse sequence.

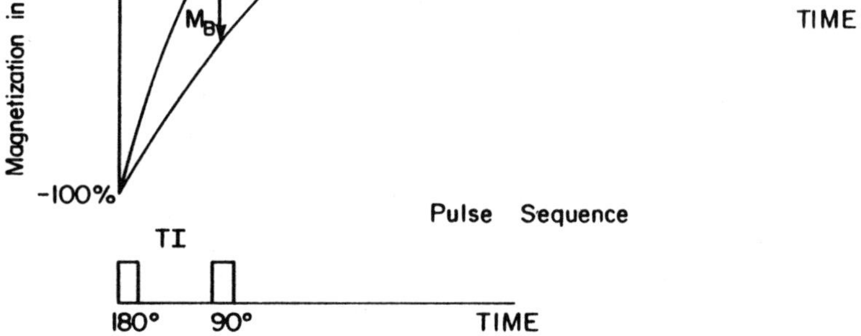

Figure 22.12. Reversal of contrast with different TI in the inversion recovery pulse sequence.

Spin Spin or T_2 Relaxation

Immediately after a 90° ($\pi/2$) pulse, all the nuclear spins are **in phase** and 90° from B_O direction. As time goes on, they get out of phase and the signal strength drops off. Figure 22.13 illustrates the loss of spin phase coherence with time.

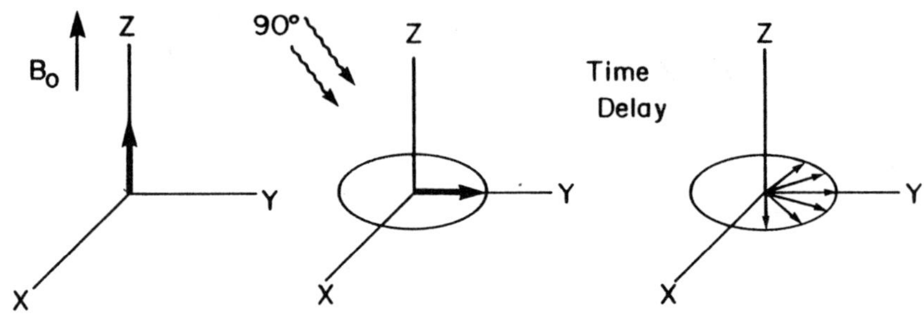

Figure 22.13. Individual spin values drop out of phase with a characteristic time T_2, the spin-spin relaxation time.

T_2 is the time for the signal to drop to .37 its original maximum value due to spin-spin interactions. T_2 is the **Spin–Spin Relaxation Time.** T_2 is always less than T_1 in solids. $T_2 = T_1$ in liquids.

T_2 is more dependent on the structure of the tissues than T_1.

Spin Echo Sequence

If a second 180° pulse (sometimes called a π pulse) is applied after a time τ, some of the phase coherence can be regained. This is known as a **Spin Echo** pulse sequence. It's as if, half way through a race, everybody had to turn around and run back to the starting line. The fastest runners would be out in front and would have to run farther to get back. Everyone should cross the finish line at the same time. Figure 22.14 illustrates the pulse sequence and spin phases in spin echo imaging.

A 180° echo pulse applied a time τ after the original 90° pulse will produce an echo 2τ later. The echo time, TE, is the time from the 90° pulse to the echo signal (TE = 2τ). TE values of 30–150 msec are common.

Figure 22.15 illustrates the formation of a spin echo signal.

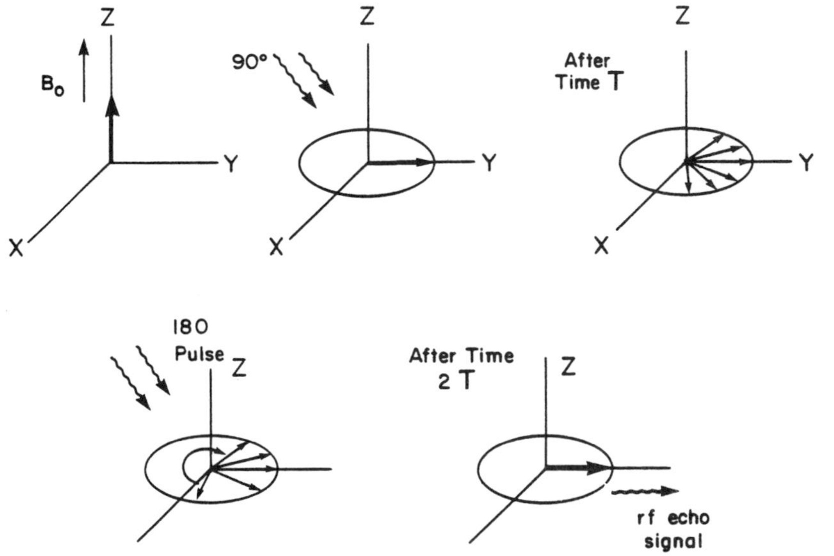

Figure 22.14. Spin echo pulse sequence for spin echo imaging.

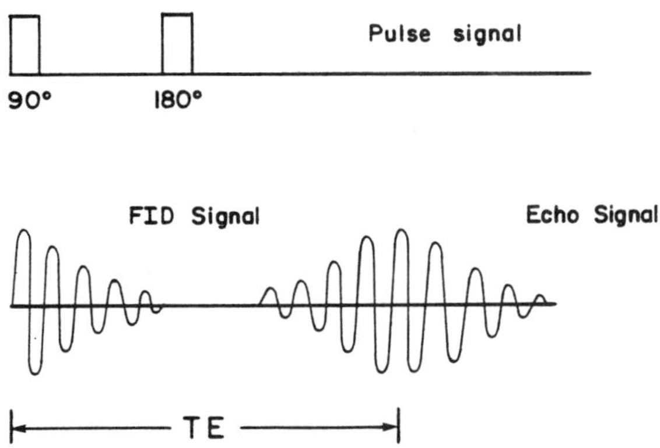

Figure 22.15. Formation of a spin echo signal a time TE after the 90° pulse.

Effect of TE on Contrast

The spin-spin relaxation time, T_2, depends on the tissue structure and so variations of TE can change the contrast between two tissues. Images which emphasize T_2 are most sensitive to changes in the surroundings of the protons being imaged. Figure 22.16 illustrates the change in signal strength from two tissues as a function of time with a spin echo pulse sequence.

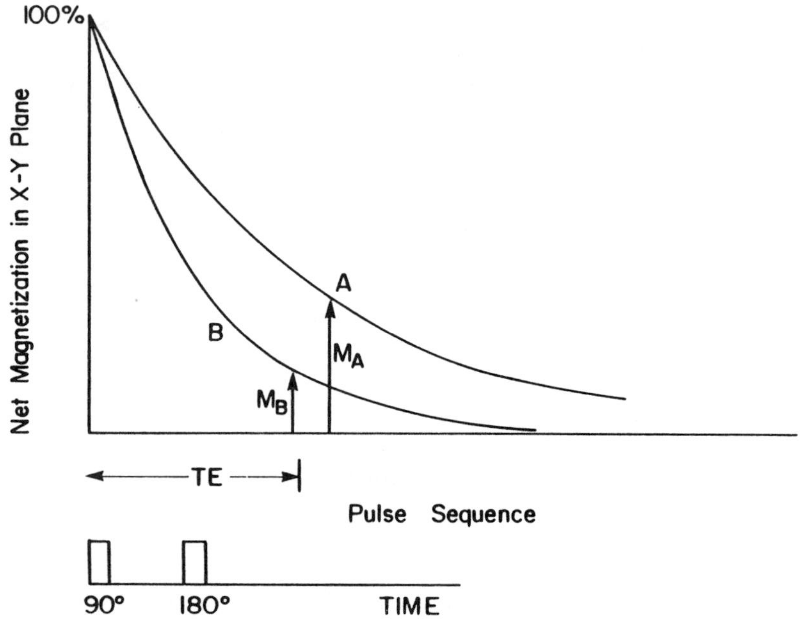

Figure 22.16. The contrast difference between two tissues depends on TE.

Note that Figure 22.16 plots the net magnetization in the X–Y plane as a function of time.

By changing TI, TE and TR, the final image can emphasize T_1, T_2 or some combination of the two. In general, it appears that T_1 images do not have as great a contrast sensitivity as T_2 images. Long TE values emphasize T_2.

Figures 22.17 and 22.18 illustrate some clinical MR scans.

Magnets

The signal to noise ratio increases with increasing field strengths. Three types of magnets have been used for Magnetic Resonance Imaging:

Permanent
Resistive
Superconducting

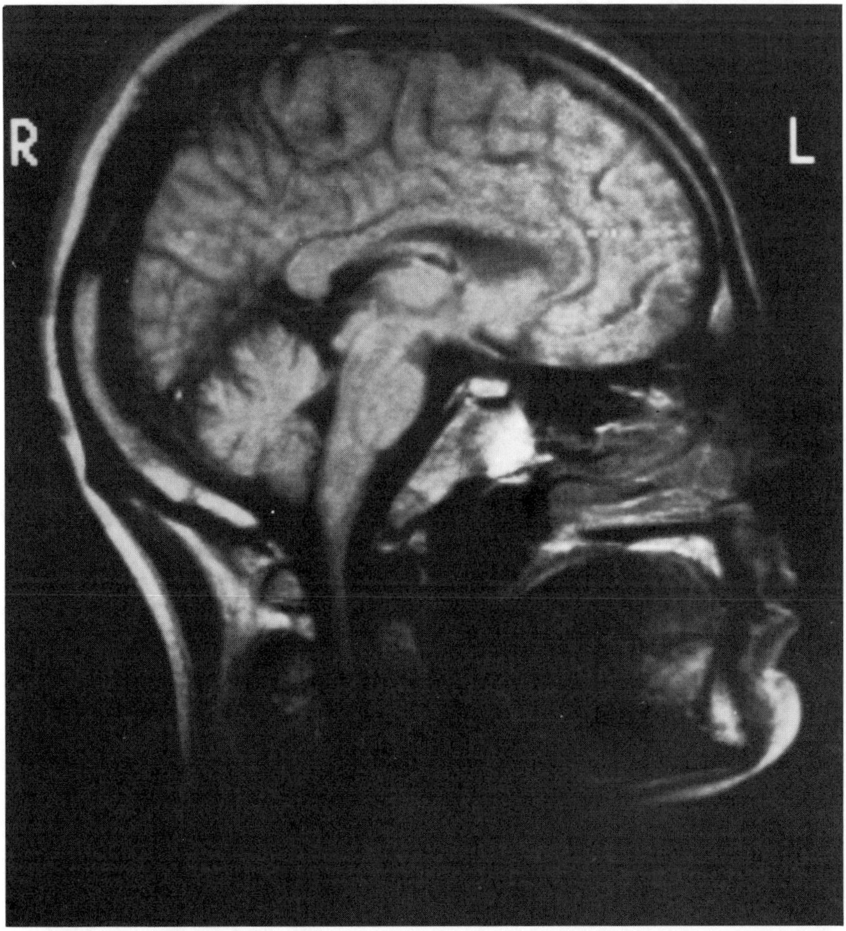

Figure 22.17. MR scan of the head. (Courtesy of Philips Medical Systems)

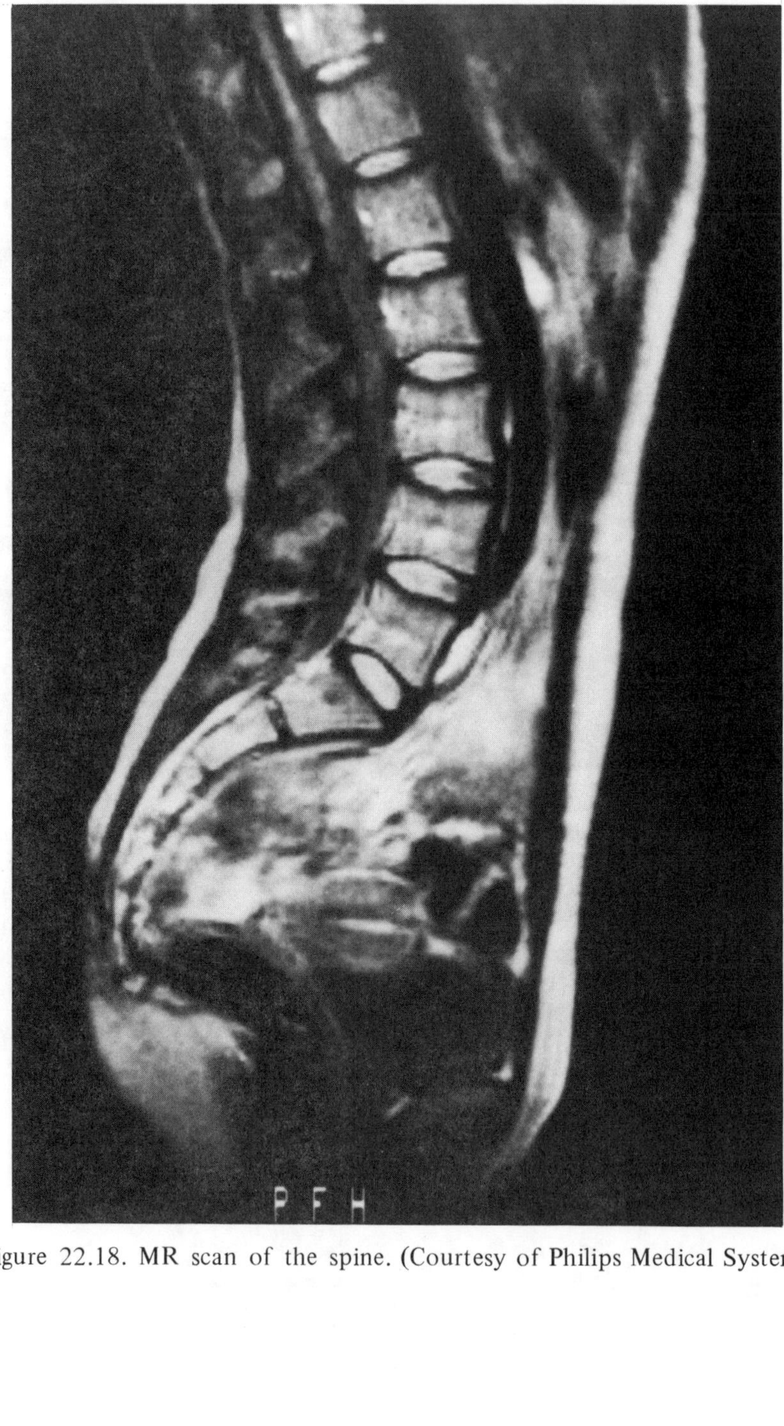

Figure 22.18. MR scan of the spine. (Courtesy of Philips Medical Systems)

Permanent Magnets

Permanent magnets are similar to the familiar bar or horseshoe magnets found in physics laboratories. Permanent magnets can produce fields up to about 0.3T (1 Tesla = 10,000 gauss). By comparison, the earth's magnetic field is about 5×10^{-5} T. Permanent magnets are heavy (100 ton) but require no maintenance once they are installed. It is difficult to obtain large fields in openings large enough for the human body (1 m diameter) with permanent magnets.

Resistive Magnets

Resistive magnets produce a magnetic field by passing current through copper or aluminum coils. Resistive heating limits the current that can be passed through the coils and the resulting magnetic fields to about 0.2T. Resistive magnets are intermediate in expense between permanent and superconducting magnets with resistive magnets with one meter diameter openings can routinely achieve 0.15–0.2T field strengths.

Superconducting Magnets

Superconductive magnets produce a magnetic field by passing current through coils made of a special mobium–titanium wire which becomes **superconducting** at about -270°C. A superconductor has **zero resistance** so the current will continue to flow in the coil forever and will not generate any heat in the coil.

Superconductive Magnet Cooling

To achieve superconductive temperatures, the magnet is surrounded by liquid helium contained in an insulated container called a **Dewar.**

Superconductive Magnet Field Strengths

Superconducting magnets have achieved 2 T fields over 1 m diameter openings. There are indications that the signal-to-noise ratio improves with increasing field strengths.

Magnetic Field Uniformity

The magnetic field must be uniform to 1 part in 10^6 over the entire opening for good signal-to-noise ratio pictures.

Nuclei

Table 22.1 presents some tissue nuclei, their abundance, sensitivity relative to protons and the Larmor frequency at 1 Tesla.

Almost all medical imaging is done using protons.

TABLE 22.1

Nucleus	*Abundance*	*Sensitivity*	*f (MHz)*
H_1	100	1	42.58
P-31	100	.066	17.24
C-13	1.1	.016	10.71
Na-23	100	.093	11.26
F-19	100	.83	40.05
O-17	0.037	.029	5.77
K-39	93	.00051	1.99

Gradient Field Position Information

In order to obtain position information a gradient field is added to the external field B_o.

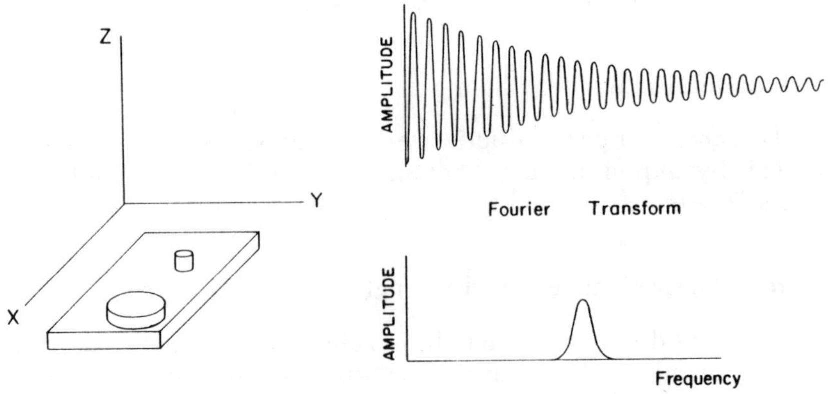

Figure 22.19. MR signal from two objects in a uniform magnetic field.

With no gradient field, both objects are in the same magnetic field and produce the same signal as shown in Figure 22.19. Adding a gradient field in the X direction.

$$B_X = KX$$

as shown in Figure 22.20 separates frequencies of the signals from the two objects.

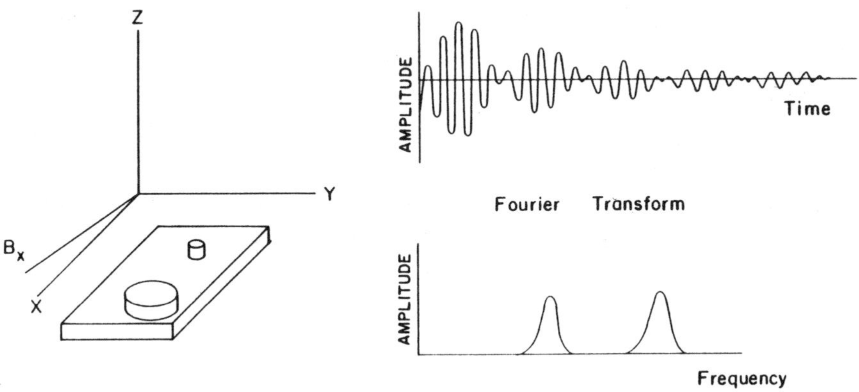

Figure 22.20. MR signals from two objects in a magnetic field with an added X gradient field.

The two objects experience different fields and the FID is made up of two frequency components. Since the precession frequency is proportional to field strength, the two objects are imaged with different frequencies. By adding gradients in the Y and Z direction and altering their relative strengths, it is possible to collect data from many angles and form a series of CT–like pictures.

RF and Surface Coils

The coils which flip the nuclear spins through 90° or 180° are placed around the inside of the magnet opening so they are as close as possible to the patient. Some MR units use the same coils to transmit and to detect the precession signals, other units use one set of coils for transmission and a separate set of surface coils for detection.

Computer and Display Systems

The computer and display systems used in MR imaging are similar to those used in digital and CT imaging.

Detection of Blood Flow

Moving blood in an MR image will appear dark because some of the nuclei with rotated spins will be carried out of the region of interest before their spins can relax back and give an rf signal.

Imaging Times

The time to form an image with a given signal to noise ratio is inversely proportional to the magnetic field strength. Higher magnetic fields can produce images in shorter times. Superior ducting magnet systems can produce images in less than one minute.

CHAPTER 22 QUESTIONS

1. Which component is **not** a part of an MR Imaging System?
   A. Magnet
   B. CPU
   C. X-ray generator
   D. RF generator

2–5, A for True, B for False

2. Every nucleus has a nuclear spin and a magnetic moment.

3. When placed in a magnetic field nuclear spins will point either along or against the field direction.

4. The net magnetization M is the average of all the nuclear spins.

5. Spins aligned along the magnetic field have higher energies than those aligned against the field.

6. The time for the magnetization vector to relax back along the external field is:
   A. TI
   B. TE
   C. T_1
   D. T_2

7. The time for the nuclear spins to lose phase is:
   A. TI
   B. TE
   C. T_1
   D. T_2

8. The Larmor precessional frequency,
   A. is the pulse repetition frequency.
   B. is the pulse echo frequency.
   C. is the pulse inversion frequency.
   D. is the nuclear spin frequency.

9. The gyromagnetic moment
   A. depends on the number of nuclei present.
   B. is the ratio of the Larmor freqeuncy to the spin lattice relaxation time.
   C. is constant for one type of nucleus.
   D. is dependent on field strength.

10. A Fourier transformer
   A. converts an rf time signal to its component frequencies.
   B. converts a MR signal into a CT signal.
   C. converts a T_1 signal into a TE signal.
   D. is used to isolate the rf transmit signal from the rf detected signal.

11. The proton density is measured by
   A. TI
   B. TE
   C. T_1
   D. T_2

12. The pulse repetition time is
   A. TI
   B. TE
   C. T_1
   D. TR

13. Partial saturation imaging uses a shorter ________.
   A. TI
   B. TE
   C. T_1
   D. TR

14. Inversion recovery imaging
   A. uses a 180° prepare pulse followed by a 90° observe pulse.
   B. uses a 180° prepare pulse followed by a 180° observe pulse.
   C. uses a 90° prepare pulse followed by a 180° observe pulse.
   D. uses a TR pulse shorter than the TI pulse.

15. In inversion recovery imaging TI

A. is the time for echo return.
B. is the time between prepare and observe pulses.
C. is the time between pulse sequences.
D. is the time between two tissue signals.

16. A 90° pulse

A. can start an imaging sequence.
B. is a $\pi/2$ pulse.
C. is the observe pulse in inversion recovery imaging.
D. All of the above.

17. In spin echo imaging

A. the signal is measured as soon as the spins have lost phase coherence.
B. TE equals the delay time between initial and the π pulse.
C. the echo signal returns at a time equal to twice the delay time between the initial pulse and the π pulse.
D. the FID signal is enhanced by TR.

18. The Dewar

A. surrounds the rf transmitter to improve the signal-to-noise ratio.
B. is a vacuum insulated container surrounding a superconducting magnet.
C. surrounds the resistive magnet to provide insulation and cooling.
D. provides support for the large permanent magnet pole faces.

19. Resistive magnets for NMR

A. are limited by the rf heating in the magnet coils.
B. are limited by the I^2R power loss in the magnet coils.
C. can provide noise free signals by phase locking the rf and magnet coils together.
D. All of the above.

20. Position information in MR imaging is obtained
    A. by adding gradient fields to the external fields.
    B. by adding an xyz grid to the magnet frame.
    C. by accepting only rf signals from a specified plane.
    D. by slowly moving the patient through the magnet.

21. Moving blood will appear dark in an MR image because
    A. the red blood cells selectively absorb the rf radiation.
    B. the moving blood carries the nuclei out of the detection region before the spins relax.
    C. the red blood cells Doppler shift the emitted radiation.
    D. the moving blood washes away the rf signal before it reaches the nuclei.

CHAPTER 23

RISK FACTORS IN DIAGNOSTIC RADIOLOGY

Introduction

Radiation effects are classified as either somatic or genetic. Somatic effects deal with radiation effects to the irradiated individual; genetic effects are expressed in future generations. Irradiation to a fetus in utero is classified as a somatic effect.

Somatic Effects

Major somatic effects of radiation exposure are cancer induction, leukemia induction and cataract induction. At one time, there was a belief that radiation also produced a generalized life shortening due to debilitation and loss of disease fighting abilities. There is currently no evidence of a generalized life shortening due to radiation.

Sources of Data

Data on the risk of various somatic effects are based on animal studies at low doses and animal and human effects observed at high radiation doses. Human have been exposed to high radiation doses resulting from nuclear weapon explosions both in Japan and from the test fallout in the South Pacific, from accidents involving radioactive sources and from some medical treatments. Table 23.1 lists the acute radiation symptoms and effects and mean survival time for relatively high doses. The mean survival time is extremely dose dependent.

TABLE 23.1
EARLY AND ACUTE RADIATION EFFECTS
FROM SINGLE WHOLE BODY EXPOSURE

Dose (CentiGrays)	*Effect*	*Mean Survival Time Days*
50	Reduced Blood Count	
200–1000	Hematologic	45
1000–5000	Gastrointestinal	7
$>$ 5000	Central Nervous System	1.5

High Exposure Effects

The prodromal syndrome appears within hours of a radiation exposure of more than about 100 cGy (1 cGy = 1 rad). It includes nausea, diarrhea and a drop in the white blood count. After the prodromal syndrome, which may last from a few hours to a few days, the latent period occurs. The latent period may last days or weeks depending on the dose. It is a period of apparent recovery with no symptoms of radiation sickness.

Hematological Syndrome

Following the latent period, doses from about 200–1000 cGy produce a repeat of the prodromal symptoms together with a feeling of malaise, fever and lethargy. Recovery, if it occurs, will begin in about 3 weeks but may require as much as 4–6 months depending on dose. At doses higher than about 400 cGy, the depletion of blood cells will continue until the body's defenses against infection is completely exhausted. Death is a result of generalized infection. The dose to kill 50% of an irradiated population within 30 days is known as the $LD_{50/30}$, For humans, the $LD_{50/30}$ is approximately 400 cGy to the whole body.

Gastrointestinal Syndrome

Radiation doses between about 1000–5000 cGy produce death by killing all the stem cells of the intestinal lining. The turnover time for the cells of the intestinal lining is about 5 days. When all the intestinal lining cells have died and are not replaced, the intestines can no longer retain body fluids and the victim dies of dehydration, electrolyte imbalance and uncontrolled infection.

CNS Syndrome

Radiation doses greater than 5000 cGy damage the brain and nervous system so badly that death always occurs within a few days.

Radiation Risk Estimates

Estimates of the risk of radiation are based on data collected at high doses (100 cGy or greater) with extrapolation to the lower doses encountered in medical or occupational exposures.

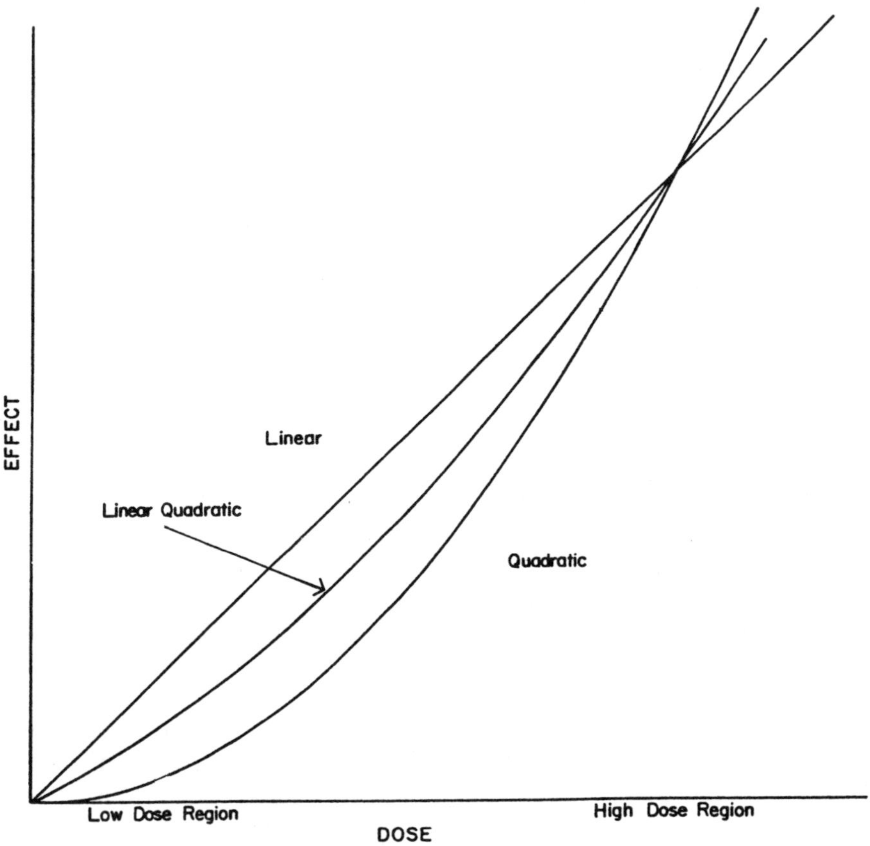

Figure 23.1. Linear, quadratic and linear quadratic response to dose.

Extrapolation Hypothesis

The question of how to extrapolate the high dose effects back to low radiation doses has not been solved completely. Figure 23.1 presents three possible methods of extrapolating the high dose effects into the low dose region.

The linear hypothesis is the simplest and most straightforward. It assumes a linear relationship between dose and effect. The linear quadratic hypothesis and the quadratic hypothesis are two other methods of extrapolating the high dose data into the low dose region. Radiobiology data indicate the linear quadratic hypothesis is probably correct. The linear hypothesis has been used in making risk estimates and setting regulations because it is more conservative. That is, the linear hypothesis predicts more effects than the radiobiological data and the linear quadratic hypothesis indicate will appear.

Threshold Dose Level

If biological systems showed a threshold response there would be some dose, the **threshold dose** that must be exceeded in order to observe any response. This would mean low doses, below the threshold, would produce no damage. There is no evidence for a threshold dose level. Regulatory agencies do not use the threshold hypothesis in setting limits.

Cancer Induction

The best estimate of cancer induction is 300 cancers per 10^6 per cGy over a lifetime. About half the cancers will result in death. This means that if a million people received a whole body radiation dose of one cGy there would be 300 cancers induced and about 150 cancer deaths due to radiation during the lifetime of the million people. This should be contrasted with the expected 165,000 cancer deaths from a similar group of million people who did not receive the radiation. The "extra" 150 deaths are known as excess deaths. The risk of leukemia is approximately equal to the risk of cancer induction for irradiated individuals over about 10 years of age. These numbers indicate why it is so difficult to predict exactly the effects of low doses. Statistical fluctuations in the normal incidence of cancer and leukemia can completely mask low dose effects.

Cataract Induction

Cataract induction occurs at dose levels of approximately 500 rads. There is no evidence of cataract formation at doses of less than about 200 cGy.

In Utero Exposure

Table 23.2 presents the periods of pregnancy.

TABLE 23.2
STAGES OF PREGNANCY

Days Since Menses	*Stage*
14	Conception
26	Implantation
30–75	Organogenesis
75–284	Fetal Development

Current evidence indicates that irradiation effects during the first two weeks of pregnancy are an "all or nothing" phenomenon. If there is radiation damage, the result is spontaneous abortion, if there is not, the fetus develops normally. Animal studies indicate radiation during the first trimester results in microcephaly and mental retardation at fetal doses above 100 cGy. No effects were observed at doses of 10 cGy. Irradiation during the early fetal stages (75–170 days) can result in growth retardation. Fetal irradiation during the last two trimesters increases the risk of leukemia and other cancers. The risk of leukemia death from fetal irradiation is approximately 300 per 10^6 live births per cGy. The risk of deaths from other radiation induced cancers is approximately the same.

Ten Day Rule

The concensus of opinion is against postponing abdominal examinations of potentially pregnant females until the 10 day period immediately following the onset of menses. A potentially pregnant female who presents for an abdominal examination either is or isn't pregnant. If she isn't pregnant, there is no purpose in postponing the examination. If she is pregnant the examination will either have to be postponed until the end of term, performed immediately or delayed until the pregnancy is confirmed. If it can be postponed until the end of term, it probably shouldn't be ordered regardless of the pregnancy. If it can't be postponed for nine months, it should be performed during the "all or nothing" period if possible.

Abortion

The American College of Radiology has stated that interruption of pregnancy is never justified because of radiation risk to the embryo/fetus from a diagnostic x-ray examination.

Genetic Effects

Genetic effects on future generations can be described in terms of a doubling dose. The **doubling dose** is defined as that radiation dose which produces twice the genetic mutation in a population as seen without the radiation. The doubling dose for humans is estimated to lie in the 50–100 cGy range.

Genetically Significant Dose

The genetically significant dose (GSD) measures the effect of relatively high doses of radiation to a few members of the population on the total genetic pool. The GSD is defined as that dose which, if delivered to every member of the population, would produce the same genetic effect as produced by the actual doses to the individual members of the population. The GSD depends on the radiation dose delivered, the age of the individual, the sex and the possible number of future children. For example, a radiation dose delivered to a male with a vasectomy would contribute nothing to the GSD because he could have no future offspring. Medical exposures contribute about 200 μGy (10 μGy = 1 mrad) to the GSD in the United States.

Risk to the Patient

Table 23.3 presents a series of typical radiographic procedures together with their entrance exposures and gonadal dose per film.

TABLE 23.3
RADIATION DOSES PER FILM
FROM DIAGNOSTIC EXAMINATIONS

Examination	*Entrance Dose μGy*	*Gonadal Dose μGy* male	*Gonadal Dose μGy* female
Skull	3000	–	–
Breast Low Dose Film Screen	5000	–	–
Chest	250	–	–
Thoracic Spine	10000	100	250
Lumbar Spine	14000	2000	7000
Abdomen	6000	1000	3000
Pelvis	4500	750	1500
IVP	7000	1000	4000
Barium Enema*	15000	2000	9000
Upper GI*	7000	1500	5560
Extremity	1500	–	–
Dental	3000	–	–
CT Scans Head	20000		
Abdomen	40000		

*Does not include fluoroscopy
BE Fluoro Dose ≃ 15000 μGy
UGI Fluoro Dose ≃ 22000 μGy

Comparison of Relative Risks

Lee and Cohen (Health Physics 36, 1979) have estimated the relative risks of radiation compared with other well-known and accepted risks in everyday life.

These risks are presented in terms of days of life shortening. For example, they estimate that life shortening due to being overweight is about 30 days per pound overweight. A summary of some of their data is presented in Table 23.4.

Many x-ray examinations are compared with chest x-rays to give the patient some idea of relative risk. Most patients consider a chest x-ray to be harmless. The chances of contracting a cancer

TABLE 23.4
RELATIVE RISK OF SOME MODERN ACTIONS FROM LEE AND COHEN

Activity	*Life Shortening Days*
Smoking 1 pack/day	2400
20% Overweight	985
Auto Accidents	200
Exposure to 1 cGy	1

from a single chest x-ray is about 1 in a million. This is about the same risk as smoking 5 cigarettes or driving 60 miles. That is, driving 100 miles is equivalent in risk to smoking 8 cigarettes or an exposure of about 500 μGy.

The conclusion of most experts who have studied the problem is that risks from radiation are well documented and are not significantly greater than other everyday risks in modern life.

CHAPTER 23 QUESTIONS

1. Radiation effects on future generations are _______ effects.
   A. Somatic
   G. Genetic
   C. Quadratic
   D. Linear

2. Radiation effects on the irradiated individual are ________ effects.
   A. Somatic
   B. Genetic
   C. Quadratic
   D. Linear

3-6, Match the dose ranges and biological effects.

3. Hematological Damage	A. 50-100 cGy
4. Reduced Blood Counts	B. 200-1000cGy
5. Central Nervous System	C. 1000-5000cGy
6. Gastrointestinal Damage	D. $>$5000 cGy

7. The ________ syndrome appears within hours of a radiation exposure and may include nausea, diarrhea and a drop in white blood count.
   A. Latent
   B. Quadratic
   C. CNS
   D. Prodromal

8. The period of wellbeing with apparent recovery from radiation sickness is the ____________ period.
   A. Latent
   B. Quadratic
   C. CNS
   D. Prodromal

9. Hematological Syndrome death occurs
   A. due to loss of red blood cells.
   B. due to loss of intestinal stem cells.
   C. from generalized infection.
   D. from weight loss and dehydration.

10. The current best estimate of the relation between dose and effect is
    A. Linear Hypothesis
    B. Quadratic Hypothesis
    C. Linear-Quadratic Hypothesis
    D. The Quasi Threshold Hypothesis.

11. The current best estimate of cancer induction is ________ per 10^6 per cGy.
    A. 50
    B. 1000
    C. 500
    D. 300

12. A threshold dose
    A. is the dose which will always produce an effect.
    B. is the dose level at which an effect will first be observed.
    C. is the dose level to produce an effect in 37% of the population.
    D. is the dose which will cause death in 50% of the population in 30 days.

13. The genetically significant dose
    A. is that dose which when averaged over all members of the genetic pool greater than child bearing age will produce an effect equal to that actually produced.
    B. is that dose which is actually delivered to the gonads of the members in the genetic pool.
    C. is that dose which would produce the same genetic effect as observed if delivered to all the members of the population.
    D. is that dose which would produce the same population if delivered to the gonads of the genetic pool.

14. An abortion should be recommended following a diagnostic examination if the dose to the fetus exceeds

A. 2 cGy
B. 5 cGy
C. 10 cGy
D. Never

CHAPTER 24

RADIATION PROTECTION

Dose Reduction

There are three techniques to reduce radiation exposure:

1. time
2. distance
3. shielding

Time

Reduction in exposure time reduces the radiation exposure by a corresponding amount.

Example 24.1:
What is the exposure reduction when the fluoroscopic "on" time is reduced from three minutes to two mintues if the table side exposure rate is 2.3 μC/kg (9 mR) per minute?

$$\text{Exposure for 3 min} = 3 \times 2.3 = 7\ \mu\text{C/kg}$$

$$\text{Exposure for 2 min} = 2 \times 2.3 = 4.7\ \mu\text{C/kg}$$

$$\text{Reduction} = 2.3\ \mu\text{C/kg}$$

Distance

The patient is the major source of scattered radiation during fluoroscopy. Scattered radiation falls off wih the square of the distance to the patient. Even one step backward away from the fluoroscopic table can significantly reduce the exposure level.

Example:
If the exposure rate at table side 20 cm from patient is 143 μC/kg–hr (550 mR) per hour what is the exposure rate one step (1 meter) away from the table side?

at 20 cm:

$$E = 143\ \mu C/kg\text{-}hr$$

at 120 cm:

$$E = 143 \times \left(\frac{20}{120}\right)^2$$

$$= 4\ \mu C/kg\text{-}hr$$

A factor of 36 reduction!

Shielding

Shielding can be contained in the walls of the room in the control panel, in the lead aprons, in gloves worn during fluoroscopy or in lead drape hung from the image intensifier mount. All shielding is effective in reducing radiation dose to the occupationally exposed personnel.

Lead Aprons

Lead aprons are equivalent to either 1/4 or 1/2 mm lead shielding. The transmission of scattered radiation through lead aprons is 10% or less depending on the energy of the primary radiation.

Occupational Limits

Table 24.1 summarizes the annual limits for occupationally exposed individuals. The maximum permissible dose (MPD) is given in sievert or rems.

$$1\ Sv = 1\ Gy \times QF$$
$$1\ rem = 1\ rad \times QF$$

where QF is a Quality Factor that depends on the type of radiation and its biological effectiveness. The QF for x–rays, gamma rays and beta particles encountered in Radiology is always 1.

TABLE 24.1
LIMITS FOR OCCUPATIONALLY EXPOSED WORKERS

	Annual		*Quarterly*	
Whole body, gonads, eyes, blood forming organs	50 mSv	5 rem	12.5 mSv	1.25 rem
Hands and feet	750 mSv	75 rem	187.5 mSv	18.75 rem
Thyroid	300 mSv	30 rem	75.0 mSv	7.50 rem
Other organs	150 mSv	15 rem	37.5 mSv	3.75 rem

The cumulative dose limit is 50(N–18) mSv [5(N–18) rem] where N is the individual's age in years.

Medical exposures to an individual are not to be included in these doses.

Individuals under 18 years old may not receive occupational exposures.

Nonoccupational Limits

Non radiation workers are limited to no more than 5 mSv/yr (500 mrem/yr). Pregnant women are recommended to limit their annual doses to that of the general public (5 mSv or 0.5 rem) because the fetus is not a radiation worker.

The general public is limited to total doses from sources other than background and medical exposures to less than 1.7 mSv (170 mrem) per year.

ALARA

All installations are currently required to adhere to the ALARA, "As Low As Reasonably Achievable" radiation protection philosophy. This requirement means the limits in Table 24.1 must be considered upper limits. Radiation workers are encouraged to reduce occupational exposures as much as reasonably possible. The word "reasonably" is added because it is always possible to reduce exposure levels by adding more shielding.

Natural Background

Natural background radiation in most parts of the United States is about 1 mSv (100 mrem) per year. In parts of the west at higher altitudes, natural background radiation levels approach 3 mSv per year. Natural background at sea level consists of approximately equal contributions from cosmic rays, internal radiation from K–40 and C–12 and natural radioactivity from the earth together with exposure from Radon gas in buildings which contributes to the dose to the lung.

Table 24.2 lists the sources and amounts of natural background.

TABLE 24.2
SOURCES AND AMOUNTS OF NATURAL BACKGROUND RADIATION

Source	*Annual Amount (mSv)*	
1. Cosmic Rays	30	
2. Internal Radiation (C–12, K–40)	30	
3. Radioactive Dirt and Building Materials	40	
4. Radon Gas in Buildings (dose to lung)	___	75
Total Body	100	

Sources 1 and 3 are twice as high in some higher altitude parts of the Western U.S.

Personnel Monitoring Requirements

Personnel monitoring is required for any individual who might receive 25% or more of the limits presented in Table 24.1. In practice, most workers are "badged" to document their non-exposure.

The purpose of personnel monitoring is documentation of occupational exposures and detection of possible defective equipment or faulty working habits which could lead to excessive radiation exposure.

Personnel Monitors

Personnel monitors are either film badge or TLD monitors. Film badges have a piece of film with several metal filters covering portions of a film (Figure 24.1).

The filters enable the company processing the film to estimate the type and the energy of the radiation striking the badge. Because film is strongly energy dependent, this information is necessary to calculate the radiation dose to the body of the wearer

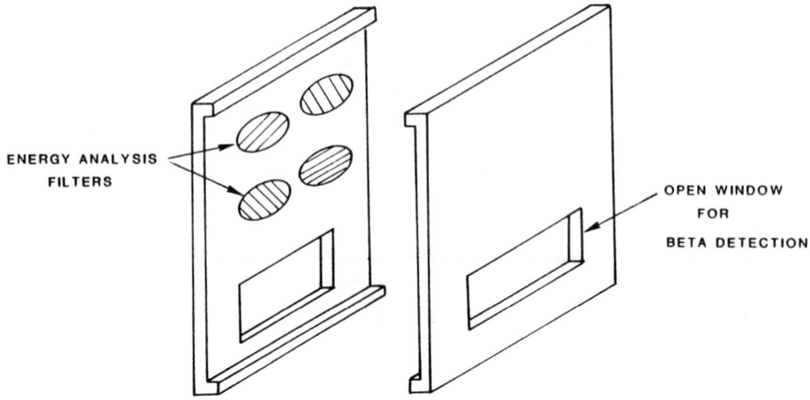

Figure 24.1. Construction of film badge and holder with filters.

of the monitoring badge. The film badges are sensitive to heat, chemical vapors and laundry soaps and are not accurate after exposure to any of these.

TLD monitors contain small TLD chips. Their energy response is very similar to tissue so no filters are required. TLD monitors are impervious to water, ordinary heat and chemical vapors. Their stability allows them to be used longer than film badges and can be changed at three month intervals.

Personnel monitors are generally worn on the belt or a pocket. During fluoroscopy, they should be worn on the collar outside the lead apron. This position will provide an indication of the thyroid and eye dose together with a knowledge that the radiation dose under the protective apron is less than 10% of the measured dose at the collar.

Shielding Calculations

Figure 24.2 illustrates a typical shielding geometry.

Calculations performed to reduce the radiation levels to the permitted radiation level depending on:

a) on how long the machine is "on" each week, (the work load W)
b) how often it is pointed at a particular wall (the use factor U)

The permitted level, **P.L.**, is given by:

$$PL = B \frac{WUT}{d^2} \qquad 24.1$$

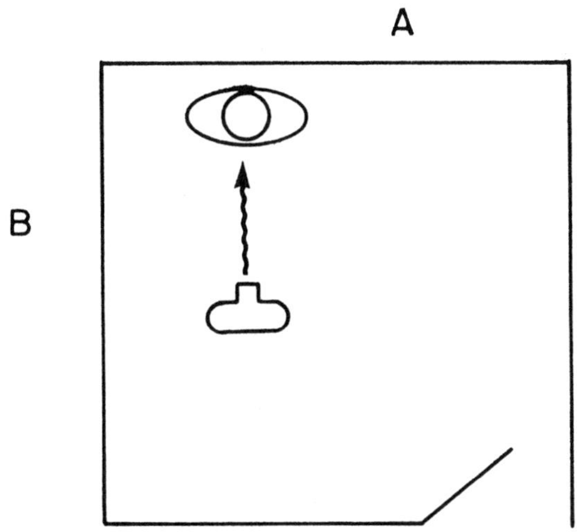

Figure 24.2. Typical x-ray shielding geometry.

where W is the workload in mA–min/week, U is the use factor which relates to how often a beam is pointed at a particular wall, T is the occupancy factor,d is the distance to the wall in meters, and B is the barrier attentuation required to reduce the radiation exposure to the permitted level. An exposure of a mA–min results in an exposure level of 260 C/kg and a dose to tissue of 1 cGy at 1 m. Permitted levels are 1 mSv (100 mrem) per week for restricted areas and 0.1 mSv (10 mrem) per week for unrestricted areas. The quality factor for medical radiations is one so mSv and mGy (or mR and mrad) are often used interchangeably.

A **restricted area** is an area under the control of the Radiation Safety Officer in which access by the general public can be restricted.

Example 24.2:
What attenuation is required in Wall A of Figure 24.2, 3 m from the tube if the workload is 1000 mA min/week and the unit is pointed at the wall 25% of the time (U = 25%). A billing office is on the opposite side of the wall (unrestricted area) and someone is in the office 40 Hrs/week (T = 1).

$$\text{For an Unrestricted Area PL} = .1 \text{ mGy/week}$$

$$\text{PL} = 10^{-4} \text{ Gy}$$

$$W = 1000 \text{ cGy/week}$$

$$= 10 \text{ Gy/week}$$

$$U = 0.25$$

$$T = 1.0$$

Calculate the barrier factor, B, from:

$$PL = B\frac{WUT}{d^2}$$

$$10^{-4} \text{ Gy} = B \times \frac{10 \times .25 \times 1}{(3)^2} \text{Gy}$$

$$10^{-4} \text{ GY} = B \times \frac{2.5 \text{ Gy}}{9}$$

$$B = \frac{9 \times 10^{-4}}{2.5}$$

$$= 3.6 \times 10^{-4} \text{ attenuation}$$

Figure 24.3 gives the attenuation of 100 kVp x–rays as a function of lead thickness. Approximately 1.8 mm lead will produce an attenuation of 3.6×10^{-4}.

Example 24.3:
What attenuation would be required if the room opposite wall A was classified as a restricted area?

PL changed to 1 mGy/week

$$W = 10 \text{ Gy/week}$$

$$U = .25$$

$$T = 1$$

$$PL = B\frac{WUT}{d^2}$$

$$PL = 1 \text{ mGy}$$

$$PL = 10^{-3} \text{ Gy}$$

$$10^{-3}\ \text{Gy} = B\frac{10 \times .25 \times 1}{(3)^2}$$

$$B = 3.6 \times 10^{-3}$$

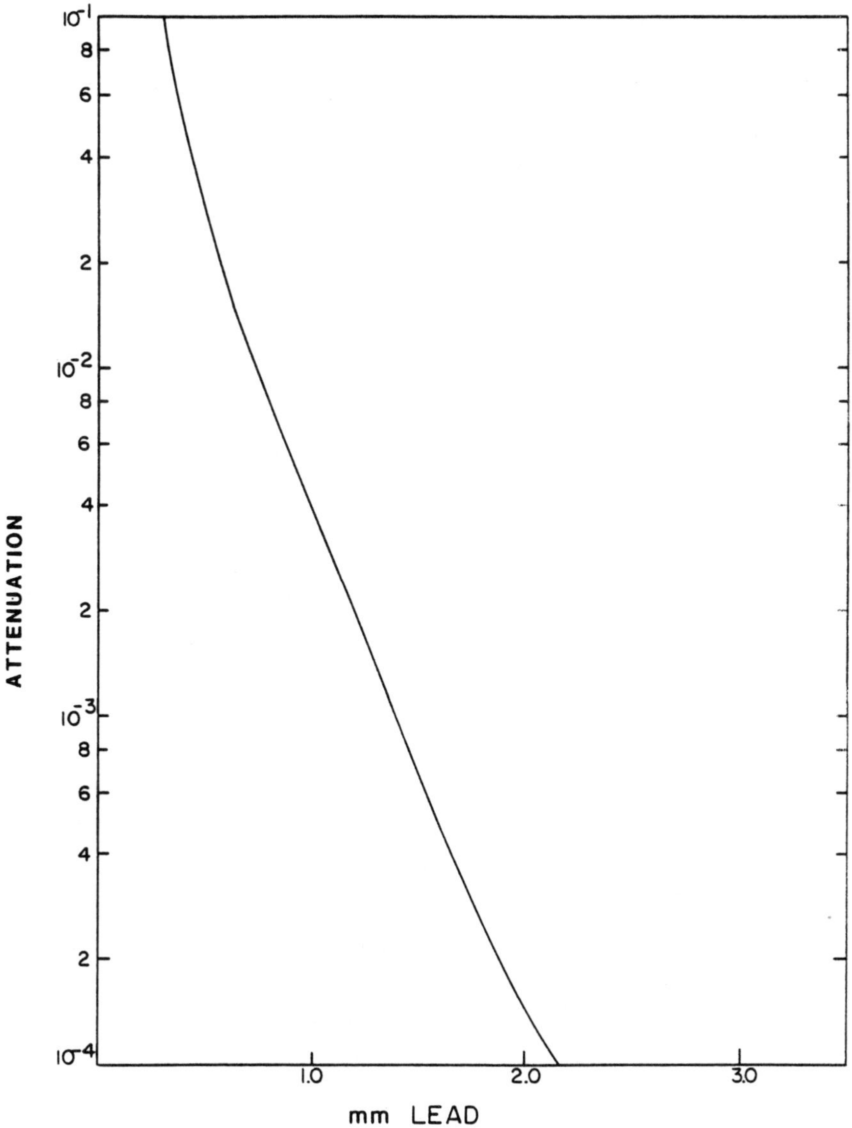

Figure 24.3. Attenuation of 100 kVp x-rays in lead.

From Figure 24.3, we see that approximately 1.1 mm lead is required for this amount of attenuation.

Shielding for Scattered Radiation

Scattered radiation 1 meter from the patient has about 1/1000th the intensity of the incident beam. The radiation is scattered in all directions so U = 1 for scattered radiation.

Example 24.4:
The x–ray beam cannot be pointed at wall B. What attenuation value is required if the wall is 2 m from the x–ray patient (source of scatter) and is an unrestricted area which is constantly occupied (T = 1)? All the other factors are the same as Example 24.3.

For an unrestricted area PL = 10^{-4} Gy/week
For scatter

$$W_S = 10^{-3}\ W$$

$$= 10^{-3} \times 10\ \text{Gy/week}$$

$$= 10^{-2}\ \text{Gy/week}$$

U = 1 because the scatter strikes all the walls no matter which way the beam is pointing.

$$T = 1$$

$$d = 2$$

$$PL = B\,\frac{W_S U T}{d^2}$$

$$10^{-4} = B\,\frac{10^{-2} \times 1 \times 1}{2^2}$$

$$B = 4 \times 10^{-2}$$

The required shielding is 1/2 mm lead.

Fluoroscopy

Entrance radiation levels in fluoroscopy are typically several cGy per minute to the patient. The limits are 2.6 mC/kg–min

(10 R/min). It is not uncommon for technical service men to turn up the exposure level in order to improve the fluoroscopic image. Fixed fluoroscopic units must have a minimum distance of 30 cm (12") between the x–ray tube and the table top.

Film Shielding

Film must be shielded to less than 0.2 mR during the storage life to avoid noticable fogging.

Leakage Radiation

The x–ray tube housing must be shielded to limit the leakage radiation to less than 26 μC/kg–hr (100 mR/hr).

Contamination Limits for Tc–99 Scans

The amount of Mo in a Tc–99 scan must be less than 0.15 μCi Mo per mCi Tc–99. There can be no more than 10 μg Al per ml of eluate and there must be less than 0.1 μCi miscellaneous activity per mCi Tc–99.

CHAPTER 24 QUESTIONS

1. What is the reduction in dose when the fluoroscopic ON time is reduced from 3.5 min to 2 min if the dose rate at table side is 4800 μGy/hr?
   A. 120 μGy
   B. 160 μGy
   C. 280 μGy
   D. 440 μGy

2. What is the reduction in dose when the fluoroscopic ON time is reduced from 4 min to 2.5 min if the table side dose rate is 3600 μGy/hr?
   A. 60
   B. 90
   C. 150
   D. 240

3. What is the dose rate in μGy/hr 90 cm from table side (20 cm from patient) if the table side dose rate is 4000 μGy/hr?
   A. 82
   B. 133
   C. 889
   D. 1273

4. If a 1/4 mm apron reduces the scattered intensity to 10% of the incident intensity, a 1/2 mm apron will reduce the scattered intensity to
   A. 5%
   B. 1%
   C. .1%
   D. Not enough information

5. The annual whole body MPD for a radiation worker is
   A. 5 Sv
   B. .5 Sv
   C. 50 mSv
   D. 5mSv

6. The maximum cumulative dose allowed for a 27-year-old radiation worker is

   A. 27 Sv
   B. .05 Sv
   C. 4.5 Sv
   D. .45 Sv

7. The maximum permissible dose for a non radiation worker is

   A. 0.5 mrem
   B. 5 mrem
   C. 0.5 rem
   D. 5 rem

8. The natural background at sea level is approximately ______ per year

   A. 1 mSv
   B. 5 mSv
   C. 1 Sv
   D. 5 Sv

9. The maximum permissible dose to the hands of a radiation worker is

   A. 7.5 mSv
   B. 75 mSv
   C. 750 mSv
   D. 7500 mSv

10. Natural background is made up of

    A. cosmic rays.
    B. radiation from dirt and building materials.
    C. internal radiation.
    D. All of the above.

11. ALARA

A. requires the radiation to be reduced below any level as reasonably achievable.
B. requires radiation to be reduced as low as reasonably achievable.
C. requires radiation alarms to be set as loud as reasonably achievable.
D. is an electronic detection and warning system designed to reduce radiation exposures to workers.

12. Personnel monitors are required for individuals

A. who may receive more than 25% of the MPD limits.
B. who are over 18 and work with radiation or radioactive materials.
C. who might receive as much as 0.5 (N–18) Sv cumulative dose.
D. who work with radiation whose QF is not equal to 1.

13. If three HVL provide adequate shielding for an x-ray room wall today how many HVL will be required if the workload is doubled?

A. 3.5
B. 4
C. 5
D. 6

14. The Quality Factor is related to ______________ of the radiation.

A. the type and biological effectiveness
B. the radiation energy
C. the HVL
D. the use factor

15. The leakage radiation through the housing of a diagnositc x-ray tube housing is limited to no more than

A. 2.6 μC/kg-hr (10 mR/hr)
B. 26 μC/kg-hr (100 mR/hr)
C. 260 μC/kg-hr (1000 mR/hr)
D. Depends on kVp setting

16. Filters are used in film badges
    - A. to filter out the low energy radiation.
    - B. to protect the wearer against high QF radiation.
    - C. to estimate the type and energy of the radiation.
    - D. All of the above.

17. During fluoroscopy film badges should be worn
    - A. at waist level.
    - B. at eye level.
    - C. inside the apron.
    - D. on the collar.

18. The use factor is related to
    - A. how long the machine is in operation.
    - B. how often the beam points at a particular wall.
    - C. what fraction of the time personnel are working on the other side of the shield.
    - D. the amount of attenuation needed to meet shielding requirements.

19. The occupancy factor is related to
    - A. how long the machine is in operation.
    - B. how often the beam points at a particular wall.
    - C. what fraction of the time personnel are working on the other side of the shield.
    - D. the amount of attenuation needed to meet shielding requirements.

20. The work load is related to
    - A. how long the machine is in operation.
    - B. how often the beam points at a particular wall.
    - C. what fraction of the time personnel are working on the other side of the shield.
    - D. the amount of attenuation needed to meet shielding requirements.

21. The scattered radiation intensity at 1 m is about _____ the incident intensity.

A. .1
B. .01
C. .001
D. .0001

22. The use factor for scattered radiation is always

A. 2
B. 1
C. .5
D. .25

23. A restricted area is an area

A. with radiation shielding.
B. which has doors and windows which can be locked.
C. where all workers wear film badges.
D. where access to the general public is restricted.

ANSWERS

CHAPTER 1

1. 48m
2. 3 m/s^2
3. 6 m/s
4. 9 m/s
5. 4 seconds
6. 2 m/s^2
7. 4 m/s^2
8. 4 kg
9. 24 N
10. 29.4 N
11. 2 slugs
12. 39.2 N
13. 4 slugs
14. F x d = w
15. 54 ft lb
16. 48 ft lb
17. 58.8 N
18. 176.4 j
19. mgh = P.E.
20. 205.8 j
21. $E = 1/2\ mv^2$
22. E = 24 j
23. E = 18 j
24. v = 4 m/s
25. 6 m/s
26. 2 m/s
27. 3.5 m/s
28. 470.4
29. 15.3 m/s
30. Convection
31. Radiation
32. Conduction
33. 12 kg m/s
34. 5/6
35. 19/30
36. 8/9
37. 5/8
38. 13/21
39. 1/5
40. 12/5 = 2 2/5
41. 10/21
42. 2
43. 1/2
44. 600000
45. 4×10^6
46. 2.05×10^{-3}
47. 1.75×10^4
48. 3.14×10^8
49. .0667
50. 30000000
51. 1.03×10^{-2}
52. 220000
53. .00732
54. 15
55. 175
56. 186
57. 99
58. 2.5

59. 3.0"
60. 2.25"
61. A car sliding on ice when the friction is reduced to almost zero.
62. 73.5 kg
63. 210 N
64. 800 ft lb
65. 36750 j
66. 15 minutes
67. 56 kg m/s
68. 11 m/s
69. convection
70. Radiation
71. 10°C
72. 122°F
73. 2.5v
74. 3 Hz
75. 1/3 second
76. 100 mR/hr
77. 225 mR/hr
78. C
79. A
80. D
81. 7 kg

CHAPTER 2

1. B
2. A
3. D
4. C
5. B
6. D
7. A
8. A
9. A
10. B
11. A
12. D
13. D
14. D
15. B
16. C
17. A
18. B
19. D
20. C
21. A
22. B
23. A
24. B
25. C
26. B

CHAPTER 3

1. D
2. B
3. B
4. A
5. C
6. A
7. C
8. D
9. C
10. B
11. A
12. A
13. B
14. A
15. B
16. A
17. B
18. D
19. C
20. C
21. B
22. D
23. D

CHAPTER 4

1. B
2. C
3. D

4. B
5. A
6. A
7. C
8. D
9. C
10. D
11. D
12. D
13. B
14. A

CHAPTER 5

1. B
2. C
3. B
4. A
5. B
6. B
7. A
8. D
9. A
10. A
11. A
12. B
13. B
14. B
15. C
16. D
17. C
18. D
19. F
20. C
21. D
22. B
23. E
24. A
25. G

CHAPTER 6

1. B
2. C
3. D
4. A
5. B
6. D
7. C
8. B
9. A
10. D
11. A
12. B
13. C
14. A
15. B
16. B
17. A
18. A
19. D
20. C
21. D
22. B
23. B
24. B
25. B
26. B
27. D
28. B
29. C

CHAPTER 7

1. B
2. D
3. D
4. A
5. B
6. B
7. A
8. A
9. A
10. A
11. B
12. B
13. B
14. C
15. B
16. C
17. A
18. B
19. D
20. D
21. D
22. B

CHAPTER 8

1. B
2. A
3. A
4. A
5. A
6. D
7. D
8. B
9. A
10. B
11. D
12. B
13. B
14. B
15. D
16. B
17. C
18. B
19. C
20. C
21. A
22. C
23. B
24. A
25. D
26. A
27. B
28. C
29. D
30. C
31. B
32. A
33. B
34. A
35. C
36. D
37. E
38. D
39. C
40. B
41. A

CHAPTER 9

1. 10
2. 31.6
3. 54.8
4. 31.0
5. 100
6. 14.1
7. 4.7
8. 29.2
9. 76.1
10. 148.3
11. 10%
12. 3.2%
13. 1%
14. 3.2%
15. 1.8%
16. 7.1%
17. 0.7%
18. 3.5%
19. 3.9%
20. 2.4%
21. 3000 cpm ± 38.7 cpm
22. 2667 cpm ± 29.8 cpm
23. 2000 ± 20 cpm
24. 2000 ± 50 cpm
25. 5000 ± 50 cpm
26. 20,000 ± 63.2 cpm
27. 1400 ± 11.8 cpm
28. 5000 ± 57.7 cpm
29. 13967 ± 68.2 cpm
30. 1467 ± 31.3 cpm
31. 3700 ± 2.1%
32. 7000 ± 1.6%
33. 4800 ± 2.1%
34. 7300 ± 1.9%
35. 940 ± 4.6%
36. 0.44 min
37. 5.93 min
38. 18.75 min
39. 8.33 min
40. 2.08 min
41. A
42. C
43. D
44. A

45. B
46. C
47. D

CHAPTER 10

1. B
2. A
3. B
4. A
5. B
6. A
7. D
8. A
9. B
10. A
11. D
12. B
13. A
14. B
15. C
16. D
17. B
18. B
19. C
20. B
21. D
22. B

CHAPTER 11

1. C
2. D
3. C
4. D
5. D
6. B
7. C
8. A
9. B
10. B
11. C
12. B
13. A
14. B
15. B
16. D
17. D
18. B
19. A
20. D
21. A

CHAPTER 12

1. A
2. B
3. B
4. Phosphorescence
5. less
6. D
7. greater
8. A
9. A
10. B
11. B
12. A
13. blue
14. B
15. A
16. B
17. C
18. C
19. A
20. A
21. C
22. C
23. B.

CHAPTER 13

1. B
2. B
3. B
4. B
5. A
6. A

7. C
8. B
9. A
10. B
11. D
12. C
13. A
14. C
15. A
16. D
17. A
18. B
19. C

CHAPTER 14

1. B
2. D
3. B
4. A
5. C
6. D
7. B
8. C
9. A
10. C
11. C
12. B
13. B
14. A
15. B
16. A
17. D
18. C
19. A
20. B
21. C
22. D
23. A
24. B
25. D

CHAPTER 15

1. B
2. A
3. A
4. B
5. C
6. B
7. B
8. A
9. B
10. A
11. A
12. B
13. A
14. C
15. B
16. D
17. C
18. C
19. D
20. C
21. A
22. B
23. B
24. C
25. A
26. B
27. A
28. B
29. C
30. A
31. A
32. A
33. A
34. C
35. C
36. B
37. A
38. A
39. B
40. A
41. A
42. D
43. B

CHAPTER 16

1. C
2. B
3. B

4. A
5. C
6. D
7. B
8. A
9. C
10. A
11. B
12. B
13. B
14. A
15. D
16. C
17. B
18. A
19. D
20. D
21. D

CHAPTER 17

1. A
2. A
3. C
4. B
5. B
6. B
7. A
8. A
9. C
10. B
11. B
12. C
13. C
14. B
15. B
16. D
17. A
18. D
19. A
20. C
21. D
22. B
23. D
24. B
25. D
26. D
27. A
28. C

CHAPTER 18

1. B
2. D
3. A
4. C
5. D
6. B
7. C
8. A
9. B
10. C
11. B
12. A
13. D
14. C
15. D

CHAPTER 19

1. D
2. C
3. B
4. D
5. A
6. D
7. B
8. D
9. C
10. A
11. B
12. C
13. C
14. A
15. B
16. A
17. B
18. D
19. C
20. C
21. C
22. D
23. B
24. A
25. D
26. A
27. A
28. B
29. D
30. B

CHAPTER 20

1. B
2. A
3. B
4. C
5. A
6. A
7. D
8. C
9. C
10. D
11. A
12. B
13. D
14. B
15. C
16. D
17. D
18. B
19. A
20. C
21. D
22. A
23. B
24. A
25. A
26. C

CHAPTER 21

1. D
2. C
3. A
4. C
5. D
6. B
7. B
8. B
9. A
10. B
11. D
12. C
13. A
14. B
15. A
16. C
17. D
18. C
19. C
20. B
21. D
22. C
23. A
24. B
25. C
26. A
27. D
28. A
29. D
30. C
31. B
32. B
33. C
34. A
35. B
36. C
37. A
38. D
39. D
40. D
41. B
42. A
43. C
44. B
45. C
46. B
47. A
48. C

CHAPTER 22

1. C
2. B
3. A
4. A
5. B
6. C
7. D
8. D
9. C
10. A
11. C
12. D
13. D
14. A
15. B
16. D
17. C
18. B
19. B
20. A
21. B

CHAPTER 23

1. B
2. A
3. B
4. A
5. D
6. C
7. D
8. A
9. C
10. C
11. D
12. B
13. C
14. D

CHAPTER 24

1. A
2. B
3. B
4. D
5. C
6. D
7. C
8. A
9. C
10. D
11. B
12. A
13. B
14. A
15. B
16. C
17. D
18. B
19. C
20. A
21. C
22. B
23. D

ABBREVIATIONS

A	Activity
A	Amplitude
Å	Angstrom (10^{-10} m)
A	Atomic weight
$\tilde{A}$	Cumulative activity
A_o	Original activity
AC	Alternating current
ADC	Analog–to–Digital Converter
ALARA	As low as reasonably achievable
amp	Amperes
AMU	Atomic mass unit
B	Background count rate
B	Barrier factor
B	Bucky factor
B	Magnetic field
BE	Barium enema
BGO	Bismuth germinate
B_o	Original magnetic field
Bq	Becquerel
B_x	Gradient magnetic field in x direction
C	Celsius
C-	Centi
C	Contrast
C	Coulomb
C	Velocity of light
CD	Contrast detail
cGy	Centigray
Ci	Curie
cm	Centimeters
CNS	Central nervous system
CoI	Cesium iodide
cps	Cycles per second
CPU	Central processing unit

cr	Count rate
CRT	Cathode ray tube
c/s	Cycles per second
CT	Computed tomography
$\overline{D}$	Average absorbed dose
D	Density
D	Diameter
d	Distance
d_m	Minimum separation
DAC	Digital-to-Analog Converter
db	Decibel
DC	Direct current
DF	Duty factor
DSA	Digital subtraction angiography
e	Base of natural logarithms
e	Electron
E	Energy
E	Exposure
E_b	Binding energy
E_γ	Gamma ray energy
EC	Electron capture
ECT	Emission computed tomography
E_e	Electron energy
ev	Electron volt
F	Fahrenheit
f	f-Factor, rad to Roentgen ratio
f	f-Number of lens
f	Frame
f	Frequency
FID	Free induction decay
FN	False negative
FNF	False negative fraction
FP	False positive
FPF	False positive fraction
FPR	False positive rate
f/s	Frames per second
ft	Foot
g	Gram

G	Gross count rate
G	Number of gray levels
GI	Gastrointestinal
GM	Geiger Mueller
G_m	Minification gain
GR	Grid ratio
GSD	Genetically significant dose
Gy	Gray
h	Planck's constant
$h\nu$	Photon energy
H & D	Hurter and Driffield
hp	Horsepower
Hz	Hertz
HU	Heat units
HVL	Half value layer
I	Current
I	Intensity
I_p	Current in transformer primary circuit
I_s	Current in transformer secondary circuit
I^2R	Power loss due to current in a resistor
IVP	Intravenous pyelogram
j	Joule
JND	Just noticeable difference
K	Contrast improvement factor
k	Kilo
KeV	Kiloelectron volts
kg	Kilogram
kHz	Kilohertz
kV	Kilovolts
kVp	Kilovoltage potential
lb	Pound
$LD_{50/30}$	Lethal dose to 50% of the population within 30 days
LET	Linear energy transfer
Log	Logarithm to the base 10
ln	Natural logarithm
lp/mm	Line pairs per mm
LSF	Line spread function

M	Magnetization
M	Magnification
M	Mega
m	Meter
m	Milli
mA	Milliamperes
MAS	Milliamp seconds
mC/kg	Millicoulomb per kilogram
MeV	Million electron volts
mGy	Milligray
MHz	Megahertz
mm	Millimeters
MP	Melting point
MPD	Maximum permissible dose
MR	Magnetic resonance
mR	Milliroentgen
MRI	Magnetic resonance imaging
M_t	Total mass
$M\nu$	Momentum
MTF	Modulation transfer function
mw/cm^2	Milliwatts per square centimeter
$\overline{N}$	Average value of N
n	Nano
N	Newton
N	Number of atoms
N	Number of counts
n	Number of millicuries
N	Number of neutrons
N	Number of turns in a transformer winding
NaI	Sodium iodide
nC/kg	Nanocoulombs per kilogram
ni	Fraction of times a disintegration produces the ith radiation
N_p	Number of turns in the transformer primary
N_s	Number of turns in the transformer secondary
OD	Opitcal density
OID	Object image distance
P	Momentum
p-	Pico

PD	Pulse duration
PET	Positron emission tomography
PL	Permitted radiation exposure level
PRF	Pulse repetition frequency
PZT	Lead zirconium titanate
Q	Charge
Q	Q factor, ratio of resonant frequency to band width
QF	Quality factor
r	Radius
R	Count Rate
R	Reflection coefficient
R	Resistance
R	Resolution
R	Roentgen
rad	Rad
RAM	Random access memory
R_c	Collimator resolution
rem	Rem
R_{eq}	Equivalent resistance
RF	Radio frequency
R_i	Intrinsic resolution
ROC	Receiver operating characteristic
ROM	Read only memory
rpm	Revolutions per minute
R_T	Total resolution
S	Mean dose per cumulative activity
s	Second
SCR	Silicon controlled rectifier
SI	Systeme Internationale
SID	Signal to noise ratio
SNR	Signal to noise ratio
SOD	Source to object distance
SPECT	Single photon emission computed tomography
Sv	Sievert
T	Half life
T	Occupancy factor
T	Period

T	Tesla
T	Time
T	Transmission
T_1	Spin–lattice relaxation time
T_2	Spin–spin relaxation time
T_{Avg}	Average half time
TE	Echo time
T_b	Biological half life
T_d	Daughter half life
T_{eff}	Effective half life
TGC	Time gain compensation
TI	Inversion time
TLD	Thermoluminescent dosimeter
TN	True negative
TNF	True negative fraction
T_p	Parent half life
T_p	Physical half life
TP	True positive
TPF	True positive fraction
TPR	True positive rate
TR	Pulse repetition time
TV	Television
TVG	Time varied gain
U	Use factor
UGI	Upper gastrointestinal
v	Velocity
V	Volt
V	Voltage
W	Watt
W	Work
W	Workload in mA min/week
wt	Weight
Z	Acoustic impedence
Z	Atomic number
$(ZnCd)_S$	Zinc cadmium sulfide
α	Alpha particle

β	Beta particle
γ	Gamma ray
γ	Gyromagnetic ratio
Γ	Radioisotope gamma factor
Γ	Slope of film characteristic curve
ΔI	Change in intensity
ΔX	Change in thickness
ΔV	Change in voltage
$\Delta\lambda$	Change in wavelength
Δ_i	Equilibrium absorbed dose constant for the ith radiation
λ	Wavelength
λ_{min}	Minimum wavelength
μ	Linear attenuation coefficient
μ_m	Mass attenuation coefficient
μ	Micro
μC/kg	Microcoulomb per kilogram
ν^*	Antineutrino
ν	Neutrino
Ω	Ohm
ω	Larmor precessional frequency
ϕ_i	Absorbed fraction for the ith radiation
ρ	Physical density gm/cm^3
$\%\sigma$	Percent standard deviation
σ_q	Quantum noise
σ	Standard deviation
Σ	Sigma, symbol for summation
τ	Dead time
θ_i	Angle of incidence
θ_r	Angle of reflection
θ_t	Angle of transmission

INDEX

A

A, Mass Number, 35
Abbreviations - Powers of Ten, 8
A Mode Display, 377
Abortion, 418
Absorbed Fraction, 348
Absorption Blur, 170
Absorption Efficiency, 201
Absorption, Photoelectric, 128, 201
Absorption, Ultrasound, 365
Acceleration, 13
Acoustic Impedence, 367
Activity, 326, 348
Acuity, Visual, 244
Acute Radiation Effects, 414
ADC, 266, 277
AET, 82
Afterglow, 285
Air, 136
Air Gap, 222, 310
ALARA, 426
Algorithm, 282
Aliasing, 296
Alpha Particle, 25, 35
Alpha Decay, 317
Alternating Current 64
Aluminum Filtration, 117, 123, 296
Ammeter, 56
Amplification, Gas, 229
Amplitude, of Wave, 23, 358
AMU, 35
Angle
  Anode, 92
  Incidence, 369
  Reflection, 369
  Refraction, 369
Analog-to-Digital Converter, 266, 272
Analog Signal, 266
Angiography, 272
Angstrom Unit, 24
Annihilation, Positron, 329
Anode
  Angle, 92
  Construction, 91
  Cooling, 97
  Heat Limits, 97, 99, 285
  Rotating, 95
  Stationary, 91
Answers, 439
Antineutrino, 323
Aperture, 250
Apparent Focal Spot Size, 93
Armature, 67
Array, Transducer, 379
Artifacts, in CT Scanning, 296
Atomic
  Mass, 35
  Number, 35
  Orbits, 37
  Structure, 34
  Weight, 35
Attenuation, 122, 431
  of Iodine, 130
  of Tissue, 133
  Variation with Energy, 129, 132, 159
  Variation with Atomic Number, 130, 159
  Variation with Thickness, 159
  Variation with Density, 159
  Variation with Electrons/gm, 132
  of Ultrasound, 365
Attenuation Coefficient, Linear, 123
Attenuation Coefficient, Mass, 124, 201, 282
Atomic Orbits, 34
Auger Electron, 40
Automatic Exposure Terminator, 82, 206
Automatic Brightness Control 251
Autotransformer, 77
Average Current, 80

Average Energy of X-ray Beam, 115
Average Life, 324
Average Value, 144
Axial Resolution, 372
Azimuthal Resolution, 374

B

B Mode Display, 377
BGO Detector, 237, 285
Background Count Rate, 151
Backscatter Peak, 235
Backing, of Ultrasound Transducers, 360
Band Pass, TV, 260
Band Width
  TV, 260
  Ultrasound, 360
Bar Magnet, 48
Barrier, Shielding
  Primary, 428
  Secondary, 432
Base Fog, 187
Battery, 54
Beam Hardening Artifact, 296
Beam Width, 374
Becquerel, 326
Beta Decay, 320
Beta Particles, 25
Biological Half Life, 325
Binary Numbers, 268
Binding Energy, 38
Bit, 268
Bloodflow, Detection, 379, 408
Blooming, Focal Spot, 90
Blur, 165
  in Tomography, 308
Bohr Model of the Atom, 34
Bone, Attenuation, 134
Boost Voltage, 91
Breast
  Cancer, 307
  Compression, 304
Bremsstrahlung, 111
Bridge Circuit, 69
Brightness
  Automatic Control, 254
  Film, 186
  Gain, 246
Bucky Grid, 218
Bucky Factor, 219
Byte, 268

C

CaWO4, 201
CNS Syndrome, 415
CT Scanning, 282
Calcium Tungstate Screens, 201
Camera
  Cine, 255
  Gamma, 340
  Lens, 255
  Scintillation, 340
  TV 258
Cancer Induction, 307, 416
Candela, 249
Capacitor, 56
Capacitive Discharge Generator, 82
Capture, Electron, 330
Carbon, 36, 317
Carcinogenesis, 416
Cardiac Motion, 170
Cataract Induction, 417
Cathode, 89
Cavitation, 380
Celsius Temperature Scale 20
Center Tap Transformer, 77
Central Processing Unit, 266
Cesium Decay, 310
Cesium Iodide, 246, 285
Charge, 46
Characteristic Curve, 187
Characteristic X-rays, 111
Cine Camera, 255
Circuit
  AET, 82
  Bridge, 69
  Digital Subtraction, 272
  Electrical, 49, 64
  Full Wave, 69
  Half Wave, 68
  High Voltage, 71, 77
  Parallel, 53
  Scintillation, 340
  Series, 51
  Single Phase, 68
  Six Pulse, 69
  Three Phase, 69
  Twelve Pulse, 72
  X-ray, 77

Circular Tomographic Motion, 310
Classical Scattering, 127
Coherent Scattering, 127
Coincidence Detection, 347
Collimator, 342
  CT, 285
  Converging, 343
  Diverging, 343
  Efficiency, 342
  Gamma Camera, 342
  Lens, 251
  Multihole, 343
  Parallel Hole, 345
  Pinhole, 343
  Resolution, 344
  Septa, 344
Compensation, Space Charge, 82
Compounds, 42
Compton
  Attenuation Coefficient, 127, 130
  Edge, 235
  Electrons, 131
  Scattering, 131, 211, 233
  Wavelength Shift, 131
Computer CPU, 266
Computer Hardware, 267
Computer Software, 267
Computed Tomography, 282
  Artifacts, 284, 296
  Display, 290
  Filtration, 296
  Geometry, 284
  Heat Load, 285
  Operation, 282
  Patient Exposure, 299
  Scanning Motion, 284
  Spatial Resolution, 297
Conductor, 47, 64
Conduction, 19
Confidence Limits, 148
Cone Vision, 244
Contamination Limits, TC-99, 433
Contrast Detail Test, 174
Contrast
  Amplification, 296
  Display, 157, 164
  Film, 189
  Image, 287
  Long Scale, 160
  Media, 272
  Perception, 288
  Radiographic, 157
  Resolution, 287
  Scale, 160, 290
  and Scatter, 164, 211
  Short Scale, 160
  Subject, 157
Contrast Improvement Factor, 219
Converging Collimator, 345
Conversion Efficiency, Screen 201
Conversion Factor, Image Intensifier, 249
Conversion, Internal, 328
Convection, 19
Cooling, Anode, 92
Cooling, Tube, 98
Count Rate
  Background, 150
  Uncertainty in, 151
Covalent Bonding, 42
CPU, 266
Criteria, Decision, 176
Crystals
  Fluorescent, 199
  BGO, 238, 285
  CsI, 238, 245, 285
  NaI, 232, 285
  Size and Resolution, 234
  Ultrasound, 360
  ZnCds, 245
Cumulative Activity, 348
Curie, 326
Current
  Average, 80
  Electrical, 55
  Filament, 91
  Induced, 67
  Ionization, 227
  Tube, 91
Cut, Tomographic, 309
Cutoff, Grid, 215
Cycles, 23, 358

D

DAC, 266
Damping, 361
Darkroom Safe Lights, 207
Dark Adapted Vision, 244
db, 365

Dead Time, 230
Decay Constant, 324
Decay
  Alpha, 318
  Beta, 320
  Free Induction, 394
  Isomeric, 323
  Nuclear, 317
  Pulse, 237
Decentering, of Grid, 218
Decibel Scale, 365
Decision Criterion, 176
Delta Transformer Connection, 71
Density
  Difference, 159
  Optical, 184
  Photographic, 184
  Resolution, 287
  Variation of Sound Velocity, 366
Depletion Layer, 231
Depth Compensation, 371
Depth Resolution, 372
Detail Screens, 200
Detail Test, 174
Detector Blur, 171
Detectors
  BGO, 238, 285
  CsI, 238, 245, 285
  CT, 285
  Efficiency, 285
  Gas Filled, 227
  NaI, 232, 285, 341
  Radiation, 227
  Scintillation, 232, 237, 285
  Semiconductor, 231
  Sodium Iodide, 232
  Solid State, 231
  Spacing, 287
  TLD, 232
  Ultrasound, 360
  Xenon, 237, 285
Deuteron, 35, 39
Development, Film, 192
Deviation, Standard, 145
Dewar, 405
Digital to Analog Converter, 266
Digital Imaging, 266
Digital Sampling, 267
Digital Subtraction, 148, 272
Digitization Noise, 270, 276
Diode, 68
Disk Drives, Computer 267
Display
  Contrast, 164
  Level, 164, 290, 341
  TV, 259
  Ultrasound, 379
  Window, 164, 290, 341
Diverging Collimator, 345
Doppler Ultrasound, 379
Dose, Radiation, 24
Dose
  Absorbed, 24, 134
  Genetically Significant, 418
  in CT Scanning, 299
  in Digital Radiology, 277
  in Diagnostic Examinations, 419
  in Fluoroscopy, 248
  in Mammography, 307
  in Nuclear Medicine, 348
  Limits for Public, 426
  Maximum Permissible, 426
  to Gonads, 419
  Units, 24
  With Rare Earth Screens, 203
DSA, 148
Dual Filament Cathode, 90
Dual Mode Image Intensifier, 247
Duty Factor, 364
Dynode, 233

E

ECT, 347
EM Radiation, 22
Echoes, Ultrasound, 361
Edge Enhancement, 304
Effective Half Life, 325
Effective Focal Spot Size, 93
Effectiveness, Grid, 219
Efficiency
  Conversion, 201
  Detector, 285
  Electrical, 66
  Optical System, 250
  Screen Absorption, 201
  Screen Conversion, 201
Electric Field, 46
Electrical Circuits, 49, 64

Electromagnets, 67, 405
Electromagnetic Radiation, 22
Electromagnetic Spectrum, 22
Electrons, 35
  Auger, 40
  Binding Energies, 38
  Capture, 330
  Compton, 131
  Current, 50
  Energy, 322
  Mass, 35, 39
  Orbits, 37, 111
  Per Gram, 132
  Scattered, 131
  Valence, 42
  Volt, 38
Electronic Noise, 270, 276
Electrostatic
  Charging, 47
  Force, 37, 46
  Latent Image, 304
Elliptical Tomographic Motion, 310
Emission Computed Tomography, 347
Emulsion, 184
Energy, 16
  Average Energy of X-ray Beam, 115
  Binding, 38
  Dependence of Photoelectric Interaction, 129
  Dependence of Compton Interaction, 132
  Kinetic, 17
  Level Diagrams, 40, 112, 323, 392
  Potential, 17
  Resolution, 236
  Shells, 34
  Spectra, 235, 322
Equilibrium Absorbed Dose Constant, 350
Equilibrium, Secular, 331
Equilibrium, Transient, 331
Equivalent Resistance, 52
Errors, Combination of, 149
Escape Peak, 236
ev, 38
Exact Framing, 256
Exposure, 24, 135
  Cine, 257
  Film, 188
  Image Intensifier, 248
  Occupational Limits, 426
  Radiation, 24
  Spot Film, 258
  Timer, 81
Eye
  Brightness Response, 186, 244
  Integration Time, 244

F

Fahrenheit Temperature Scale, 20
Falling Load Generator, 105
False Negative Fraction 176
False Positive Fraction, 176
Fan Beam, 283
Far Zone, 376
Fat, 136
Ferromagnets, 49
Fetal Irradiation, 417
f Factor, 135
FID, 394
Field Emission X-ray Tube, 103
Field, TV, 259
Field of View, 345
Filament
  Boost Voltage, 91
  Circuit, 78
  Coating, 91
  Current, 78, 91
  Transformer, 78
Film
  Badge, 427
  Base Fog, 187
  Characteristic Curve, 187
  Chemistry, 191
  Construction, 184
  Contrast, 189
  Density, 184
  Development, 192
  Exposure, 188
  Gamma, 188
  Latitude, 190
  Panchromatic, 203
  Orthochromatic, 203
  Single Emulsion, 184
  Speed, 190
  Transport, 256
  X-ray, 184
Filter
  Attenuation, 115

Wedge, 297
Filtration, 117
Fission, 334
Fixer, Film, 192
Fluence, 24
Fluorescence, 199
Fluoroscopy, 243
Dual Mode, 247
Exposure Rate, 244
Image Intensified, 245
MTF, 173
System, 249
Flux Gain, 246
FNF, 176
f Number, 250
Focal Spot
Blooming, 90
Dual, 90
Effective, 93
Line Focus Principle, 92
Penubra, 169
Size, 95
Focal Zone, Ultrasound, 375
Focused
Collimator, 343
Grid, 217
Transducer, 375
Ultrasound Beam, 375
Focusing
Cathode Cup, 90
Dynodes, 233
Electrodes, 245
Fog, 187
Force
Electrostatic, 37, 46
Gravitational, 15, 37
Magnetic, 48
Nuclear, 37
Fourier Transform, 394
Fovea, 244
FPF, 176
Fractions, 5
Frame, TV, 259
Framing, Cine, 256
Fraunhoffer Zone, 376
Free Induction Decay, 394
Frequency, 23, 394
Bandpass, 260
Larmor, 394
Resonance, 394
Response, 360
Ultrasound, 358
of Wave, 23, 358
Fresnel Zone, 375
Full Wave Rectification, 71
Full Width at Half Maximum, 236

G

Gain
Brightness, 246
Flux, 246
of Image Intensifier, 246
Minification, 246
Time Varied, 371
Gamma
Camera, 240
Factor, 333
Film, 188
Rays, 25, 322
Gas Amplification, 229
Gas Filled Detector, 227, 285
Gastrointestinal Syndrome, 414
Gauss, 405
Gaussian Distribution, 144
Geiger-Meuller Counter, 229
Gelatin, 184
General Population Exposure Limits, 426
Generator
Electrical, 54, 65
Falling Load, 105
Ratings, 80
X-ray, 77, 80
Genetic Effects, 418
Genetically Significant Dose, 418
Geometry, 8
Geometric Magnification, 10, 250
Glare, Veiling, 251
GM Counter, 229
Gonads, Dose to, 419
Gradient Coils, in MR Imaging, 391, 406
Gravity, 15, 37
Gray, 24, 417
Gray Levels, 271
Grid
Antiscatter, 213
Bucky, 218
Construction, 214
Controlled X-ray Tube, 91

Cutoff, 215
Effectiveness, 219
Focused, 217
Linear, 215
Lines per inch, 214
Moving, 218
Parallel, 215
Ratio, 213
Scatter Reduction, 213
GSD, 418
Gyromagnetic Ratio 394

H

H & D Curve, 187
Hardware, Computer, 247
Half Life, 324
Biological, 325
Effective, 325
Physical, 324
Half Value Layer, 124
Half Wave Rectification, 69
Halo, 305
Heat, 19
Heat Limits, Anode, 99, 285
Heat Units, 98
Heel Effect, 93
Helium, 35
Hematologic Syndrome, 414
Hertz, 261
Heterogeneous X-ray Beam, 126
High Voltage Transformer, 71, 77
Horizontal Resolution, 260
Hounsfield Unit, 283
Housing, X-ray Tube, 433
HU, 283
HVL, 124, 297
Hydrogen, 37, 391
Hypocycloidal Tomographic Motion, 309

I

Image Intensifier
Automatic Brightness Control, 254
Construction, 245
Conversion Factor, 249
Dual Field, 247
Exposure Rate, 248
Gain, 246
Input Phosphor, 246
MTF, 175
Noise, 252
Opitcal System, 249
Output Phosphor, 246
Resolution, 260
Size, 247, 256
Image
Contrast, 157
Intensifier, 245
Latent, 192
Noise, 146, 252
Quality, 171
Impedence, Acoustic, 367
Inherent Filtration, 115
Inert Gases, 38
In Utero Exposure, 417
Incidence, Angle, 369
Induced Current, 67
Induction, 47
Information Density, 345
Input Phosphor, 246
Insulator, 47
Integration Time, of Eye, 244
Internal Dosimetry, 348
Intrinsic Resolution, 347
Intensification Factor, 200
Intensifying Screens, 199
CaWO, 200
Construction, 199
Rare Earth, 201
Intensity, 24
Ultrasound, 365
Variation Due to Heel Effect, 94
vs Filtration, 115
vs kVp, 114
vs mA, 114
Interface, Acoustic, 368
Internal Conversion, 328
Inverse Square Law, 27
Inversion Recovery, 398
Iodine, 130, 191, 333, 349
Ion Pair, 227
Ionic Bonding, 42
Ionization, 227
Ionization Chamber, 227
Isobar, 36
Isomer, 323
Isomeric Transitions, 323
Isotone, 37,
Isotope, 36, 317

Isotope Production, 334
Isotropic Scattering, 211

J

JND, 271
Joule, 4, 16, 25, 38
Just Noticeable Difference, 271

K

K Absorption Edge, 130, 201
K Shell, 38, 40, 112
KeV, 38
Kilowatt Rating, 80
Kinetic Energy, 17
kVp, 38, 205

L

L Shell, 38, 112
Lag, Vidicon, 259
Larmor Precessional Frequency, 394
Latent Image
  Film, 192
  Electrostatic, 304
Lateral Decentering, 218
Lateral Resolution, 374
Latitude, Display, 165
Latitude, Film, 190
Latitude, Radiographic, 160
Lead Aprons, 425
Lead Glass, 243
Lead Zirconium Titanate, 360
Leakage Radiation, 433
Length, 3
Lens
  Focal Length, 250
  f Number, 250
LET, 26
Leukemia, 416
Level, Display, 165, 290, 341
Life Shortening, 419
Light, Velocity of, 22
Line Focus Principle, 92
Line Pairs per mm, 165, 269
Line Spread Function, 172
Lines Per Inch, 214
Linear
  Attenuation Coefficient, 123
  Array, 379
  Grid, 215
  Energy Transfer, 26
  Quadratic Risk Hypothesis, 415
  Risk Hypothesis, 415
  Tomographic Motion, 310
Log Relative Exposure, 188
Logarithms, 185, 365
Logarithmic Brightness Scale, 186
Logarithmic Repsonse of Eye, 186
Long Contrast Scale, 160
Longitudinal Recovery Time, 394
Longitudinal Resolution, 372
LSF, 172

M

MAS, 79, 98, 115
M Mode Display, 377
Magnets
  Permanent, 48, 405
  Resistive, 405
  Superconducting, 405
Magnetic Domains, 49
Magnetic Resonance Imaging, 390
Magnetism, 48
Magnetization Vector, 392
Magnification, 13, 247, 310
Mammography, 303
Mammography, Tube, 104
Mask, Subtraction, 272
Mass, 3, 14
  Atomic, 35
  Atomic Units, 35
  Attenuation Coefficient, 123, 201
  Defect, 39
  Electron, 35, 39, 329
  Energy Equivalence, 38
  Number, 35
Matrix, 147, 266, 283, 286
Matter, 42
Maximum Permissible Dose, 425
Mean Dose per Cumulative Activity, 351
Mean Value, 144
Median Value, 144
Memory Size vs Gray Levels, 271
Meta Stable State, 353
Minimal Detectable Contrast, 271, 388
Minification Gain, 246
Minimum Wavelength, 111
M Mode, 377
Modal Value, 144

Modulation Transfer Function, 172
Molybdenum, 96, 104, 303, 323
Momentum, 19
Monoenergetic Radiation, 123
Motion Artifacts, 298
Motion Blurring, 170
Motor, 65
Mottle, Quantum, 206, 252, 273
Moving Grid, 218
Moving Slit Scatter Reduction, 223
MPD, 425
MTF, 172, 306
Muscle, 136, 367

N

NaI Detector, 232, 285
Natural Background, 426
Near Zone, 375
Neutron, 25, 35
Neutrino, 323
Newton's Laws of Motion, 13
Noble Gases, 36
Noise
  Digital, 270
  Digitization, 270, 276
  Electronic, 270, 276
  Statistical, 147, 206, 252, 270
Nonoccupational Exposure Limits, 426
Normal Distribution, 144
Nuclear
  Energy Levels, 318
  Fission, 334
  Force, 37
  Magnetic Resonance, 390
  Particles, 35
  Reactor, 334
  Spins, 390
Nucleon, 35
Nucleus, of Atom, 35
Number System, Binary, 268
Number
  Atomic, 35
  Mass, 35
  CT, 283

O

Object-Image Distance, 12, 310
Observe Pulse, 398
Observer Performance Tests, 174
Occupancy Factor, T, 429
Occupational Exposure Limits, 425
Ohms, 58
Ohm's Law, 51
Open Circuit, 50
Optical Density, 184
Orbital Shells, 34, 37
Orthochromatic Film, 203
Output Phosphor, 246
Overframing, 256

P

p–n Detector, 231
Pair Production, 127, 132
Panchromatic Film, 203
Par Speed Screens, 200
Parallel
  Circuit, 51
  Grid, 215
  Hole Collimator, 345
Parallax, 312
Paramagnetism, 48
Partial Saturation Recovery, 397
Partial Volume Effect, 295
Patient Dose, 248, 277, 299, 307, 348, 419
Penetration, of Ultrasound, 365
Penetration, X-rays in Tissue, 127
Penubra, 169
Percent Standard Deviation, 144
Percentages, 8
Perception, Image, 288
Period, of Wave, 23, 358
Periodic Table, 35
Peripheral Devices, Computer, 267
Permanent Magnet, 49, 405
Personnel Monitoring, 427
Phased Array, 379
Phosphor, 246
Phosphorescence, 199
Photocathode, 233, 245
Photoconductive Layer, 258
Photodisintegration, 127
Photoelectric
  Attenuation Coefficient, 127
  Effect, 128
Photoelectric Peak, 235
Photographic Density, 185
Photographic Emulsion, 184
Photomultiplier Tube, 233

Photons, 24, 131, 329
Phototimers, 82, 206
Phototopic Vision, 244
Physical Half Life, 324
Piezoelectric Effect, 360
Pileup, Pulse, 238
Pinhole Collimator, 345
Pixel, 144, 268, 282, 285
Planck's Constant, 22
Plumbicon TV Camera, 259
Positron Decay, 329
Potential Energy, 17
Power, 58
Powers of Ten, 8
Precession, 393
Precessional Frequency, Larmor, 394
Prepare Pulse, 398
Primary
  Barrier, 429
  Radiation, 211, 428
  Transformer, 68, 77
Proportional Counter, 229
Protection, Radiation, 428
Protective Barrier, 429
Proton, 25, 35
Public, Radiation Dose Limits, 426
Pulse
  Decay Time, 236
  Duration, 362
  Echo, 361
  Height, 236
  Length, 362
  Pile Up, 238
  Rate, 151, 237
  Repetition Frequency, 363
PZT, 360

Q

Q Value, 360
QF, 26
Quadratic Risk Hypothesis, 416
Quality Factor, 26
Quantum Mottle, 206, 252
Quantum Noise, 146, 206, 252, 272
Quantum Sink, 206, 252, 272

R

R, 24
rf Pulse, 393
rad, 24
Radiation
  Background, 426
  Barrier, 429
  Characteristic, 40, 112
  Detectors, 227
  Dose, 24, 248, 277, 299, 307, 348, 419
  Electromagnetic, 22
  Exposure, 24
  Exposure Limits, 426
  Ionizing, 23
  Leakage, 433
  Limits, 426
  Protection, 424
  Risk, 413
  Scattered, 211
  Shielding, 425, 428
Radiation of Heat, 19
Radio Waves, 22
Radioactive Decay, 324
Radium, 318
RAM, 268
Random Access Memory, 268
Random Noise, 146, 206, 252, 272, 288
Rare Earth Screen, 201
Rayls, 367
Reactor, 334
Read Only Memory, 268
Receiver Operating Characteristic Test, 175
Reciprocity Law, 191
Recoil Electron, 131
Rectifier, 68, 79
Reflection Coefficient, 367
Reflections, Ultrasound, 368
Refraction, 369
Relative Risk, 419
Relaxation Time, in MR Imaging, 393, 400
rem, 26, 426
Resistance, 51
Resolution
  Axial, 372
  Azimuthal, 372
  Collimator, 344
  Contrast, 287
  Density, 287
  Depth, 372
  Energy, 237
  of Eye, 244
  Horizontal, 260

Intrinsic, 347
Lateral, 374
in Magnification Radiography, 311
and Scatter, 211
Spatial, 165, 201, 260, 268, 297
TV Stop Action, 261
Vertical, 260
Resonant Frequency, 360, 394
Restricted Area, 429
Ring Artifact, 285, 298
Ripple, 72
Risk Factors, 413, 420
ROC Test, 174
Rod Vision, 244
Roentgen, 24
ROM, 268
Rotating Anode, 95
Rotor, 96
Rotor Heat Load, 103

S

SCR, 93
SNR, 271, 288
Safe Light, Darkroom, 207
Sampling Frequency, 267
Saturation Recovery, 397
Saturation Voltage of Detector, 228
Scan Field Size, 287
Scan Lines, 259
Scan Time, 288
Scatter, 211
and Contrast, 164, 212
and Field Size, 213
Scattering,
Coherent, 127
Compton, 131, 211
Thompson, 127
Scientific Notation, 6
Scintillation Detector, 232
Scotopic Vision, 244
Screen
Absorption, 201
Construction, 199
Conversion Efficiency, 201
Second Half Value Layer, 125
Secondary
Barrier, 432
Radiation, 211, 432
of transformer, 68, 77
Secular Equilibrium, 331
Selenium, 304
Semiconductor Detector, 53, 55, 231, 285
Sensitivity, 176, 228
Sensitivity Speck, 192
Septal Penetration, 344
Series Circuit, 51
Shielding, 428
Shoulder Region, 188
Short Contrast Scale, 160
Shutter, 255
Sievert, 26, 426
Signal to Noise Ratio, 270
Silver Halide, 184, 191
Similar Triangles, 9, 27
SI Units, 3
Six Pulse Rectified Circuit, 72
Slice Thickness, 282, 309
Slit Radiography, 223
Snell's Law, 370
Sodium, 329, 406
Sodium Iodide Detector, 232, 285
Soft Tissue, Attenuation, 132, 371
Software, Computer, 267
Solid State Detector, 231, 285
Somatic Effects, 413
Sound Intensity, 365
Source Image Distance, 10, 311
Source Object Distance, 10, 311
Space Charge, 82
Spatial
Frequency, 165, 172
Resolution, 165, 201, 260, 268, 297
SPECT, 347
Specific Activity, 327, 334
Specificity, 176
Spectra
Beta, 322
Energy, 235, 322
Gamma Ray, 235, 322
Pulse Height, 235
Speed
Film, 190
Intensifying Screen, 200
Spin-Echo Relaxation, 400
Spin-Lattice Relaxation, 393
Spin, Nuclear, 391
Spin-Spin Relaxation, 400
Spot Film Camera, 257

Standard Deviation, 145
Star Artifact, 298
Static Electricity, 46
Statistical Noise, 146
Statistics, 144, 252
Stator, 96
Step Down Transformer, 68
Step Up Transformer, 68
Streak Artifact, 298
Stereoradiography, 312
Stereoradiographic Tube, 103, 312
Stop Action Resolution 261
Subject
  Contrast, 157
  Contrast, Variation with kVp, 159
  Contrast, Variation with Scatter, 164
Substance, 42
Subtraction Image - and Noise, 149
Subtraction Mask, 272
Surface Coils, in MR Imaging, 391
Superconducting Magnet, 405
Synchronization, 256

T

T, Occupancy Factor, 428
T-1 Relaxation Time, 394
T-2 Relaxation Time, 400
Target Material, 92
TE, 400
Technecium, 323
Television
  Bandwidth, 260
  Camera, 258
  Display, 259
  System, 258
Temperature, 20
Temporal Averaging, 277
Ten Day Rule, 417
Tesla, 405
Test Pattern, Contrast Detail, 174
Thermionic Emission, 91
Thermoluminescent Dosimeter, 232, 427
Thickness
  of Intensifying Screens, 200
  of Ultrasound Crystals, 360
Thompson Scattering, 127
Three Phase AC, 69, 79
Three Phase Generator, 79
Threshold Dose, 416
Threshold Value, 176
TI, 398
Time, 3
Time to Count, 152
Time Varied Gain, 371
Tissue Attenuation, 127, 132
TLD, 232, 427
TNF, 176
Toe Region of Film, 187
Tomography, Conventional, 308
Tomographic Angle, 309
Toner, 305
TPF, 176
TR, 397
Transducer, Ultrasound, 360
Transformer, 67
  Auto-, 77
  Filament, 78
  High Voltage, 77
  Turns Ratio, 67
Transmission, Optical, 186
Transient Equilibrium, 331
Transport, Cine Film, 256
True Negative Fraction, 176
True Positive Fraction, 176
Tube Current, 91
Tungsten, 40, 112
Turns Ratio, of a Transformer, 67
Twelve Pulse Rectified Circuit, 72
TV Frame, 259
TV Field, 259
TV System, 258

U

U, Use Factor, 428
Ultrasound
  A-Mode, 377
  Amplitude, 358
  Attenuation, 365
  Beam, 365
  B-Mode, 377
  Doppler, 379
  Far Zone, 376
  Frequency, 358
  Fresnel Zone, 374
  Fraunhoffer Zone, 376
  Intensity, 365
  M-Mode, 377
  Near Zone, 374

Penetration, 374
Pulses, 373
Reflections, 367
Refraction, 369
Resolution, 372
Transducer, 360
Transmission, 368
Velocity, 359
Uncertainties
Combination of, 148, 270
in Count Rate, 151
in Digitization, 276
in Gray Levels, 273
Unit(s)
Atomic Mass, 35
Derived, 3
English, 3
Fundamental, 3
Hounsfield, 283
Radiation, 24
SI, 3
Unsharpness, 165
Upside Down Grid, 217
Use Factor, U, 428
Utero, Exposure in, 417

V
Valence Electrons, 42
Veiling Glare, 251
Velocity, 13
of Light, 24
of Ultrasound, 367
of Wave, 23, 358
Vertical Resolution - TV, 260
Video Signal, 258
Vidicon TV Camera, 259
Vignetting, 251
Visibility of Objects in Noise, 149
Visual Acuity, 244
Voltage
Electrical, 51
Filament, 78, 91
Gain, 246
Primary, 78
Saturation, 228
Secondary, 78
Voltmeter, 56
Volume, Partial, 295
Voxel, 282

W
W, Workload, 428
Water, 267
Watt, 58
Wave, 23, 358
Wave Form Factor, 115
Wavelength, 23, 358
Wedge Filter, 297
Weight, 14
Window, Display, 165, 237, 290, 341
Word, 268
Work, 16
Workload W, 428
Wye Transformer Connection, 71

X
Xenon Detector, 237, 285
Xeroradiography, 304
X-ray
Attenuation, 122
Barrier, 429
Detectors, 227
Film 184
Filters, 115, 297
Generator, 77, 80
Interactions, 122
Production, 110
Variation with filtration, 115
Variation with mA, 114
Variation with kVp, 114
Variation with Current, 114
Scatter, 212
Spectra, 111, 113, 114, 116
Tube, 89

Z
Z, Acoustic Impedence, 367
Z, Atomic Number, 35
ZnCds, 245
Zone
Far, 376
Fresnel, 376
Fraunhoffer, 376
Near, 374